T0176967

Management of Dental Emergencies in Children and Adolescents

Management of Dental Emergencies in Children and Adolescents

Edited by

PD Dr. med. dent. Klaus W. Neuhaus, MMA MAS
Clinic of Periodontology, Endodontology and Cariology
University Center for Dental Medicine Basel
University of Basel, Basel, Switzerland;
Private dental office, Herzogenbuchsee, Switzerland

Prof. em. Dr. med. dent. Adrian Lussi, dipl. Chem.Ing. ETHZ
Department of Preventive, Restorative and Pediatric Dentistry
School of Dental Medicine
University of Bern, Bern, Switzerland

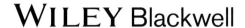

This edition first published 2019
© 2019 John Wiley & Sons Ltd

All rights reserved. No part of this publication may be reproduced, stored in a retrieval system, or transmitted, in any form or by any means, electronic, mechanical, photocopying, recording or otherwise, except as permitted by law. Advice on how to obtain permission to reuse material from this title is available at http://www.wiley.com/go/permissions.

The rights of Klaus W. Neuhaus and Adrian Lussi to be identified as the authors of the editorial material in this work has been asserted in accordance with law.

Registered Office
John Wiley & Sons, Inc., 111 River Street, Hoboken, NJ 07030, USA

Editorial Office
111 River Street, Hoboken, NJ 07030, USA
9600 Garsington Road, Oxford, OX4 2DQ, UK
For details of our global editorial offices, customer services, and more information about Wiley products visit us at www.wiley.com.

Wiley also publishes its books in a variety of electronic formats and by print-on-demand. Some content that appears in standard print versions of this book may not be available in other formats.

Limit of Liability/Disclaimer of Warranty
The contents of this work are intended to further general scientific research, understanding, and discussion only and are not intended and should not be relied upon as recommending or promoting scientific method, diagnosis, or treatment by physicians for any particular patient. In view of ongoing research, equipment modifications, changes in governmental regulations, and the constant flow of information relating to the use of medicines, equipment, and devices, the reader is urged to review and evaluate the information provided in the package insert or instructions for each medicine, equipment, or device for, among other things, any changes in the instructions or indication of usage and for added warnings and precautions. While the publisher and authors have used their best efforts in preparing this work, they make no representations or warranties with respect to the accuracy or completeness of the contents of this work and specifically disclaim all warranties, including without limitation any implied warranties of merchantability or fitness for a particular purpose. No warranty may be created or extended by sales representatives, written sales materials or promotional statements for this work. The fact that an organization, website, or product is referred to in this work as a citation and/or potential source of further information does not mean that the publisher and authors endorse the information or services the organization, website, or product may provide or recommendations it may make. This work is sold with the understanding that the publisher is not engaged in rendering professional services. The advice and strategies contained herein may not be suitable for your situation. You should consult with a specialist where appropriate. Further, readers should be aware that websites listed in this work may have changed or disappeared between when this work was written and when it is read. Neither the publisher nor authors shall be liable for any loss of profit or any other commercial damages, including but not limited to special, incidental, consequential, or other damages.

Library of Congress Cataloging-in-Publication Data
Names: Neuhaus, Klaus W., editor. | Lussi, Adrian, editor.
Title: Management of dental emergencies in children and adolescents / edited
    by Klaus W. Neuhaus, Adrian Lussi.
Description: Hoboken, NJ : Wiley-Blackwell, 2019. | Includes bibliographical
    references and index. |
Identifiers: LCCN 2019005874 (print) | LCCN 2019006936 (ebook) | ISBN
    9781119372660 (Adobe PDF) | ISBN 9781119372639 (ePub) | ISBN 9781119372646
    (pbk.)
Subjects: | MESH: Emergencies | Dental Care–methods | Tooth
    Diseases–therapy | Tooth Injuries–therapy | Child | Adolescent
Classification: LCC RK51.5 (ebook) | LCC RK51.5 (print) | NLM WU 105 | DDC
    617.6/026–dc23
LC record available at https://lccn.loc.gov/2019005874

Cover Illustration and Layout: BernadetteRawyler
Cover Images: © Meinzahn/Getty Images, © wScottLoy/Getty Images, © Image Source/Getty Images,
© knape/Getty Images, Photo Credit (FOR 3 INSET PHOTOGRAPHS) Klaus W. Neuhaus

Set in 10/12pt Warnock by SPi Global, Pondicherry, India
Printed and bound in Singapore by Markono Print Media Pte Ltd

10 9 8 7 6 5 4 3 2 1

Contents

Contributors

Julia Amato
Department of Periodontology,
Endodontology and Cariology,
University Center for Dental Medicine Basel,
University of Basel, Basel, Switzerland

Wolfgang H. Arnold
Department of Biological and Material
Sciences in Dentistry, School of Dentistry,
Faculty of Health, Witten/Herdecke
University, Witten, Germany

Dick S. Barendregt
Department of Periodontology,
ACTA, Amsterdam, Netherlands;
Private dental office Proclin Rotterdam,
Netherlands

Michael M. Bornstein
Oral and Maxillofacial Radiology,
Applied Oral Sciences, Faculty of Dentistry,
The University of Hong Kong, Hong Kong,
China

Thiago Saads Carvalho
Department of Restorative,
Preventive and Pediatric Dentistry,
School for Dental Medicine,
University of Bern, Bern, Switzerland

Renata Chałas
Department of Conservative Dentistry
and Endodontics, Medical University of
Lublin, Lublin, Poland

Vivianne Chappuis
Department of Oral Surgery and
Stomatology, School of Dental Medicine,
University of Bern, Bern, Switzerland

Karl Dula
Department of Oral Surgery and
Stomatology, School for Dental Medicine,
Bern, Switzerland; Private dental office,
Chiasso, Switzerland

Edwin Eggink
Private dental office Proclin Rotterdam,
Netherlands

Andreas Filippi
Department of Oral Surgery and
Center of Dental Traumatology,
University Center for Dental
Medicine Basel,
University of Basel, Basel, Switzerland

Vlasios Goulioumis
Department of Operative and Preventive
Dentistry, School of Dentistry, Faculty of
Health, Witten/Herdecke University,
Witten, Germany

Stefan Hänni
Department of Preventive,
Restorative and Pediatric Dentistry,
School for Dental Medicine, University
of Bern, Bern, Switzerland; Private
endodontic office, Bern, Switzerland

Roswitha Heinrich-Weltzien
Department of Preventive and Paediatric Dentistry, Jena University Hospital, Jena, Germany

Nicola P. Innes
Department of Paediatric Dentistry, School of Dentistry, University of Dundee, Dundee, United Kingdom

Samira Helena João-Souza
Department of Restorative, Preventive and Pediatric Dentistry, School for Dental Medicine, University of Bern, Bern, Switzerland

Hrvoje Jurić
Department of Paediatric and Preventive Dentistry, School of Dental Medicine, University of Zagreb, Zagreb, Croatia

Gabriel Krastl
Department of Conservative Dentistry and Periodontology and Center of Dental Traumatology, University Hospital of Würzburg, Würzburg, Germany

Jan Kühnisch
Department of Conservative Dentistry and Periodontology, Ludwig-Maximilians-University, Munich, Germany

Rafael Lazarin
Department of Oral Surgery and Stomatology, School of Dental Medicine, University of Bern, Bern, Switzerland

Maria Lessani
School of Dentistry, Birmingham, United Kingdom; Private dental office, London, United Kingdom

Manfred Leunisse
Clinic for Orthodontics, Rotterdam, Netherlands

Marcel L. E. Linssen
Private dental office Proclin Rotterdam, Netherlands

Adrian Lussi
Department of Preventive, Restorative and Pediatric Dentistry, School of Dental Medicine, University of Bern, Bern, Switzerland

Birte Melsen
Department of Orthodontics, University of Western Australia, Perth, Australia

Joana Monteiro
Department of Paediatric Dentistry, Eastman Dental Hospital, London, United Kingdom

Ella A. Naumova
Department of Biological and Material Sciences in Dentistry, School of Dentistry, Faculty of Health, Witten/Herdecke University, Witten, Germany

Klaus W. Neuhaus
Clinic of Periodontology, Endodontology and Cariology, University Center for Dental Medicine Basel, University of Basel, Basel, Switzerland; Private dental office, Herzogenbuchsee, Switzerland

Jakob Passweg
Department of Hematology, University Hospital Basel, Basel, Switzerland

Isabelle Portenier
Department of Endodontics, Dental Faculty, University of Oslo, Oslo, Norway; Private dental clinic, Nyon, Switzerland and Oslo, Norway

Adrian M. Ramseier
Department of Oral Health & Medicine, University Center for Dental Medicine Basel, University of Basel, Basel, Switzerland

Dan-Krister Rechenberg
Clinic of Preventive Dentistry, Periodontology and Cariology, Center of Dental Medicine, University of Zurich, Zurich, Switzerland

Nadja Rohr
Department of Reconstructive Dentistry,
University Center for Dental Medicine
Basel, University of Basel, Basel, Switzerland

Markus Schaffner
Department of Preventive, Restorative
and Pediatric Dentistry, School of Dental
Medicine, University of Bern, Bern,
Switzerland

Nathalie Scheidegger Stojan
Private dental office, Biel, Switzerland

Falk Schwendicke
Department of Operative and Preventive
Dentistry, Charité Centre for Dental
Medicine, Berlin, Germany

Richard Steffen
Clinic of Orthodontics and Paediatric
Dentistry, University Center for Dental
Medicine Basel,
University of Basel, Basel, Switzerland;
Private dental office, Weinfelden,
Switzerland

Eirini Stratigaki
Clinic of Orthodontics and Pediatric
Oral Health, University Center for Dental
Medicine Basel, University of Basel, Basel,
Switzerland

Valerie G. A. Suter
Department of Oral Surgery and
Stomatology, School of Dental Medicine,
University of Bern, Bern, Switzerland

Hubertus van Waes
Clinic of Orthodontics and Pediatric
Dentistry, Center of Dental Medicine,
University of Zurich, Zurich,
Switzerland

Carlalberta Verna
Department of Orthodontics and Paediatric
Dentistry, University Center for Dental
Medicine Basel, University of Basel, Basel,
Switzerland

Tuomas Waltimo
Department of Oral Health & Medicine
University Center for Dental
Medicine Basel,
University of Basel, Basel, Switzerland

Cynthia K. Y. Yiu
Paediatric Dentistry, Faculty of Dentistry,
The University of Hong Kong,
Hong Kong, China

Nicola U. Zitzmann
Department of Reconstructive Dentistry,
University Center for Dental Medicine
Basel, University of Basel, Basel,
Switzerland

Andrea Zürcher
Department of Oral Surgery and
Center of Dental Traumatology,
University Center for Dental
Medicine Basel,
University of Basel, Basel,
Switzerland

Preface

Dear readers,

Dental emergency situations are often demanding due to the patient's pain, or due to time constraints on the dentists' side. When children or adolescents suffer dental emergencies, the situation might be even more challenging because of the patients' age, the worried patients, not rarely accompanied by loud screaming. In this setting it is demanding for the dental team to remain quiet and provide the necessary and considerate treatment.

This book aims at providing some assistance to dental practitioners in order to better manage potentially stressful situations with children and adolescents in the dental office.

The focus lies on the management of therapeutic demands.

The content of this book is not totally new. Knowledge can be obtained from books on dental traumatology, cariology, pediatric dentistry, endodontology, or orthodontics. However, this is the first time that a textbook particularly emphasizes how to manage emergency situations with young patients only, and which treatments potentially could be offered once the acute emergency is over.

While the first section of the book recapitulates the biologic and developmental differences between treatment of adults vs. children/adolescents, the following chapters emphasize how to manage tooth substance loss, how to deal with endodontic problems in deciduous teeth or in teeth with an open apex. Furthermore, general dental practitioners should be aware of the long-term consequences of early tooth loss, and of methods to deal with that.

Because teeth are not the only possible cause for emergencies in the dental office, other chapters focus on oral health related problems and on the management of non-infective conditions.

We are happy about the more than competent team of contributing authors. We chose authors that deal with young to very young patients every day in order to guarantee as much practical relevance as possible. At the same time the authors are experienced lecturers and have up-to-date theoretical knowledge included in their chapters.

We hope that reading this book help the readers to acquire a higher level of confidence while coping with demanding emergency situations of children and adolescents during daily work.

Klaus W. Neuhaus
Adrian Lussi

Invited Preface

Dental emergencies in children and adolescents are 'grist for the mill' for paediatric dentists and endodontists. However, during our initial dental training, we are mostly taught by individual disciplines, and therefore it is easy to miss the interdisciplinary nature of the care required for paediatric and adolescent emergencies that provides the best outcome for the patient.

To have a book that brings the elements of comprehensive emergency care together is of great benefit to clinicians. The editors have brought together a host of dental clinicians as authors who have a wealth of relevant experience that is shared in the text.

Emergencies in children are different to those for older individuals. As development is still occurring, this has great influence on treatment planning, as well as the ability to provide the best care for the child. Development includes both physical, psychological and behavioural aspects, and these need to be considered in both immediate and long-term definitive care.

Treatment of emergencies has evolved over the years as the evidence has improved, however, there is still much to learn regarding the most appropriate care for the individual patient. For example, the chapter on management of deep carious lesions illustrates the vast changes that have evolved as the related evidence-base increases in size and validity – treatment of the deep carious lesion is far less aggressive than in previous decades, as the importance of maintenance of pulpal health and 'sealing' of the lesion has become preeminent.

Another example is the chapter on regenerative endodontics, an area of clinical care that was non-existent 25 years ago. The use of MTA, and now including newer calcium silicate-based materials, has revolutionised endodontics. The ability to encourage healthy tissue to re-establish itself in a root canal system previously filled with necrotic tissue creates the possibility of continued root development in a partially developed tooth and has wide-ranging clinical consequences.

In paediatric and adolescent emergencies, treatment decisions often need to be made immediately, therefore a sound understanding of the short- and long-term consequences of treatment options is vital, and the following text provides the clinician with a sound base to inform these decisions. The decision may be as dichotomous as whether to replant an avulsed permanent incisor or not – leading to the thought process which may include – how long has the extra-oral time been? How long was the 'dry time'? What storage medium has been used? How developed is the tooth? Is the soft tissue and/or bony socket damaged? Is the child capable of accepting care in the dental chair, or will sedation or a general anaesthesia be necessary? Will this change my treatment options or recommendations? What do I talk to the parents about? Do I have informed consent? Should I extirpate the pulpal tissue – now or later, or at all? When and how often is follow-up? What tests should I undertake? All leading to the question – what is the best option for the individual patient?

This contextually broad but concise text provides the clinician with ample information on how to deal with emergencies, from pulpotomies to facial swellings to post-trauma orthodontic tooth movement. The comprehensive nature of the text covering treatment of both the primary and permanent dentitions makes it a valuable reference text that should be in all dental clinics.

Prof. David Manton
The University of Melbourne
Melbourne, Australia

Acknowledgements

We would like to thank the following persons:

Bernadette Rawyler, ZMK Bern, for her wonderfully clear yet artistic figures in this book. You deserve the best!

Jessica Evans, Wiley, for encouraging to pursue the idea of compiling this book.

Jayadivya Saiprasad, Wiley, for her constant support and her prompt help whenever it was needed.

Monisha Swaminathan, Wiley, for her assistance in the production process.

Tim West, Wiley, for a tremendous job in copyediting the manuscript.

Susan Engelken, Wiley, for organizing the layout.

About the Companion Website

This book is accompanied by a companion website:

www.wiley.com/go/neuhaus/dental_emergencies

Scan this QR code to visit the companion website

The website includes multiple choice questions.

Unit 1

General Considerations for Emergency Management in Children and Adolescents

1.1

Developmental and Histological Aspects of Deciduous and Young Permanent Teeth

Markus Schaffner and Adrian Lussi

Department of Preventive, Restorative and Pediatric Dentistry, School of Dental Medicine, University of Bern, Bern, Switzerland

Differences between Deciduous and Permanent Teeth

The most noticeable difference between deciduous and permanent teeth is related to their anatomy: deciduous teeth are generally smaller than their permanent counterparts and have a significantly thinner enamel layer (Grine, 2005; Mahoney, 2013) (Figure 1.1.1a,b). Additionally, histological differences may influence their susceptibility to dissolution.

Deciduous teeth have an outermost layer of aprismatic (prismless) enamel, with a thickness varying from 15 to 30 µm (Kodaka et al., 1989; Ripa, 1966; Ripa et al., 1966). The aprismatic layer is significantly thicker on the labial than the lingual surfaces of anterior deciduous teeth, but no significant differences have been found between the surfaces of deciduous molars (Shellis, 1984a).

A prismatic enamel layer has been observed in both deciduous and permanent teeth, with a variable thickness of between 10 and 30 µm (Horsted et al., 1976; Kodaka et al., 1991). In relation to the enamel crystals, the arrangement of enamel prisms is fairly similar in both deciduous and permanent teeth (Radlanski et al., 2001); they reach the surface at an almost perpendicular angle in both dentitions (Horsted et al., 1976). Shellis (1984a) was able to trace the prisms in permanent teeth all the way to the surface, but the prisms in deciduous teeth are distinctly different – more gently curved, with slightly more pronounced Hunter–Schreger bands (Shellis, 1984b) (Figure 1.1.2a,b). Furthermore, the prisms in deciduous teeth are smaller, with more complete boundaries, and are more widely spread out than those in permanent teeth (Shellis, 1984b), which is suggestive of more porous enamel in deciduous than in permanent teeth. The interprismatic fraction and prism-junction density are also greater in the enamel of deciduous teeth than in that of permanent teeth (Shellis, 1984a).

The organic content of enamel also varies according to the kind of tooth. It has been shown to range between 0.7 and 12.0% in deciduous teeth, as compared to 0.4–0.8% in permanent ones (Stack, 1953). Studies of the inorganic content have found that a mineralisation gradient from the surface to the amelo-dentinal junction is clearly observable in both dentitions: a more mineralised layer of enamel is present nearer to the tooth surface and decreases towards the amelo-dentinal junction. In general,

Management of Dental Emergencies in Children and Adolescents, First Edition.
Edited by Klaus W. Neuhaus and Adrian Lussi.
© 2019 John Wiley & Sons Ltd. Published 2019 by John Wiley & Sons Ltd.
Companion website: www.wiley.com/go/neuhaus/dental_emergencies

(a)   (b)

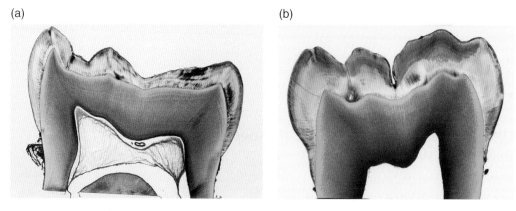

Figure 1.1.1 (a) Deciduous teeth have a significantly thinner enamel layer than (b) permanent teeth. Note: The enamel - cementum border in the deciduous teeth is more coronal compared to permanent teeth.

(a)   (b)

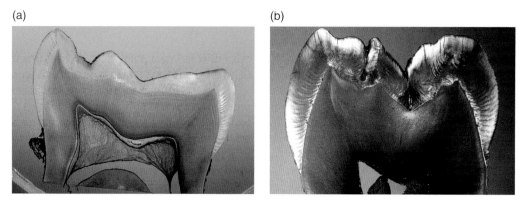

Figure 1.1.2 The prisms in deciduous teeth are more curved than those in permanent teeth. Therefore (a) deciduous teeth show more pronounced Hunter–Schreger bands than (b) permanent teeth.

deciduous enamel is considerably less mineralised than permanent enamel (Wilson and Beynon, 1989). Moreover, Sønju Clasen and Ruyter (1997) observed that deciduous enamel has a greater total carbonate content than permanent enamel. The carbonate ion can occupy the position either of the hydroxyl (OH–) groups (type A carbonated hydroxyapatite) or of the phosphate (PO_4^{3-}) groups (type B carbonated hydroxyapatite) in the hydroxyapatite crystal. The same authors noted that there is more type A carbonated hydroxyapatite in deciduous enamel than in permanent enamel.

Although the carbonate ion can cause distortion of the apatite crystal lattice in both positions, when it is in the position of type A,

it is assumed to be less tightly bound and to contribute to greater solubility of the enamel.

All of the preceding histological differences between deciduous and permanent enamel may be related to the fact that deciduous enamel has significantly lower surface microhardness (Lussi et al., 2000; Johansson et al., 2001; Magalhães et al., 2009) and elasticity (Lippert et al., 2004). This, in turn, could render deciduous teeth more susceptible to dissolution. In vitro studies of deciduous teeth have shown them to be more susceptible to caries-like acid dissolution than permanent teeth (Shellis, 1984a), and artificial caries lesions have been shown to progress 1.5 times faster in deciduous than in permanent enamel (Featherstone and Mellberg, 1981).

Tooth Development and Structural Characteristics of Dental Hard Tissue

Tooth development in the human embryo begins at between 28 and 40 days of gestation. Epithelial cells grow in the ectomesenchymal (mesectodermal) parts of the jaw. A protruberance of the oral epithelium is formed, derived from the inner and outer enamel epithelium of the enamel organ (bud stage; Figure 1.1.3a). The dental papilla is formed by the further penetration of the epithelial cells into the ectomesenchyme (cap and bell stage;

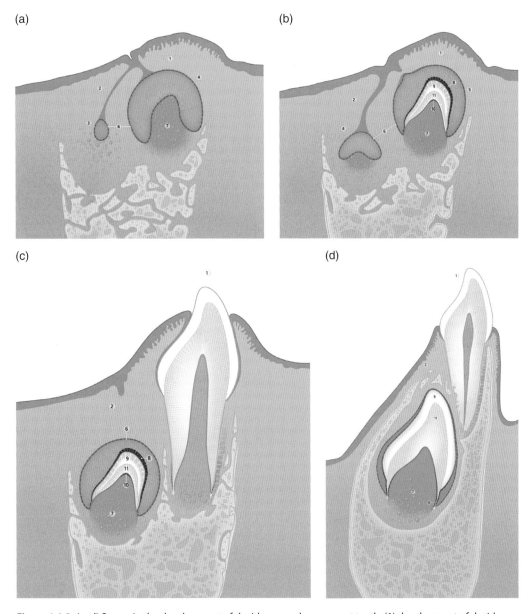

(a)

(b)

(c)

(d)

Figure 1.1.3 (a–d) Stages in the development of deciduous and permanent teeth: (1) development of deciduous tooth; (2) development of permanent teeth; (3) bud stage; (4) cap stage; (5) bell stage; (6) enamel epithelium; (7) dental papilla; (8) ameloblasts; (9) enamel; (10) odontoblasts; (11) dentin; (12) Hertwig epithelial root sheath.

Figures 1.1.3b, 1.1.4–1.1.6). At this time, cell differentiation for the formation of the dental hard tissue occurs. Ameloblasts arise from the ectodermal cells, whilst odontoblasts arise from the adjoining ectomesenchymal cells of the dental papilla, as part of a mutual induction chain. The formation of the dental hard tissue does not start simultaneously in the ectodermal parts and the dental papilla along the entire contact surface. In the case of front teeth, the first layers of enamel and dentin are formed in the middle of the later incisal edge; with lateral teeth, this occurs in the region of the later cusp tips (Figures 1.1.3b–d). With continued growth, the various areas of tooth formation fuse, forming the occlusal surface.

Through further penetration of the epithelial cells into the ectomesenchyme, the double-layered Hertwig's epithelial root sheath is produced (Figures 1.1.3d and 1.1.7). This determines the size, shape and number of the resulting tooth roots. In multirooted teeth, tongue-like extensions grow from the circular edge of the Hertwig's epithelial root sheath over the apical edge of the dental papilla. These projections fuse into the bi- or trifurcation. The resulting dentin layers will later form the base of the crown cavity. The Hertwig's epithelial sheaths proliferate apically and form the tooth roots (Figure 1.1.8a–d). The remnants of the Hertwig's epithelial sheaths are responsible for the formation of true enamel pearls or cementum-free root parts. These remnants are known as epithelial cell rests of

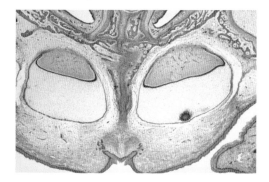

Figure 1.1.5 Tooth germ at the early bell stage.

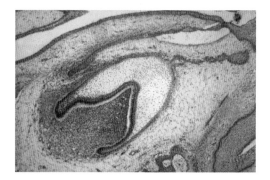

Figure 1.1.6 Tooth germ at the bell stage.

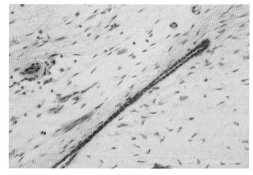

Figure 1.1.7 Hertwig epithelial root sheath with outer and inner enamel epithelium.

Malassez, and play a role in the formation of odontogenic cysts.

Structural Features of the Enamel

Light microscopy reveals brown lines in the enamel, which run obliquely to the occlusal direction from the enamel–dentin border.

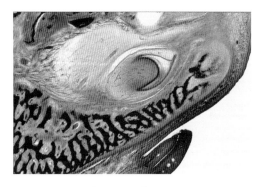

Figure 1.1.4 Tooth germ at the cap stage.

(a)

(b)

(c)

(d)

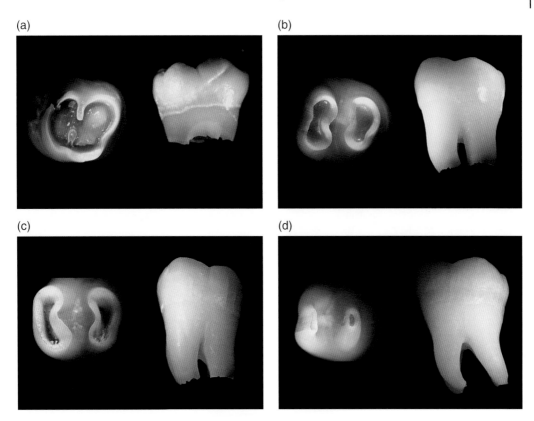

Figure 1.1.8 Apical view (left) and view from the side (right) of the developing tooth roots. (a) The tongue-like projections meet in the region of the later bifurcation, fuse there and form new epithelial sheaths for the development of two tooth roots. (b–d) With increasing root development, there is a narrowing of the root canals until the apex is reached. The root growth accelerates the tooth eruption.

These are the cross-striations and striae of Retzius, which reflect the cyclical deposition of the enamel in the developing teeth (Figure 1.1.9). In a horizontal cross-section, these stripes resemble the annual rings of a tree. Where the striae of Retzius meet the surface of the enamel, imbrication lines are formed. Between the imbrication lines are the perikymata, which are easily recognisable in newly erupted teeth (Figure 1.1.10).

Structural Defects and Paraplasia of the Enamel

In most teeth, structural defects of the enamel are visible under the light microscope. A large proportion of these defects occur during enamel development. Examples include enamel spindles and enamel tufts.

Enamel spindles are formed by odontoblast projections, which extend from the enamel–dentin boundary into the enamel matrix and are enclosed by the enamel during fusion (Figure 1.1.11). Enamel tufts are produced by incompletely mineralised matrix-enriched areas, which extend along the enamel prisms (Figure 1.1.12a,b). Enamel tufts can be a weak spot with regard to caries spread.

An enamel pearl is a developmental anomaly whereby enamel occurs in an atypical localisation. Enamel pearls come in two types: real and composite. The real ones are composed only of enamel. They are up to 0.3 mm in size and are often covered with cementum (Figure 1.1.13). The remains of Hertwig's epithelial root sheaths are responsible for their formation. These epithelial sheath residues can give rise to the differentiation of

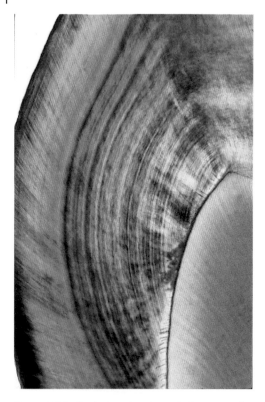

Figure 1.1.9 Vertical section through the crown of a permanent tooth. The cyclical pattern of enamel formation is reflected in the striae of Retzius.

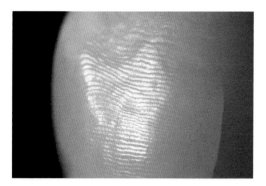

Figure 1.1.10 Enlargement of the tooth surface, clearly showing the perikymata and the imbrication lines between them.

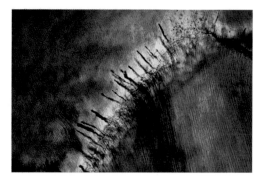

Figure 1.1.11 Columnar and piston-like enamel spindles extending from the dentinoenamel junction into the enamel.

(a)   (b)

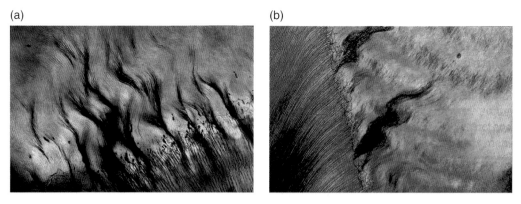

Figure 1.1.12 (a,b) Enamel buds unfold like grass tufts from the dentinoenamel junction into the enamel. The figure clearly shows the incompletely mineralized matrix-enriched enamel components running along the enamel prisms.

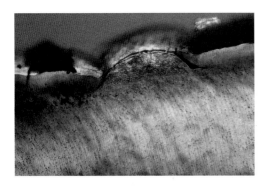

Figure 1.1.13 A real enamel pearl lies on the dentin in the root area. It is surrounded and overlaid by acellular cementum.

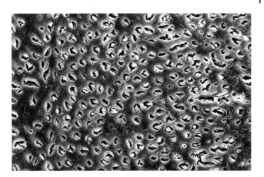

Figure 1.1.15 Scanning electron micrograph (SEM) image of cross-sectioned dentinal tubules with odontoblast extensions.

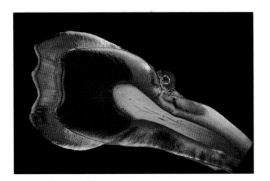

Figure 1.1.14 On the root surface of a permanent tooth, a composite enamel pearl with a dentin core is clearly recognisable.

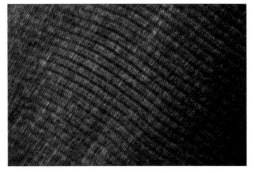

Figure 1.1.16 Light microscope image of dentin with incremental lines of von Ebner running perpendicular to the dentinal tubules.

ameloblasts, which deposit enamel on the root surface. Composite enamel pearls can be several millimetres in size. They consist of enamel and dentin, and can have pulp fractions (Figure 1.1.14). They can cause isolated periodontitis in the furcation area or interdental space. The cause of their development is not known.

Structural Features of Dentin

A mature odontoblast is a long, columnar cell with a process on the secretory side. Odontoblasts secrete predentin, which is later calcified in the process of mineralisation. Odontoblast processes, together with dentinal tubules, become longer as dentin formation progresses (Figure 1.1.15).

The development of the circumpulpal dentin, which makes up most of the dentin layer, is a cyclical process with active-secretion and resting phases. This cyclical dentin deposition can be observed by light microscopy. During the resting phases, von Ebner's lines are formed (Figure 1.1.16). These correspond to the Retzius striae of the enamel. Broadened and hypomineralised growth lines called Owen lines are caused by a disturbance of the dentin mineralisation, which may occur during childbirth or as a result of illness.

The mineralisation of the circumpulpal dentin proceeds from centres in the area of the mineralisation front, the so-called calcospherites (Figure 1.1.17). These can be detected by electron microscopy after removal of the predentin (Figure 1.1.17).

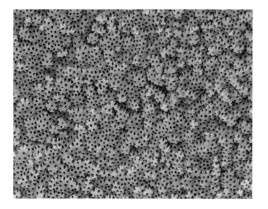

Figure 1.1.17 After removal of the predentin, the calcospherites facing the pulp wall and the many entrances of the dentinal tubules in the SEM are clearly visible.

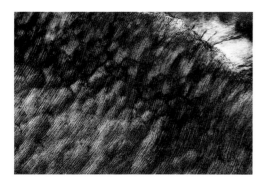

Figure 1.1.18 Light microscope image of the dentinoenamel boundary (upper right) and arc-shaped interglobular dentin in the region of the crown.

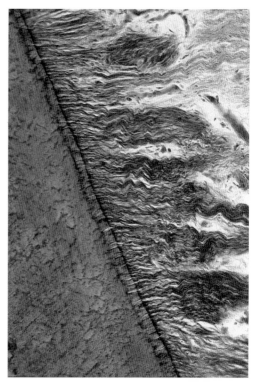

Figure 1.1.19 Sharpey fibre bundles anchored in a thin layer of acellular extrinsic fibre cementum. The dentin structures are recognisable under the acellular cementum layer.

In the crown, they remain partly as interglobular dentin (Figure 1.1.18).

Structural Features of the Cementum

Cementum is a mineralised connective tissue covering the entire tooth root surface that anchors the periodontal fibres to the tooth (Figure 1.1.19). Cellular cementum bears a certain resemblance to bone tissue. However, bone is vascularised, whereas cementum is not. Cementum develops further after tooth eruption. As a result, it has reparative properties, which can play an important role in tooth trauma and root resorption (Figure 1.1.20).

The cementoblasts, cementocytes and fibroblasts of the periodontal ligament (PDL) are responsible for the formation of the cementum. These are cells of the ectomesenchyme. The cementoblasts form and secrete the cementum matrix. Cementocytes are formed from cementoblasts, which are trapped in the cementum during cementation (Figure 1.1.21). Fibroblasts, which are found adjacent to the cementum layer, form the acellular extrinsic fibre cementum. Their structure is very similar to that of the cementoblasts.

Four types of cementum can be distinguished: acellular afibrillar cementum (Figure 1.1.20), acellular extrinsic fibre cementum (Figure 1.1.19), cellular intrinsic fibre cementum (Figure 1.1.20) and cellular mixed fibre cementum (Figures 1.1.22 and 1.1.23).

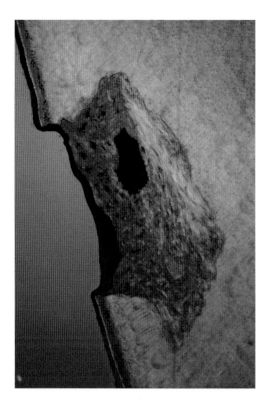

Figure 1.1.20 Repair of superficial root resorption by intrinsic cellular cementum. Above and below the cementum repair, a thin layer of acellular-afibrillar cementum covers the dentin.

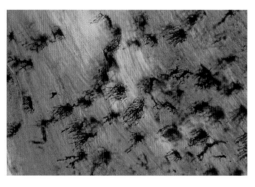

Figure 1.1.21 During the development of cementum, cementoblasts are enclosed within it. This results in cementocytes, which are clearly recognisable with long processes.

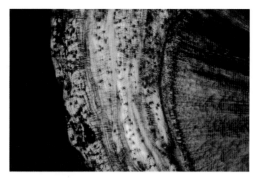

Figure 1.1.22 Cellular mixed-fibre cementum consisting of superposed layers of acellular extrinsic fibre and intrinsic cellular cementum. The granular layer of Tomes is also recognisable.

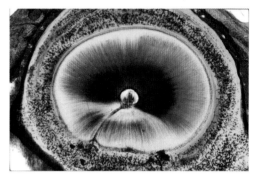

Figure 1.1.23 Horizontal section through the middle of a tooth root. The root dentin is coated with a thick layer of cellular mixed-fibre cementum. The excessive formation of cellular mixed-fibre cementum is called hypercementosis. A lateral channel, which runs from the pulp towards the root surface, is clearly visible.

Acknowledgements

The histological pictures and sections were made by Dr H. Stich and Mrs I. Hug. Some of the text has been taken from Carvalho and Lussi (2014) and Lussi and Schaffner (2012).

References

Carvalho, T. S., Lussi, A., Jaeggi, T., Gambon, D. 2014. Erosive tooth wear in children. *Monographs in Oral Science*, **25**, 262–3.

Featherstone, J. D., Mellberg, J. R. 1981. Relative rates of progress of artificial carious lesions in bovine, ovine and human enamel. *Caries Research*, **15**, 109–14.

Grine, F. E. 2005. Enamel thickness of deciduous and permanent molars in modern Homo sapiens. *American Journal of Physical Anthropology*, **126**, 14–31.

Horsted, M., Fejerskov, O., Larsen, M. J., Thylstrup, A. 1976. The structure of surface enamel with special reference to occlusal surfaces of primary and permanent teeth. *Caries Research*, **10**, 287–96.

Johansson, A. K., Sorvari, R., Birkhed, D., Meurman, J. H. 2001. Dental erosion in deciduous teeth – an in vivo and in vitro study. *Journal of Dentistry*, **29**, 333–40.

Kodaka, T., Nakajima, F., Higashi, S. 1989. Structure of the so-called "prismless" enamel in human deciduous teeth. *Caries Research*, **23**, 290–6.

Kodaka, T., Kuroiwa, M., Higashi, S. 1991. Structural and distribution patterns of surface "prismless" enamel in human permanent teeth. *Caries Research*, **25**, 7–20.

Lippert, F., Parker, D. M., Jandt, K. D. 2004. Susceptibility of deciduous and permanent enamel to dietary acid-induced erosion studied with atomic force microscopy nanoindentation. *European Journal of Oral Scienes*, **112**, 61–6.

Lussi, A., Schaffner, M. 2012. Structure and pathology of the tooth. In: Lussi, A., Schaffner, M. (eds). *Advances in Restorative Dentistry*. London: Quintessence, pp. 3–16.

Lussi, A., Kohler, N., Zero, D., Schaffner, M., Megert, B. 2000. A comparison of the erosive potential of different beverages in primary and permanent teeth using an in vitro model. *European Journal of Oral Scienes*, **108**, 110–14.

Magalhães, A. C., Rios, D., Honório, H. M., Delbem, A. C., Buzalaf, M. A. 2009. Effect of 4% titanium tetrafluoride solution on the erosion of permanent and deciduous human enamel: an in situ/ex vivo study. *Journal of Applied Oral Science*, **17**, 56–60.

Mahoney, P. 2013. Testing functional and morphological interpretations of enamel thickness along the deciduous tooth row in human children. *American Journal of Physical Anthropology*, **151**, 518–25.

Radlanski, R. J., Renz, H., Willersinn, U., Cordis, C. A., Duschner, H. 2001. Outline and arrangement of enamel rods in human deciduous and permanent enamel. 3D-reconstructions obtained from CLSM and SEM images based on serial ground sections. *European Journal of Oral Sciences*, **109**, 409–14.

Ripa, L. W. 1966. The histology of the early carious lesion in primary teeth with special reference to a "prismless" outer layer of primary enamel. *Journal of Dental Research*, **45**, 5–11.

Ripa, L. W., Gwinnett, A. J., Buonocore, M. G. 1966. The "prismless" outer layer of deciduous and permanent enamel. *Archives of Oral Biology*, **11**, 41–8.

Shellis, R. P. 1984a. Relationship between human enamel structure and the formation of caries-like lesions in vitro. *Archives of Oral Biology*, **29**, 975–81.

Shellis, R. P. 1984b. Variations in growth of the enamel crown in human teeth and a possible relationship between growth and enamel structure. *Archives of Oral Biology*, **29**, 697–705.

Sønju Clasen, A. B., Ruyter, I. E. 1997. Quantitative determination of type A and type B carbonate in human deciduous and permanent enamel by means of Fourier transform infrared spectrometry. *Advances in Dental Research*, **11**, 523–7.

Stack, M. V. 1953. Variation in the organic content of deciduous enamel and dentine. *Biochemical Journal*, **54**, xv.

Wilson, P. R., Beynon, A. D. 1989. Mineralization differences between human deciduous and permanent enamel measured by quantitative microradiography. *Archives of Oral Biology*, **34**, 85–8.

1.2

Pulp Biology of Deciduous and Permanent Teeth

Wolfgang H. Arnold[1], Ella A. Naumova[1] and Vlasios Goulioumis[2]

[1] Department of Biological and Material Sciences in Dentistry, School of Dentistry, Faculty of Health, Witten/Herdecke University, Witten, Germany
[2] Department of Operative and Preventive Dentistry, School of Dentistry, Faculty of Health, Witten/Herdecke University, Witten, Germany

Introduction

Dental pulp morphology and biology were ignored in the scientific literature until the beginning of the 20th century (Stanley, 1962). Currently, the dental pulp is considered a pulp organ with a complex morphological structure and diverse functions supporting tooth vitality, such as nutrition (James, 1955; Provenza, 1958; Klingsberg et al., 1959), restoration (regeneration) (Sayegh and Reed, 1968; Klinge, 2001; Han et al., 2013) and immunology (Zachrisson, 1971; Marchetti et al., 1992; Oehmke et al., 2003; Berggreen et al., 2009). The pulp organ has been described as a sensory organ (Uchizono and Homma, 1959; Pischinger and Stockinger, 1968; Egan et al., 1999) and the source of stem cells (Kerkis and Caplan, 2012; Isobe et al., 2016). The pulp tissue of deciduous and permanent teeth is embryologically derived from the ecto-mesenchyme of the neural crest. Therefore, it might be assumed that there are no differences in their structures. Comparative studies of the morphology of the pulp in deciduous and permanent teeth are scarce (Stanley, 1962; Herlesova, 1968; Sahara et al., 1993). However, distinct differences have been described (Bardellini et al., 2016).

It is the aim of this chapter to describe structural and functional similarities and differences in the pulp between the deciduous and permanent teeth.

Architecture of the Dental Pulp

The pulp organ is divided into the coronal chamber pulp and root canal pulp, with central and peripheral portions. The central portion of the pulp mainly contains the pulpoblasts (fibroblasts) embedded within a loose reticular meshwork and blood vessels, lymphatic vessels and nerves. The reticular meshwork appears to be denser in deciduous than in permanent teeth (Figure 1.2.1). The peripheral portion of the pulp contains three layers: the cell-rich zone of odontoblasts, the cell-free zone of Weil and the bipolar zone containing the nerve plexus (Raschkow plexus), located beneath the cell-free zone (Pischinger and Stockinger, 1968) (Figure 1.2.2). The cell-rich zone is thicker in permanent than in deciduous teeth (Figure 1.2.3), which may indicate a higher

Management of Dental Emergencies in Children and Adolescents, First Edition.
Edited by Klaus W. Neuhaus and Adrian Lussi.
© 2019 John Wiley & Sons Ltd. Published 2019 by John Wiley & Sons Ltd.
Companion website: www.wiley.com/go/neuhaus/dental_emergencies

(a)

(b)

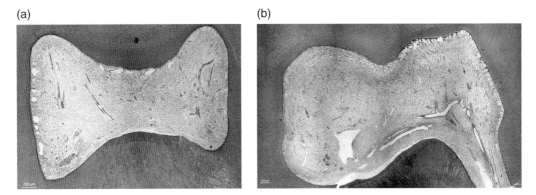

Figure 1.2.1 Histologic overview (Gomori staining) of the pulp chamber of (a) a deciduous molar and (b) a permanent molar. The pulp architecture is similar in both.

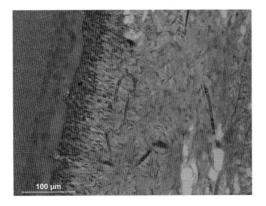

Figure 1.2.2 Histologic section (HE staining) of the pulp periphery, showing (a) the cell-rich zone with odontoblasts; (b) the cell-free zone of Weil; and (c) the bipolar cell zone containing the Raschkow plexus.

regenerative potential for new dentin formation in permanent teeth. The architecture of the root canal pulp is different from that of the coronal chamber pulp. The core of the root canal pulp mainly contains dense collagenous connective tissue (Figure 1.2.4a). At the root canal wall, the pulp consists of loose connective tissue adjacent to the odontoblastic layer (Figure 1.2.4b). The odontoblastic layer in the root canal pulp contains fewer odontoblasts than that in the coronal chamber pulp. The odontoblasts in the root canal pulp are cubic or flat, whilst those in the coronal chamber pulp are prismatic. Specific differences in the root canal pulp between deciduous and permanent teeth have not been described.

(a)

(b)

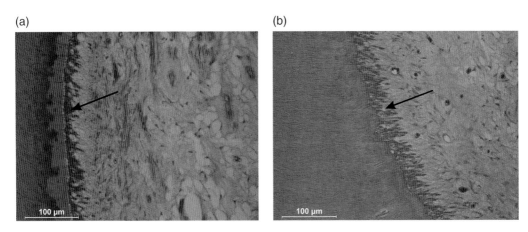

Figure 1.2.3 Histologic section (HE staining) of the cell-rich zone of the odontoblast layer (arrows) in (a) deciduous teeth and (b) permanent teeth. In deciduous teeth, this layer is much thinner.

(a)

(b)

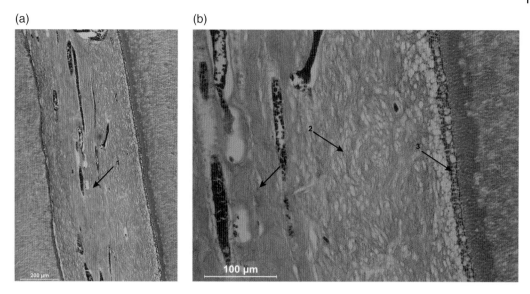

Figure 1.2.4 Histologic section (Azan staining) of the root pulp. (a) The central core of the pulp shows dense collagen with blood vessels (1). (b) The connective tissue in the periphery is loose (2), and the odontoblasts are cubic (3).

Dental Pulp Cells and Extracellular Matrix

Within the pulp organ, four different cell types can be found: pulpocytes, dental pulpal stem cells (DPSCs), immunocompetent cells and odontoblasts. The most common type is the pulpocytes, which are derived from their precursors, pulpoblasts or pulpal stem cells (Gronthos et al., 2000, 2002). These form a reticular network (Figure 1.2.5a) and are embed-

ded in a gelatinous extracellular matrix of proteoglycan, glycosaminoglycan, fibronectin, ncollagenous proteins and various types of collagen (Bergenholtz et al., 1985; Linde, 1985). In deciduous teeth, the meshwork of reticular fibres is rather dense, but in permanent teeth it is loose, condensing around the central and peripheral blood vessels (Figure 1.2.5b). The second most common cell type is the DPSC (Gronthos et al., 2002), which can differentiate into three

(a)

(b)

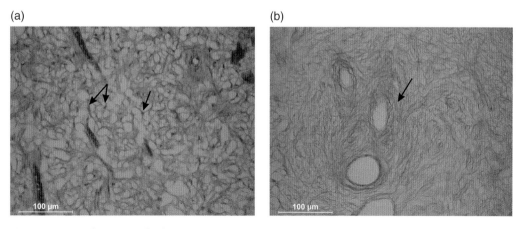

Figure 1.2.5 Histologic view of pulp connective tissue (a) with reticular cells (arrows) and a loose meshwork of reticular fibres (HE staining) and (b) with dense reticular fibres around the blood vessels (arrow) (Gomori staining).

subpopulations: adipocytes, nervous cells and odontoblast-like cells. Odontoblast-like cells produce primary dentin (Gronthos et al., 2000, 2002) and are important for the regeneration of pulp tissue and dentin. Relatively immature dental pulp stem cells (IDPSCs) have been isolated from exfoliated deciduous teeth; these show a higher potential than DPSCs to differentiate into various cell subtypes (Kerkis et al., 2006; Kerkis and Caplan, 2012) and may be a major source for regenerative tooth therapy in the future (Gronthos et al., 2002; Kerkis and Caplan, 2012). The third cell type is immunocompetent cells, such as mast cells, macrophages and plasma cells (Figure 1.2.6). These are normally located in the periarterial connective tissue sheet. Lymphocytes and granulocytes migrate into the pulp connective tissue during pulp inflammation. The fourth cell type is the odontoblasts. Odontoblasts are post-mitotic cells derived from neural crest cells that are not capable of regeneration. They produce predentin during their entire life and are responsible for secondary dentin development adjacent to the pulp camber wall. The odontoblastic layer of permanent teeth contains more odontoblasts than that of deciduous teeth, where it is much thinner (Figure 1.2.3).

Blood Vessels

The central pulp artery, derived from the root canal artery, is a branch of the subodontoblastic capillary plexus (James, 1955; Provenza, 1958; Klingsberg et al., 1959; Kramer, 1960) and is responsible for the nutrition of odontoblasts. The pattern of the vascular and nervous architecture is similar between deciduous and permanent teeth (James, 1955; Provenza, 1958; Klingsberg et al., 1959; Egan et al., 1996, 1999).

Lymphatic Vessels

The capillaries of the lymphatic system of the pulp begin near the zone of Weil. They merge into larger lymphatic vessels in the coronal chamber pulp and exit the pulp together with the blood vessels through the apical foramen of the tooth root (Bernick, 1972; Marchetti et al., 1992; Oehmke et al., 2003; Radlanski, 2011).

Pulp Nerves

The nerve enters the pulp through the apical foramen of the tooth root and branches within the coronal chamber pulp to build a

(a)

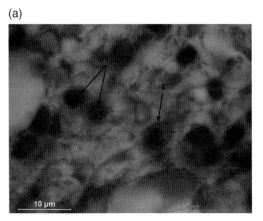

(b)

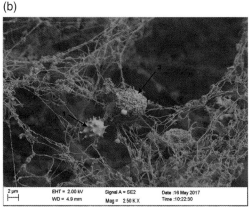

Figure 1.2.6 Higher-magnification images of immunocompetent cells within the pulp tissue: (a) histologic view (HE staining) demonstrating leucocytes (1) and macrophages (2); and (b) a scanning electron micrograph showing a leucocyte (1) and a pulp fibrocyte (3).

nerve plexus (Raschkow plexus) beneath the cell-free zone of Weil. Most nerves are nonmyelinated nerves of the autonomous nervous system that regulate the blood flow in the pulp. Myelinated nerves are branches of the trigeminal nerve and are somatosensible (Radlanski, 2011). Thus far, no differences between deciduous and permanent teeth have been reported in terms of the innervation pattern (Rapp et al., 1967; Itoh, 1976).

Pulp Regeneration

The regenerative capacity of the pulp tissue is limited. The main source for pulp regeneration is the pulpal stem cells. The pulp tissue contains pre- and postnatal stem cells. As already noted, stem cells are capable of differentiating into four cell types (Gronthos et al., 2000; Kerkis and Caplan, 2012; Maxim et al., 2015), chief amongst them pulpocytes, which are the cells of the reticular meshwork, and odontoblasts, which produce various types of intrapulpal dentin. Primary odontoblasts produce secondary dentin adjacent to the pulp wall following external stimulation. This process is similar in deciduous and permanent teeth. Newly differentiated secondary odontoblasts from pulpal stem cells produce various kinds of intrapulpal calcifications, such as denticles, fibrodentin and osteodentin (Figure 1.2.7), which are summarised as

(a)

(b)

(c)

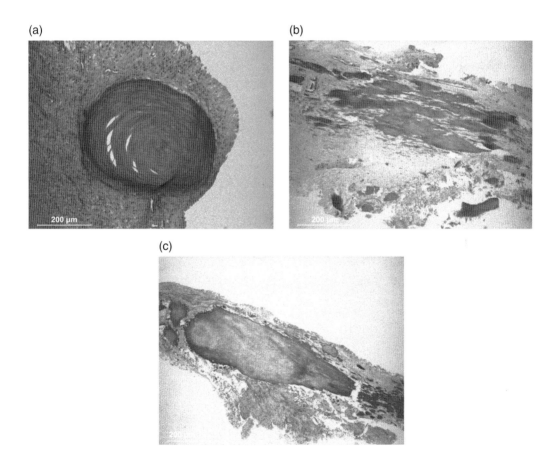

Figure 1.2.7 Histologic sections (HE staining) demonstrating various intrapulpal calcifications, including (a) a denticle, (b) fibrodentin and (c) osteodentin.

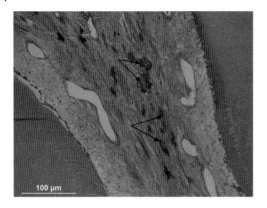

Figure 1.2.8 Histologic section (HE staining) of a deciduous root canal pulp with calcifications (arrows) prior to root resorption.

tertiary dentin. Tertiary dentin is produced as a response of the pulp to external stimuli, inflammation or trauma and may therefore be regarded as cicatrix of the pulp tissue. Pulp capping produces a reaction of the pulp, beginning with chronic inflammation and followed by fibrous proliferation, alignment of the pulp cells, differentiation of the odontoblasts and tertiary dentin synthesis (Glass and Zander, 1949). In permanent teeth, pulp calcifications become increasingly common with age (Sayegh and Reed, 1968). In deciduous teeth, they are less common, perhaps because their lifespan is much shorter. However, before the onset of deciduous root resorption, calcifications can be found in the root canal (Figure 1.2.8).

Pulp Resorption

There are two types of pulp resorption: physiologic resorption of the pulp and dental hard tissue in deciduous teeth and pathologic resorption in permanent teeth. Physiologic root resorption occurs during the exfoliation of deciduous teeth. The cells

of the stellate reticulum of the developing permanent teeth pulp secrete parathyroid hormone-related protein (PTHrP) and interleukin-1α, which activate the cells of the dental sac (Philbrick, 1998). The dental sac cells are stimulated by PTHrP and interleukin-1α to produce colony-stimulating factor and monocyte chemotactic protein. Monocytes that have migrated from the blood vessels into the pulp tissue fuse and differentiate into odontoclasts, which resorb dentin, resulting in deep resorption lacunae (Figure 1.2.9). Then, B and T lymphocytes migrate into the pulp tissue, which is replaced by granulated tissue and resorbed by macrophages (Soskolne and Bimstein, 1977) (Figure 1.2.10). The odontoblasts also degenerate (Figure 1.2.11).

Trauma to the teeth may result in pathologic pulp degeneration and hard-tissue resorption of the tooth (Gassmann and Arnold, 2015). This eventually results in an internal granuloma that destroys the whole tooth crown. The pulp tissue is replaced with fibrous connective tissue and infiltrated by leucocytes (Figure 1.2.12). Numerous odontoclasts are found at the wall of the pulp coronal chamber, resorbing dentin (Figure 1.2.12).

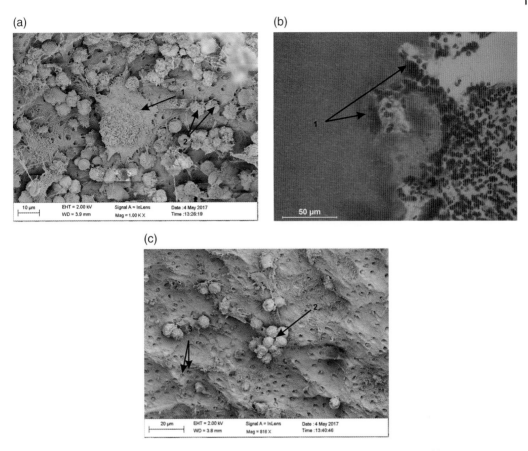

Figure 1.2.9 (a) Scanning electron micrograph of an odontoclast (1) surrounded by odontoblasts (2). (b) Histologic section (HE staining) of resorption lacunae of dentin with odontoclasts (1). (c) Scanning electron micrograph of resorption lacunae, with a few odontoblasts (2) and remnants of odontoblast processes within the dentin tubules (3).

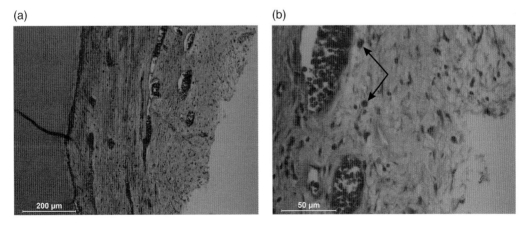

Figure 1.2.10 Histologic section (HE staining) of the pulp resorption area of a deciduous incisor tooth with (a) granulated tissue and (b) macrophages (arrows), which are responsible for tissue degradation.

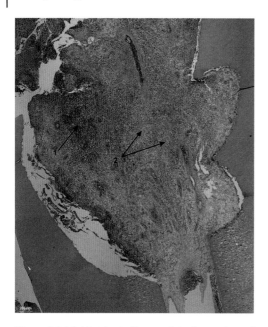

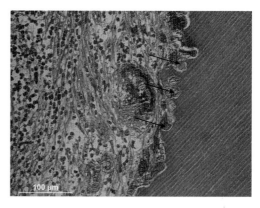

Figure 1.2.12 Higher-magnification image of odontoclasts (arrows) resorbing dentin in an internal granuloma.

Figure 1.2.11 Histologic (Azan staining) overview of an internal granuloma following tooth trauma with infiltration of leucocytes (1) into the pulp tissue and fibrous degeneration (2) of the pulp tissue.

References

Bardellini, E., Amadori, F., Santoro, A., Conti, G., Orsini, G., Majorana, A. 2016. Odontoblastic cell quantification and apoptosis within pulp of deciduous teeth versus pulp of permanent teeth. *Journal of Clinical Pediatric Dentistry*, **40**, 450–5.

Bergenholtz, G., Mjor, I. A., Cotton, W. R., Hanks, C. T., Kim, S., Torneck, C. D., Trowbridge, H. O. 1985. The biology of dentin and pulp. Consensus report. *Journal of Dental Research*, **64**(Spec. No.), 631–3.

Berggreen, E., Haug, S. R., Mkonyi, L. E., Bletsa, A. 2009. Characterization of the dental lymphatic system and identification of cells immunopositive to specific lymphatic markers. *European Journal of Oral Sciences*, **117**, 34–42.

Bernick, S. 1972. Vascular and nerve changes associated with the healing of the human pulp. *Oral Surgery Oral Medicine Oral Pathology*, **33**, 983–1000.

Egan, C. A., Bishop, M. A., Hector, M. P. 1996. An immunohistochemical study of the pulpal nerve supply in primary human teeth: evidence for the innervation of deciduous dentine. *Journal of Anatomy*, **188**(Pt 3), 623–31.

Egan, C. A., Hector, M. P., Bishop, M. A. 1999. On the pulpal nerve supply in primary human teeth: evidence for the innervation of primary dentine. *International Journal of Paediatric Dentistry*, **9**, 57–66.

Gassmann, G., Arnold, W. H. 2015. Case report of an internal granuloma investigated by light and scanning electron microscopy. *Head & Face Medicine*, **11**, 20.

Glass, R. L., Zander, H. A. 1949. Pulp healing. *Journal of Dental Research*, **28**, 97–107.

Gronthos, S., Mankani, M., Brahim, J., Robey, P. G., Shi, S. 2000. Postnatal human dental pulp stem cells (DPSCs) in vitro and in vivo. *Proceedings of the National Academy of Science USA*, **97**, 13 625–30.

Gronthos, S., Brahim, J., Li, W., Fisher, L. W., Cherman, N., Boyde, A., Denbesten, P., Robey, P. G., Shi, S. 2002. Stem cell properties of human dental pulp stem cells. *Journal of Dental Research*, **81**, 531–5.

Han, G., Hu, M., Zhang, Y., Jiang, H. 2013. Pulp vitality and histologic changes in human dental pulp after the application of moderate and severe intrusive orthodontic forces. *American Journal of Orthodontics and Dentofacial Orthopedics*, **144**, 518–22.

Herlesova, J. 1968. Histology of dental pulp in clinically intact deciduous and permanent teeth in children. *Acta Universitatis Carololinae. Medica (Praha)*, **14**, 229–34.

Isobe, Y., Koyama, N., Nakao, K., Osawa, K., Ikeno, M., Yamanaka, S., Okubo, Y., Fujimura, K., Bessho, K. 2016. Comparison of human mesenchymal stem cells derived from bone marrow, synovial fluid, adult dental pulp, and exfoliated deciduous tooth pulp. *International Journal of Oral Maxillofacial Surgery*, **45**, 124–31.

Itoh, K. 1976. The distribution of nerves in human deciduous and permanent teeth. *Archivum Histologicum Japonicum*, **39**, 379–99.

James, W. W. 1955. The blood capillary system of the odontoblast layer of the dental pulp. *Journal of Anatomy*, **89**, 547–9.

Kerkis, I., Caplan, A. I. 2012. Stem cells in dental pulp of deciduous teeth. *Tissue Engineering. Part B, Reviews*, **18**, 129–38.

Kerkis, I., Kerkis, A., Dozortsev, D., Stukart-Parsons, G. C., Gomes Massironi, S. M., Pereira, L. V., Caplan, A. I., Cerruti, H. F. 2006. Isolation and characterization of a population of immature dental pulp stem cells expressing OCT-4 and other embryonic stem cell markers. *Cells Tissues Organs*, **184**, 105–16.

Klinge, R. F. 2001. Further observations on tertiary dentin in human deciduous teeth. *Advances in Dental Research*, **15**, 76–9.

Klingsberg, J., Cancellaro, L., Butcher, E. O. 1959. A capillary network in the odontoblastic layer of developing teeth. *Journal of Dental Research*, **38**, 419.

Kramer, I. R. 1960. The vascular architecture of the human dental pulp. *Archives of Oral Biology*, **2**, 177–89.

Linde, A. 1985. The extracellular matrix of the dental pulp and dentin. *Journal of Dental Research*, **64**(Spec. No.), 523–9.

Marchetti, C., Poggi, P., Calligaro, A., Casasco, A. 1992. Lymphatic vessels of the human dental pulp in different conditions. *Anatomical Record*, **234**, 27–33.

Maxim, M. A., Soritau, O., Baciut, M., Bran, S., Baciut, G. 2015. The role of dental stem cells in regeneration. *Clujul Medical*, **88**, 479–82.

Oehmke, M. J., Knolle, E., Oehmke, H. J. 2003. Lymph drainage in the human dental pulp. *Microscopy Research and Technique*, **62**, 187–91.

Philbrick, W. M. 1998. Parathyroid hormone-related protein is a developmental regulatory molecule. *European Journal of Oral Sciences*, **106**(Suppl. 1), 32–7.

Pischinger, A., Stockinger, L. 1968. The nerves of the human dental pulp [German]. *Zeitschrift für Zellforschung und Mikroskopische Anatomie*, **89**, 44–61.

Provenza, D. V. 1958. The blood vascular supply of the dental pulp with emphasis on capillary circulation. *Circulation Research*, **6**, 213–18.

Radlanski, R. J. 2011. *Orale Struktur- und Entwicklungsbiologie*. Berlin: Quintessenz.

Rapp, R., Avery, J. K., Strachan, D. S. 1967. The distribution of nerves in human primary teeth. *Anatomical Records*, **159**, 89–103.

Sahara, N., Okafuji, N., Toyoki, A., Ashizawa, Y., Yagasaki, H., Deguchi, T., Suzuki, K. 1993. A histological study of the exfoliation of human deciduous teeth. *Journal of Dental Research*, **72**, 634–40.

Sayegh, F. S., Reed, A. J. 1968. Calcification in the dental pulp. *Oral Surgery Oral Medicine Oral Pathology*, **25**, 873–82.

Soskolne, W. A., Bimstein, E. 1977. A histomorphological study of the shedding process of human deciduous teeth at various chronological stages. *Archives of Oral Biology*, **22**, 331–5.

Stanley, H. R. 1962. The cells of the dental pulp. *Oral Surgery Oral Medicine Oral Pathology*, **15**, 849–58.

Uchizono, K., Homma, K. 1959. Electron microscopic studies on nerves of human tooth pulp. *Journal of Dental Research*, **38**, 1133–41.

Zachrisson, B. U. 1971. Mast cells in human dental pulp. *Archives of Oral Biology*, **16**, 555–6.

1.3

Management of Odontogenic Infections: Indications for Antibiotics

Rafael Lazarin and Vivianne Chappuis

Department of Oral Surgery and Stomatology, School of Dental Medicine, University of Bern, Bern, Switzerland

Introduction

One in four children has their first encounter with a dentist due to an emergency situation (Agostini et al., 2001). Depending on the child's age and the appointment setting (e.g. hospital or dental clinic), the emergency may be related to pain (82%), dental caries (40–79%), soft-tissue disease (4–20%), disease of the pulp and periapical tissue (40%), dental trauma (6–51%) or cellulitis and abscess of the mouth (3%) (Rowley et al., 2006; Shqair et al., 2012; Allareddy et al., 2014). Many of these conditions are caused by an odontogenic infection, which may require antibiotic therapy in order to control infection and prevent bacterial spread. However, as childhood is a period of continuous growth and development, administration of antibiotics in children should be carefully evaluated. Long-term administration may cause peculiar neurologic and physical abnormalities such as neurodevelopmental dysfunction, enamel hypo- and dysplasia, discoloration of teeth and dysfunction in bone growth (Reed and Besunder, 1989; Alcorn and McNamara, 2003; Sánchez et al., 2004). Further, dosages in paediatric patients must be adjusted for their lower weight and body size (Agarwal et al., 2014). Dentists have raised questions about the risks and benefits of antibiotic administration for prophylactic or therapeutic purposes due to the development of resistant microbial strains, doubts over the efficacy of prophylactic regiments, possible adverse reactions and poor compliance by patients (Agarwal et al., 2014).

The scientific literature includes a number of guidelines on whether to administer antibiotics (Palmer, 2006; Agarwal et al., 2014; Caviglia et al., 2014; AAPD, 2016a,b,c). One of the best-accepted is that from the American Academy of Pediatric Dentistry (AAPD, 2016a,b,c). However, studies reveal a low adherence to these guidelines, varying between 6 and 33% (Coutinho et al., 2009; Cherry et al., 2012; Yesudian et al., 2015). A recent study showed that dentists are overprescribing antibiotics for children, and that at least 21% of the dosages recommended for children were inappropriate (Michael and Hibbert, 2014). Fortunately, dentists are aware that antibiotic resistance is a growing problem (Sivaraman et al., 2013). Studies have shown that following educational measures, the percentage of appropriate recommendations can increase (Palmer et al., 2001; Palmer and Dailey, 2002; Yesudian et al., 2015). Therefore, the aim of this chapter is to summarise the current literature in order to assist clinicians in their decision-making process.

Management of Dental Emergencies in Children and Adolescents, First Edition.
Edited by Klaus W. Neuhaus and Adrian Lussi.
© 2019 John Wiley & Sons Ltd. Published 2019 by John Wiley & Sons Ltd.
Companion website: www.wiley.com/go/neuhaus/dental_emergencies

Antibiotic Resistance, Misuse and Adverse Drug Events

Dental professionals are responsible for 10% (almost 25 million) of all antibiotic prescriptions worldwide (Hicks et al., 2015; CDC, 2017). Thus, they must be responsible in their recommendations, in order to minimise the risk of adverse events and reduce the spread of antibiotic-resistant bacteria (Fluent et al., 2016). According to the literature, six events can occur when antibiotics are applied (Pallasch, 2000):

1) The antibiotic may aid the immune system to gain control of the infection.
2) Toxicity or allergy may occur.
3) Already resistant microbes may be selected for, and a superinfection may result.
4) The antimicrobial may promote microbial chromosomal mutations.
5) Gene transfer from resistant to nonresistant microbes may be encouraged.
6) Latent resistance genes may be expressed.

Antibiotic Resistance

Antibiotic resistance is a major global health threat. Every year in the United States alone, at least 2 million people became infected with antibiotic-resistant bacteria, and about 23 000 die as a direct result of these infections (CDC, 2017). A study performed in adults with isolated microorganisms from orofacial infections found significant rates of antibiotic-resistant bacteria: 32.5% showed resistance to penicillin, 29.3% to clindamycin and 30% to erythromycin (Kim et al., 2017). Clinicians and patients play a fundamental role in the development of antibiotic resistance. Clinicians should avoid overprescription, whilst patients should be aware that antibiotics should not be applied for every type of pain or problem. According to Pallasch (2000), the main reasons for the inappropriate use of antibiotics are:

- Insufficient training in infectious diseases and proper antibiotics therapy.
- Empirical use.

- Lack of culture and sensitivity tests.
- Inadequate diagnosis.
- Inappropriate choice of drug, dose and duration.
- Need for self-assurance.
- Patient demand.
- Fear of litigation.

Antibiotic resistance may be prevented through a few strategies aimed at minimising the emergence of resistant bacteria (AAPD, 2016b; CDC, 2017), including improving clinician training and providing patients with information on antibiotic therapy (Palmer et al., 2001; Palmer and Dailey, 2002; Jain et al., 2015; Yesudian et al., 2015; CDC, 2017). Patient compliance is a key factor in order in reducing the emergence of resistant bacteria. Patients should be aware of when antibiotics will and won't help. They should only take antibiotics exactly as prescribed, and shouldn't save them for later or share them with others (CDC, 2017).

In summary, the most important aspect in minimising the emergence of antibiotic resistance is improving prescription of antibiotics by means of the education of clinicians and patients. The key is to prescribe the right antibiotic, at the right dosage and drug interval, for the right time period and at the right time point, according to well-accepted guidelines. The development of antibiotic resistance can thus be reduced.

Misuse of Antibiotics in Dentistry

The key to avoiding misuse of antibiotics in dentistry is to correctly diagnose patient complaints. A detailed medical and dental history, an extraoral/intraoral clinical examination and a radiographic analysis are necessary for an adequate diagnosis, and the subsequent provision of a treatment plan (with or without the use of antibiotic medication). The misuse of antibiotic drugs in dentistry involves their application in inappropriate clinical situations, their administration for too short or too long a period of time and further situations such as

(Pallasch, 2000; Palmer, 2006; Michael and Hibbert, 2014):

- Giving antibiotics after a dental procedure is completed in an otherwise healthy patient in order to "prevent" an infection (that is, to prevent a lawsuit, in many cases), which in all likelihood will not occur.
- Using antibiotics as "analgesic."
- Employing antibiotics for prophylaxis in a patient not at risk for metastatic bacteraemia.
- Using antimicrobials to treat chronic adult periodontitis.
- Using antimicrobial therapy in lieu of mechanical therapy in periodontitis management.
- Using antibiotics instead of surgical incision and drainage of infections.
- Using antibiotic to "prevent" claims of negligence.

Adverse Drug Events

Adverse drugs events (ADEs) are the most common cause of iatrogenic harm in health care and have recently received attention in national patient safety initiatives (Shehab et al., 2016). Amongst children, ADEs related to antibiotics are the most frequent cause of emergency department visits (CDC, 2017): 27.5% of ADEs affect children aged 0–18 years (Bourgeois et al., 2009). In a study based on more than 42 500 ADE cases, it was found that 46.4% were related to antibiotics at age 5 years and younger, and 31.8% at ages 6–19 (Shehab et al., 2016). The most commons ADEs include dermatologic, gastrointestinal, neurological, psychological, endocrine, respiratory and cardiovascular symptoms, general malaise/fever, oedema/swelling and sensory or motor disturbance (syncope/dizziness/muscular weakness) (Bourgeois et al., 2009; Shehab et al., 2016).

Patients should be aware that the following ADEs may occur during antibiotic therapy: rash, diarrhoea (including Pseudomembranous colitis or *Clostridium difficile* infection), abdominal pain, gastrointestinal disturbance, nausea/vomiting, drug fever, joint pain, weakness, taste alterations, tooth discoloration in children <8 years, jaundice, dizziness, drowsiness, headache, insomnia, metallic mouth taste and hypersensitivity reactions (Table 1.3.1). In the drug class of penicillins – the first choice of antibiotic for dental treatment – hypersensitivity is one of the most frequent ADEs. Reactions can range from a simple rash or urticaria in 1–7% of cases (Palmer, 2006) to a life-threatening, severe anaphylactic reaction in 0.004–0.2% (Caviglia et al., 2014).

Indications for Antibiotic Therapy

Indications for Using Antibiotic Therapy

Antibiotics should always be applied in addition to causative dental treatment and should never be used as the exclusive therapy of choice. Antibiotics cannot serve as a substitute for surgical or endodontic treatment, for the following reasons (Pallasch, 1993, 1996, 2000): antibiotics do not diffuse well into infected areas; blood supply to abscesses is usually compromised; due to the acidic environment and low pH level within dentoalveolar infections, some antibiotics are ineffective; high levels of antibiotic inhibitors (beta-lactamases) may be present in infections; and the efficacy of penicillins and cephalosporins is reduced in infections where microorganisms are dividing slowly or not at all.

The use of antibiotics in dentistry is indicated for two major reasons: to control oral infection and to prevent bacteraemia precipitated by dental manipulations from causing severe systemic sequelae (Agarwal et al., 2014). In general, consideration should be given to the patient's systemic condition, the patient's symptoms, the intraoral localisation, the extension of the inflammation, the type of wound and the progression of the disease. In 2016, the AAPD revised its guidelines concerning indications for antibiotic therapy in paediatric dental patients with the

Table 1.3.1 The main antibiotics used in paediatric dental patients (according to Palmer, 2006; Agarwal et al., 2014; Caviglia et al., 2014; and Donaldson et al., 2015).

Name	Oral dosage – drug interval				Side effects (most common)	Additional information
	Agarwal et al. (2014)	Caviglia et al. (2014)	Donaldson et al. (2015)			
Amoxicillin	50–90 mg/kg/day 08–12 h	20–50 mg/kg/day 08 h	20–90 mg/kg/day 08–12 h		Nausea/vomiting, abdominal pain, diarrhoea, drug fever, hypersensitivity reaction	First choice in dentistry – broad-spectrum penicillin
Amoxicillin– Clavulanate potassium	45–50 mg/kg/day 08 h	40–80 mg/kg/day 08 h	25–90 mg/kg/day 12 h		Nausea/vomiting, abdominal pain, diarrhoea, drug fever, hypersensitivity reaction	Indicated in cases of late untreated infection or bad evolution after treatment with first choice
Ampicilin	50–100 mg/kg 06 h	–	–		Nausea/vomiting, abdominal pain, diarrhoea, drug fever, hypersensitivity reaction, fever, headache, weakness	Preferred to be administered parenterally
Azithromycin	–	–	5–10 mg/day Once day × 4 days		Nausea/vomiting, abdominal pain, diarrhoea, dizziness, taste alterations	Alternative to amoxicillin, similar to erytromycin
Clarithromycin	–	7.5–15 mg/kg/day 12 h	7.5 mg/kg 12 h		Nausea/vomiting, abdominal pain, headache, insomnia, taste alterations	Useful for patient allergic to penicillin – good soft-tissue diffusion
Clindamycin	–	10–30 mg/kg/day 06 h	10 mg/kg 08 h		Nausea/vomiting, abdominal pain, diarrhoea (pseudomembranous colitis), joint pain, jaundice	Useful for patients allergic to penicillin – good bone-tissue diffusion
Doxycycline[a]	–	–	2–4 mg/kg/day 12 h		Nausea/vomiting, abdominal pain, diarrhoea, discoloration of permanent teeth	–
Erytromycin	30–50 mg/kg 06 h	–	7.5–12.5 mg/kg 06 h		Nausea/vomiting, abdominal pain, diarrhoea, dizziness	Useful for patient allergic to penicillin
Metronidazole	30–50 mg/kg 06 h	–	30 mg/kg/day 06 h		Nausea/vomiting, taste alterations, gastrointestinal disturbances, drowsiness, dizziness, headache	Usually indicated in periodontal diseases, in association with penicillin
Penicillin	25–50 mg/kg 06–12 h	–	25–50 mg/kg/day 06–08 h		Nausea/vomiting, abdominal pain, diarrhoea, drug fever, hypersensitivity reaction	Alternative to amoxicillin
Tetracycline[a]	–	–	25–50 mg/kg/day 06 h		Nausea/vomiting, diarrhoea, discoloration of permanent teeth, swollen tongue	First systemic choice in cases of avulsion of permanent teeth Alternative in cases of treatment of AP

[a] Not recommended for children younger than 8 years, because this is the period in which tooth enamel is being formed (Shetty, 2002). AP, agressive periodontitis.

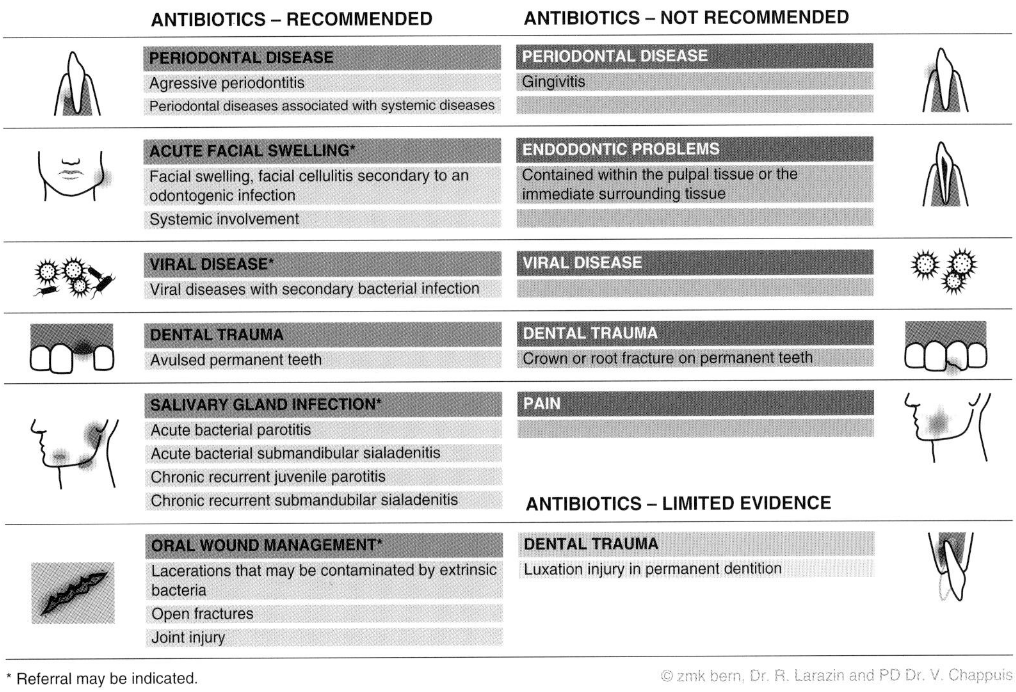

ANTIBIOTICS – RECOMMENDED	ANTIBIOTICS – NOT RECOMMENDED
PERIODONTAL DISEASE	**PERIODONTAL DISEASE**
Agressive periodontitis	Gingivitis
Periodontal diseases associated with systemic diseases	
ACUTE FACIAL SWELLING*	**ENDODONTIC PROBLEMS**
Facial swelling, facial cellulitis secondary to an odontogenic infection	Contained within the pulpal tissue or the immediate surrounding tissue
Systemic involvement	
VIRAL DISEASE*	**VIRAL DISEASE**
Viral diseases with secondary bacterial infection	
DENTAL TRAUMA	**DENTAL TRAUMA**
Avulsed permanent teeth	Crown or root fracture on permanent teeth
SALIVARY GLAND INFECTION*	**PAIN**
Acute bacterial parotitis	
Acute bacterial submandibular sialadenitis	
Chronic recurrent juvenile parotitis	**ANTIBIOTICS – LIMITED EVIDENCE**
Chronic recurrent submandubilar sialadenitis	
ORAL WOUND MANAGEMENT*	**DENTAL TRAUMA**
Lacerations that may be contaminated by extrinsic bacteria	Luxation injury in permanent dentition
Open fractures	
Joint injury	

* Referral may be indicated.

© zmk bern, Dr. R. Larazin and PD Dr. V. Chappuis

Figure 1.3.1 Clinical situations in which antibiotic therapy is and is not indicated for paediatric dental patients.

following recommendations (AAPD, 2016b) (Figure 1.3.1):

A) **Oral wound management**
- Facial lacerations may require topical antibiotic agents.
- Intraoral lacerations that may be contaminated by extrinsic bacteria, open fractures and joint injury should be covered with antibiotics.

B) **Pulpitis/apical periodontitis/draining sinus tract/localised intraoral swelling**
- Antibiotic therapy usually is not indicated if the dental infection is contained within the pulpal tissue or the immediate surrounding tissue.
- Antibiotics may be an option for cases of advanced nonodontogenic bacterial infection such as staphylococcal mucositis, tuberculosis, gonococcal stomatitis and oral syphilis.

C) **Acute facial swelling of dental origin**
- Children with facial swelling, facial cellulitis secondary to an odontogenic infection and any signs of systemic involvement should receive immediate dental attention.

D) **Dental trauma**
- Antibiotics are recommended for avulsed permanent incisors with open or closed apex.
- Antibiotics are generally not indicated for cases of luxation involving the primary dentition.

E) **Pediatric periodontal diseases**
- Cases of periodontal diseases associated with systemic diseases (e.g. severe congenital neutropenia, Papillon–Lefèvre syndrome, leukocyte adhesion deficiency) may require adjunctive antibiotic therapy.

F) **Viral diseases**
- Conditions of viral origin should not be treated with antibiotics unless there is strong evidence that a secondary bacterial infection exists.

G) **Salivary gland infection**
- If there is confirmation of bacterial aetiology, some salivary gland infection

and acute bacterial parotitis and chronic recurrent juvenile parotitis, antibiotic therapy is recommended.

- In cases of acute bacterial submandibular sialadenitis and chronic recurrent submandibular sialadenitis, the use of antibiotics is already included as part of the treatment.

Complementing the topic of dental trauma, the International Association of Dental Traumatology (IADT) provides a series of guidelines for the management of traumatic dental injuries (TDIs) in the primary and permanent dentition (Andersson et al., 2012, 2016; DiAngelis et al., 2012, 2016; Malmgren et al., 2012, 2016). Together with one literature review (Andreasen et al., 2006), their conclusions about the use of antibiotics are as follows (Figure 1.3.1):

1) **Fractures and luxations of permanent teeth:** There is limited evidence for the use of systemic antibiotics in the management of luxation injury and no evidence for root-fracture teeth.
2) **Avulsion of permanent teeth:** Antibiotics are in most situations recommended after replantations of teeth (with closed or open apex). Positive effects (periodontal and pulpal healing) are observed when antibiotics are prescribed, both systemically and topically.
3) **Injuries in the primary dentition:** There is no evidence for the use of systemic antibiotics in the management of luxation injuries in the primary dentition.

In the area of periodontology, young children and adolescents may be affected by necrotising ulcerative gingivitis (NUG). If this condition is accompanied by fever, malaise or lymphadenopathy, antibiotic therapy is indicated (Agarwal et al., 2014; AAPD, 2016c). Aggressive periodontitis (AP), chronic periodontitis (CP) and periodontitis as a manifestation of systemic disease can also affect children and adolescents. During treatment of AP and periodontitis as a manifestation of systemic disease, the use of antibiotics is usually beneficial (AAPD, 2016c) (Figure 1.3.1).

The clinician should always consider whether the patient can be treated in the dental practice or should be referred to a hospital setting. Referral should always be considered in cases presenting signs of septicaemia (grossly elevated temperature, lethargy, tachycardia), spreading cellulitis, swelling compromising the airway (causing closure of the eye or difficulty in swallowing), dehydration or failure to respond to treatment, as well as with uncooperative patients (Palmer, 2006).

Indications for Not Using Antibiotic Therapy

According to the literature, antibiotic therapy should not be administered for dental treatment under the following conditions: management of dental pain, localised swelling or dental infections contained within the pulpal tissue or the immediate surrounding tissue, gingivitis and management of viral infections without secondary bacterial infections (Palmer, 2006; Agarwal et al., 2014; AAPD, 2016b). A systematic review of the literature (Matthews et al., 2003) concluded that the use of antibiotics in the management of localised dental infections is not recommended as a substitute for causative dental treatment. In addition, the effectiveness of oral antibiotics as a sole treatment for an odontogenic infection is highly questionable, due to the lack of effective circulation in a necrotic pulp or an abscess (Swift and Guiden, 2002) (Figure 1.3.1).

Time Point, Time Period, Dosage and Drug Interval of Antibiotic Therapy

Time Point and Time Period

There is a consensus that antibiotics should be administered as soon as possible for optimal results. They should continue to be applied for a minimum of 5 days beyond the point of substantial improvement of symptoms

(Agarwal et al., 2014; AAPD, 2016b). This may represent a total of 5–7 days of treatment, depending upon the specific drug selected. However, the clinician must always monitor the clinical effectiveness of the therapy. In cases of ineffectiveness before the course is completed, alteration or discontinuation should be considered (AAPD, 2016b). In addition, a lack of patient compliance should be taken into account as a potential reason for a limited response.

Dosage and Drug Interval

Two types of error in the dosage of antibiotics should be considered: underdosage and overdosage. Underdosage may produce an inadequate concentration of the drug at the infected site, fostering recurrent infections and development of resistant bacterial strains. Overdosage, on the other hand, may result in damage to the host's response, producing toxic effects and increasing the risk of ADEs (Swift and Guiden, 2002). The dosages, drug intervals and most common side effects of the main antibiotics are listed in Table 1.3.1.

Antibiotic Prophylaxis

Antibiotic prophylaxis (AP) is used in order to prevent a bacteraemia caused by dental manipulations leading to severe systemic sequelae prior to invasive dental procedures. It is recommended for patients at high risk of developing infective endocarditis (IE) and for those affected by several immunocompromised conditions (Donaldson et al., 2015) (Table 1.3.2).

Infective Endocarditis

IE is a microbial infection of intracardiac structures. It often occurs on previously damaged or congenitally malformed cardiac valves or endocardium. It is an uncommon but serious and life-threatening disease (Wilson et al., 2007; Murdoch et al., 2009; Glenny et al., 2013). There is a controversy concerning the real efficacy and safety of AP in preventing IE in dentistry, due to a lack of prospective, randomised, placebo-controlled clinical trials to support evidence-based decisions (Glenny et al., 2013; Lockhart et al.,

Table 1.3.2 American Heart Association (AHA) antibiotic prophylaxis (AP) regimens for a dental procedure. (Wilson et al., 2007. Reprinted with permission. © 2007, American Heart Association, Inc.)

Situation	Agent	Single dose 30–60 minutes before procedure
		Children
Oral	Amoxicillin	50 mg/kg
Unable to take oral medication	Ampicillin OR cefazolin or ceftriaxone	50 mg/kg IM or IV
Allergic to penicillins or ampicillin – oral	Cephalexin[a,b] OR	50 mg/kg
	Clindamycin OR	20 mg/kg
	azithromycin or clarithromycin	15 mg/kg
Allergic to penicillins or ampicillin and unable to take oral medication	Cefazolin or ceftriaxone[b] OR	50 mg/kg IM or IV
	Clindamycin	20 mg/kg IM or IV

[a] Or other first- or second-generation oral cephalosporin in equivalent paediatric dosage.
[b] Cephalosporin should not be used in an individual with a history of anaphylaxis, angioedema or urticaria with penicillins or ampicillin.
IM, intramuscular; IV, intravenous.

2013; Baltimore et al., 2015; Donaldson et al., 2015; Cahill et al., 2017). In addition, the frequency of bacteraemia appears to be greater in daily oral hygiene and nutrition by patients, rather than cases resulting from dental procedures such as tooth extraction, periodontal surgery and others. Therefore, several IE episodes can be prevented by maintenance of good oral hygiene and access to a regular maintenance care programme (Wilson et al., 2007; Baltimore et al., 2015; Habib et al., 2015; NICE, 2015; AAPD, 2016a). The antibiotic regimens recommended by the American Heart Association (AHA) for AP are listed in Table 1.3.2.

According to the AHA and the European Society of Cardiology (ESC), AP is recommended for patients in the highest risk group before being submitted to high-risk dental procedures:

- Highest-risk patients exhibit cardiac conditions such as: cardiac valve repair with prosthetic cardiac valve or prosthetic material; previous IE; cardiac valvulopathy in a cardiac transplantation recipient; and congenital heart disease (CHD) – unrepaired cyanotic CHD (including palliative shunts and conducts), completely repaired CHD with prosthetic material or a prosthetic device (whether placed by surgery or catheter intervention during the first 6 months after the procedure), and repaired CHD with residual defects at or adjacent to the site of a prosthetic patch or prosthetic device (Wilson et al., 2007; Habib et al., 2015).
- High-risk dental procedures involve manipulation of gingival (including extractions and scaling) or periapical (including root canal) regions of the teeth or perforation of the oral mucosa. Minor procedures such as routine anaesthetic injections through noninflected tissue, treatment of superficial caries not requiring gingival manipulation, removal of sutures, taking of dental radiographs, placement of removable prosthodontic or orthodontic appliances, adjustment of orthodontic appliances, placement of orthodontic brackets, shedding of deciduous teeth and bleeding from trauma to the lips or oral mucosa do not

require AP (Wilson et al., 2007; Habib et al., 2015; Thornhill et al., 2016).

Regarding the controversy over AP in dental patients, the literature contains three main guidelines on prevention of IE. The AHA (Wilson et al., 2007) and ESC (Habib et al., 2015) guidelines are almost the same, recommending AP for the highest-risk patients when performing high-risk procedures, but the British guidelines (National Institute for Health and Care Excellence, NICE) do not recommend AP for any type of patient or procedure (NICE, 2015). Two recent publications, one from the AAPD (2016a) and one from the AHA (Baltimore et al., 2015), together with a systematic review with meta-analyses (Cahill et al., 2017), recommend that patients considered as high-risk should receive AP when submitted to high-risk procedures.

Clinician adherence to these guidelines is low. Research suggests that this may be because the clinicians disagree with them, or it may be that the guidelines are too vague or too difficult to remember (Jain et al., 2015). Coutinho et al. (2009), in a preliminary study, showed that only 33% of subjects interviewed said they followed the AHA guidelines. Lockhart et al. (2013) found that 70% of dentists still recommended AP for patients not considered at high risk for developing IE.

Immunocompromised Patients

Immunocompromised patients suffer from one or more defects of the immune system, exhibiting an increased risk of infection. These patients may develop a primary or secondary/acquired immunodeficiency such as cancer, need for an organ transplant, poorly controlled diabetes, HIV infection and neutrophil disorders (Fleming and Palmer, 2006; Donaldson et al., 2015). In immunocompromised patients, oral infection should be avoided. Therefore, a regular maintenance care programme, including ongoing preventative dental care, is key for these patients (Fleming and Palmer, 2006). In most cases where dental treatment is necessary, the clinician should consider working in very close collaboration with physicians or the medical team in order to decide on the best strategy for the individual case (Donaldson et al., 2015). Due to its immunosuppressive qualities, the use of AP prior to an invasive dental procedure is suggested in these patients. According to Donaldson et al. (2015), AP for immunocompromised patients should follow the same antibiotic regimens as recommended for IE (Table 1.3.2).

Conclusion

Key to the administration of an antibiotic regimen is prescribing the right antibiotic, at the right dosage and drug interval, for the right time period and at the right time point according to well-accepted guidelines. When facing a clinical situation, the clinician should find the aetiology of the patient complaint based on their medical and dental history, extra/intraoral examination and radiographic analysis, in order to reach the appropriate diagnosis. Following diagnosis, the clinician should choose an appropriate treatment plan. Several modalities can be included, such as endodontic therapy, surgical/mechanical disruption of the infectious environment and replantation of avulsed teeth. Associated with the treatment plan, and according to the guidelines presented in the literature, supportive antibiotic therapy or AP may be indicated. The clinician should monitor the patient to ensure the efficacy of the treatment. In case of persistent symptoms, the treatment plan should be revised and modified where necessary. For paediatric dental patients with any type of systemic disease, a team approach involving the clinician and the physician is important in conducting and resolving the case.

References

Agarwal, A., Panat, S. R., Anshul, Gurtu, A., Aggarwal, A. 2014. Antibiotic usage in pediatric dentistry: a comprehensive review. *Journal of Dental Sciences and Oral Rehabilitation*, **5**, 125–32.

Agostini, F. G., Flaitz, C. M., Hicks, M. J. 2001. Dental emergencies in a university-based pediatric dentistry postgraduate outpatient clinic: a retrospective study. *ASDC Journal of Dentistry for Children*, **68**(5–6), 300–11, 316–21.

Alcorn, J., McNamara, P. J. 2003. Pharmacokinetics in the newborn. *Advanced Drug Delivery Reviews*, **55**(5), 667–86.

Allareddy, V., Nalliah, R. P., Haque, M., Johnson, H., Rampa, S. B., Lee, M. K. 2014. Hospital-based emergency department visits with dental conditions among children in the United States: nationwide epidemiological data. *Pediatric Dentistry*, **36**(5), 393–9.

American Academy of Pediatric Dentistry (AAPD). 2016a. Guideline on antibiotic prophylaxis for dental patients at risk for infection. *Pediatric Dentistry*, **38**(6), 328–33.

American Academy of Pediatric Dentistry (AAPD). 2016b. Guideline on use of antibiotic therapy for pediatric dental patients. *Pediatric Dentistry*, **38**(6), 325–7.

American Academy of Pediatric Dentistry (AAPD). 2016c. Periodontal diseases of children and adolescents. *Pediatric Dentistry*, **38**(6), 388–96.

Andersson, L., Andreasen, J. O., Day, P., Heithersay, G., Trope, M., DiAngelis, A. J., et al. 2012. International Association of Dental Traumatology guidelines for the management of traumatic dental injuries: 2. Avulsion of permanent teeth. *Dental Traumatology*, **28**(2), 88–96.

Andersson, L., Andreasen, J. O., Day, P., Heithersay, G., Trope, M., DiAngelis, A. J., et al. 2016. Guidelines for the management of traumatic dental injuries: 2. Avulsion of permanent teeth. *Pediatric Dentistry*, **38**(6), 369–76.

Andreasen, J. O., Storgard Jensen, S., Sae-Lim, V. 2006. The role of antibiotics in preventing healing complications after traumatic dental injuries: a literature review. *Endodontic Topics*, **14**, 80–92.

Baltimore, R. S., Gewitz, M., Baddour, L. M., Beerman, L. B., Jackson, M. A., Lockhart, P. B., et al. 2015. Infective endocarditis in childhood: 2015 update: a scientific statement from the American Heart Association. *Circulation*, **132**(15), 1487–515.

Bourgeois, F. T., Mandl, K. D., Valim, C., Shannon, M. W. 2009. Pediatric adverse drug events in the outpatient setting: an 11-year national analysis. *Pediatrics*, **124**(4), e744–50.

Cahill, T. J., Harrison, J. L., Jewell, P., Onakpoya, I., Chambers, J. B., Dayer, M., et al. 2017. Antibiotic prophylaxis for infective endocarditis: a systematic review and meta-analysis. *Heart*, **103**(12), 937–44.

Caviglia, I., Techera, A., García, G. 2014. Antimicrobial therapies for odontogenic infection in children and adolescents. Literature review and clinical recommendations. *Journal of Oral Research*, **3**, 5–6.

Centers for Disease Control and Prevention (CDC). 2017. *Antibiotic Use in the United States 2017: Progress and Opportunities.* Atlanta, GA: US Department of Health and Human Services, CDC.

Cherry, W. R., Lee, J. Y., Shugars, D. A., White, R. P., Vann, W. F. 2012. Antibiotic use for treating dental infections in children: a survey of dentists' prescribing practices. *Journal of the American Dental Association*, **143**(1), 31–8.

Coutinho, A. C., Castro, G. F., Maia, L. C. 2009. Knowledge and practices of dentists in preventing infective endocarditis in children. *Special Care in Dentistry*, **29**(4), 175–8.

DiAngelis, A. J., Andreasen, J. O., Ebeleseder, K. A., Kenny, D. J., Trope, M., Sigurdsson, A., et al. 2012. International Association of Dental Traumatology guidelines for the management of traumatic dental injuries: 1. Fractures and luxations of permanent teeth. *Dental Traumatology*, **28**(1), 2–12.

DiAngelis, A. J., Andreasen, J. O., Ebeleseder, K. A., Kenny, D. J., Trope, M., Sigurdsson, A., et al. 2016. Guidelines for the management of traumatic dental injuries: 1. Fractures and luxations of permanent teeth. *Pediatric Dentistry*, **38**(6), 358.

Donaldson, M. Goodchild, J. H. Wrobel, M. J. 2015. Pharmacotherapy. In: Glick, M. (ed.). *Burket's Oral Medicine*, 12th edn. Raleigh, NC: PMPH USA.

Fleming, P., Palmer, N. O. 2006. Pharmaceutical prescribing for children Part 6. Dental management and prescribing for the immunocompromised child. *Primary Dental Care*, **13**(4), 135–9.

Fluent, M. T., Jacobsen, P. L., Hicks, L. A., OSAP, the safest dental visit. 2016. Considerations for responsible antibiotic use in dentistry. *Journal of the American Dental Association*, **147**(8), 683–6.

Glenny, A. M., Oliver, R., Roberts, G. J, Hooper, L., Worthington, H. V. 2013. Antibiotics for the prophylaxis of bacterial endocarditis in dentistry. *Cochrane Database of Systematic Reviews*, **9**(10), CD003813.

Habib, G., Lancellotti, P., Antunes, M. J., Bongiorni, M. G., Casalta, J. P., Del Zotti, F., et al. 2015. 2015 ESC guidelines for the management of infective endocarditis. The Task Force for the Management of Infective Endocarditis of the European Society of Cardiology (ESC). *Giornale Italiano di Cardiolgia (Rome)*, **17**(4), 277–319.

Hicks, L. A., Bartoces, M. G., Roberts, R. M., Suda, K. J., Hunkler, R. J., Taylor, T. H., Schrag, J. 2015. US outpatient antibiotic prescribing variation according to geography, patient population, and provider specialty in 2011. *Clinical Infectious Diseases*, **60**(9), 1308–16.

Jain, P., Stevenson, T., Sheppard, A., Rankin, K., Compton, S. M., Preshing, W., et al. 2015. Antibiotic prophylaxis for infective endocarditis: Knowledge and implementation of American Heart Association Guidelines among dentists and dental hygienists in Alberta, Canada.

Journal of the American Dental Association, **146**(10), 743–50.

Kim, M. K., Chuang, S. K., August, M. 2017. Antibiotic resistance in severe orofacial infections. *Journal of Oral Maxillofacial Surgery*, **75**(5), 962–8.

Lockhart, P. B., Hanson, N. B., Ristic, H., Menezes, A. R., Baddour, L. 2013. Acceptance among and impact on dental practitioners and patients of American Heart Association recommendations for antibiotic prophylaxis. *Journal of the American Dental Association*, **144**(9), 1030–5.

Malmgren, B., J. O. Andreasen, M. T. Flores, A. Robertson, A. J. DiAngelis, L. Andersson, G. et al. 2012. International Association of Dental Traumatology guidelines for the management of traumatic dental injuries: 3. Injuries in the primary dentition. *Dental Traumatology*, **28**(3), 174–82.

Malmgren, B., Andreasen, J. O., Flores, M. T., Robertson, A., DiAngelis, A. J., Andersson, L., et al. 2016. Guidelines for the management of traumatic dental injuries: 3. Injuries in the primary dentition. *Pediatric Dentistry*, **38**(6), 377–385.

Matthews, D. C., Sutherland, S., Basrani, B. 2003. Emergency management of acute apical abscesses in the permanent dentition: a systematic review of the literature. *Journal of the Canadian Dental Association*, **69**(10), 660.

Michael, J. A., Hibbert, S. A. 2014. Presentation and management of facial swellings of odontogenic origin in children. *European Archives of Paediatric Dentistry*, **15**(4), 259–68.

Murdoch, D. R., Corey, G. R., Hoen, B., Miró, J. M., Fowler, V. G., Bayer, A. S., et al. 2009. Clinical presentation, etiology, and outcome of infective endocarditis in the 21st century: the International Collaboration on Endocarditis – Prospective Cohort Study. *Archives of Internal Medicine*, **169**(5), 463–73.

National Institute for Health and Care Excellence (NICE). 2015. Prophylaxis against infective endocarditis: antimicrobial prophylaxis against infective endocarditis in adults and children undergoing interventional procedures. Clinical Guideline [CG64]. Available from https://www.nice.org.uk/guidance/cg64 (last accessed 30 January 2019).

Pallasch, T. J. 1993. How to use antibiotics effectively. *Journal of the Californian Dental Association*, **21**(2), 46–50.

Pallasch, T. J. 1996. Pharmacokinetic principles of antimicrobial therapy. *Periodontology 2000*, **10**, 5–11.

Pallasch, T. J. 2000. Global antibiotic resistance and its impact on the dental community. *Journal of the Californian Dental Association*, **28**(3), 215–33.

Palmer, N. A., Dailey, Y. M. 2002. General dental practitioners' experiences of a collaborative clinical audit on antibiotic prescribing: a qualitative study. *British Dental Journal*, **193**(1), 46–9.

Palmer, N. A., Dailey, Y. M., Martin, M. V. 2001. Can audit improve antibiotic prescribing in general dental practice? *British Dental Journal*, **191**(5), 253–5.

Palmer, N. O. 2006. Pharmaceutical prescribing for children. Part 3. Antibiotic prescribing for children with odontogenic infections. *Primary Dental Care*, **13**(1), 31–5.

Reed, M. D., Besunder, J. B. 1989. Developmental pharmacology: ontogenic basis of drug disposition. *Pediatric Clinics of North America*, **36**(5), 1053–74.

Rowley, S. T., Sheller, B., Williams, B. J., Mancl, L. 2006. Utilization of a hospital for treatment of pediatric dental emergencies. *Pediatric Dentistry*, **28**(1), 10–17.

Sánchez, A. R., Rogers, R. S., Sheridan, P. J. 2004. Tetracycline and other tetracycline-derivative staining of the teeth and oral cavity. *International Journal of Dermatology*, **43**(10), 709–15.

Shehab, N., Lovegrove, M. C., Geller, A. I., Rose, K. O., Weidle, N. J., Budnitz, D. S. 2016. US emergency department visits for outpatient adverse drug events, 2013–2014. *Journal of the American Medical Association*, **316**(20), 2115–25.

Shetty, A. K. 2002. Tetracyclines in pediatrics revisited. *Clinical Pediatrics (Philadelphia),* **41**(4), 203–9.

Shqair, A. Q., Gomes, G. B., Oliveira, A., Goettems, M. L., Romano, A. R., Schardozim, L. R., et al. 2012. Dental emergencies in a university pediatric dentistry clinic: a retrospective study. *Brazilian Oral Research,* **26**(1), 50–6.

Sivaraman, S. S., Hassan, M., Pearson, J. M. 2013. A national survey of pediatric dentists on antibiotic use in children. *Pediatric Dentistry,* **35**(7), 546–9.

Swift, J. Q., Gulden, W. S. 2002. Antibiotic therapy – managing odontogenic infections. *Dental Clinics of North America,* **46**(4), 623–33, vii.

Thornhill, M. H., Dayer, M., Lockhart, P. B., McGurk, M., Shanson, D., Prendergast, B., Chambers, J. B. 2016. Guidelines on prophylaxis to prevent infective endocarditis. *British Dental Journal,* **220**(2), 51–6.

Wilson, W., Taubert, K. A., Gewitz, M., Lockhart, P. B., Baddour, L. M., Levison, M., et al. 2007. Prevention of infective endocarditis: guidelines from the American Heart Association: a guideline from the American Heart Association Rheumatic Fever, Endocarditis and Kawasaki Disease Committee, Council on Cardiovascular Disease in the Young, and the Council on Clinical Cardiology, Council on Cardiovascular Surgery and Anesthesia, and the Quality of Care and Outcomes Research Interdisciplinary Working Group. *Journal of the American Dental Association,* **139**(Suppl.), 3S–24S.

Yesudian, G. T., Gilchrist, F., Bebb, K., Albadri, S., Aspinall, A., Swales, K., Deery, C. 2015. A multicentre, multicycle audit of the prescribing practices of three paediatric dental departments in the North of England. *British Dental Journal,* **218**(12), 681–5.

1.4

Management of Pain and Fear: Behavioural Management, Anaesthesia and Sedation

Klaus W. Neuhaus[1,2] and Nathalie Scheidegger Stojan[3]

[1] Department of Periodontology, Endodontology and Cariology, University Center for Dental Medicine Basel, University of Basel, Basel, Switzerland
[2] Private dental office, Herzogenbuchsee, Switzerland
[3] Private dental office, Biel, Switzerland

Introduction

Dental emergencies often pose specific problems to a dental office. First, they do not happen too often and, especially in trauma situations, dentists have little opportunity to train for them. Second, they cannot be foreseen. Their unexpected nature interferes with the regular schedule of a dental office, so treatment usually occurs in an environment of time constraint and increased stress. Often, emergency situations represent the first contact between a very young patient and a dentist. And where children or adolescents are involved, parents or guardians are typically involved, too, which can hamper treatment provision. Furthermore, many children have a fear of dental treatment, fear of injection, or fear of pain. Finally, some dentists feel unconfident in handling children, which can further contribute to their stress. This chapter illuminates some key factors that need to be addressed when treating young patients in emergency situations.

Behavioural Management

Not all emergency treatments are associated with pain. In a university-based survey in Houston, TX conducted over 3 years, 816 children aged between 10 days and 15 years (average 5.1 years) entered the clinic as emergencies (Agostini et al., 2001). For 25% of these patients, the emergency situation was their first encounter with a dentist. Thirty percent of the patients had pain or painful swellings associated with early childhood caries (ECC), whilst 23% had a dental trauma. In less than 20%, pain was associated with soft tissues or eruption problems. It may be speculated that in a private office, the percentage of children with caries-related pain will be far higher than for trauma cases.

If pain is associated with eruption problems, the primary focus is on calming the parents and prescribing local anaesthetics (e.g. lidocaine gel or polidocanol gel) to relieve the pain (Figure 1.4.1). Talking to the parents and reassuring them that their child's condition is not dangerous helps greatly. Sometimes, preventative measures are sufficient to handle painful conditions (Figure 1.4.2a,b). Acute trauma conditions are also often easy to handle, because the patient is frequently in a post-shock state, and the overflow of epinephrine has an analgesic effect. Necessary treatments can usually be carried out with local anaesthetic under rubber dam isolation without lack of patient compliance. The dental assistant should be instructed to keep an

Management of Dental Emergencies in Children and Adolescents, First Edition.
Edited by Klaus W. Neuhaus and Adrian Lussi.
© 2019 John Wiley & Sons Ltd. Published 2019 by John Wiley & Sons Ltd.
Companion website: www.wiley.com/go/neuhaus/dental_emergencies

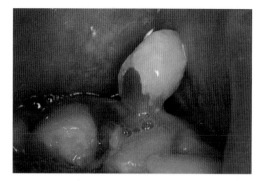

Figure 1.4.1 Sometimes, patients seek emergency treatment over trivial matters. In this case of a loosely attached tooth, 73 lidocaine gel was applied, and the tooth was extracted by the child with the help of a dental floss ligature.

eye on the accompanying parent or guardian, who may be more upset than the patient themselves. A quiet voice, together with calm and concentrated dental treatment, helps to overcome such situations.

Painful conditions due to caries are more demanding. The child will usually have had dental ache for days or weeks; they may have received analgesics, which thus will not give pain relief anymore; they will have been awake at nights, as will their parents; and there has been plenty of time for them to develop a fear of the inevitable visit to the dentist. When a patient shows up under these conditions, perhaps during after-work hours, it is unhelpful to accuse the parents of

neglecting their oral health. The goal is to relieve the patient of their pain – preferably in a way that is as nontraumatic as possible, so that the patient is inclined to return for further treatments.

Diagnosis

It is necessary to correctly diagnose the origin of the pain. The primary diagnostic instrument is the dentist's ears. If parents tell you that their child "couldn't sleep all night", "is very sensitive to temperature", "cannot sharply inhale", or "had a deep caries filled last week," they have pulpitic problems, whilst if they say the child "cannot bite on the side", "had sharp pain last week, which stopped, but now cannot chew", or "had a big pain and now has swelling", they have a periapical pathology associated with a necrotic pulp. Be aware that pulp sensitivity tests are not very reliable in children and can return false positives due to fear, response of the adjacent soft tissue, or vitality in one root canal next to pulp necrosis in another, in multirooted teeth (Gopikrishna et al., 2009). Asking the child to point to the painful tooth aids in the diagnostic process. Gently blowing with compressed air helps locate a tooth with irreversible pulpitis. It is not necessary to provoke the maximum pain response in order to be sure of the diagnosis.

(a)

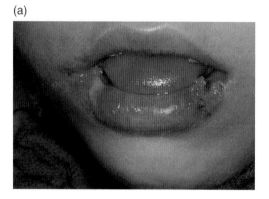

(b)

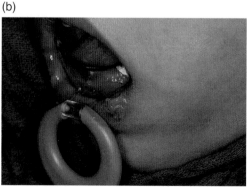

Figure 1.4.2 (a) A 5-year-old patient with disabilities was referred by a neurologist for extraction of the canines due to a painful self-injuring biting habit. (b) A vestibule protector was applied instead, preventing further biting. The habit was abandoned shortly thereafter.

If, according to the anamnesis, there is a suspicion of a symptomatic apical periodontitis, it is not necessary to knock at the suspected tooth with the handle of the mirror, because the provocation of acute pain will hamper subsequent treatment. Positive reaction to percussion may be checked with the fingers by pressing and moving the teeth. In the same diagnostic step, the fingers can be used for periradicular palpation. The dentist should always remember that his or her job is to take pain away, and not to worsen it. If visual inspection is not possible in the dental chair, which may often be the case in toddlers and infants, the patient should be positioned on the parent's lap (Figure 1.4.3a) and leaned back on to the dentist's (Figure 1.4.3b). Often, if the patient is screaming, a visual inspection will be possible. Remember that visual inspection is mandatory before setting up a treatment plan. Soft dentine lesions (Figure 1.4.4a) warrant more attention as possible origins of pain than do darkened leathery dentine lesions (Figure 1.4.4b).

(a) (b)

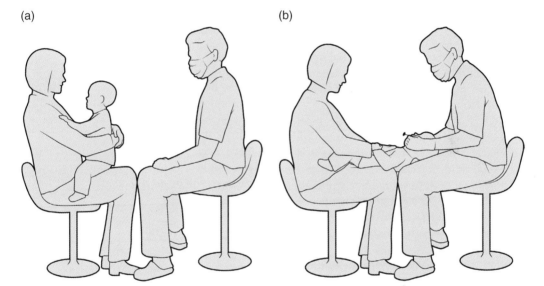

Figure 1.4.3 A safe position for inspection of toddlers and infants can be achieved when the child (a) sits in its parent's lap and (b) leans back on to the dentist's.

(a) (b)

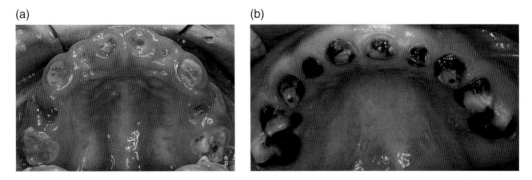

Figure 1.4.4 (a) Totally neglected oral health in a 4-year-old patient. Dentine is soft and covered with plaque, indicating active caries lesions. (b) Discoloured black dentine indicates the arrest of dentine caries. This can often be seen in patients whose parents take responsibility for their child's dental health with tooth brushing and diet control.

Fear Management/Anxiolysis

The key to paediatric management of emergency situations is trust and distraction. Roughly 40% of children referred to the School of Dental Medicine at the University of Bern as "noncompliant" or "not treatable" could be distracted by a TV screen mounted to the ceiling, allowing treatment (empiric data). Such a setting is inexpensive and may be enough to allow the handling of patients in emergency situations. Wireless headphones help reduce the sounds of dental treatment and can further distract the child. A screen in the ceiling allows the dentist to judge from the patient's pupillae how great the level of distraction is. If the sight is focused on the screen, with little eye movement and perhaps reduced responsiveness, dental treatment can be carried out with confidence. A TV screen is especially helpful in children up to the age of 5 years. Other behavioural methods such as "tell–show–do" are applicable in children aged over 5, because they require some logical operative thinking. Some knowledge of hypnosis is helpful in calming and distracting patients, and may also help the dentist remain calm and concentrated.

Other nonverbal anxiolytic methods that can be applied with success include:

- Sweet taste. Let the patient drink some syrup. The effect is via sensory fibres (*N. lingualis*) to the thalamus and amygdala, and reduces the pulse speed. The patient feels better and more confident (perhaps due to excretion of beta endorphins).
- Cold sensation. Apply a cold towel to the patient's forehead. This slows the pulse due to sympathetic thermoregulation of the thalamus, leading to centralisation of the blood.
- Cautious treatment.
- Simple images.
- Letting the patient talk.
- Making pauses.

The rationale behind these sometimes very helpful tricks, which work rapidly, is the function of the amygdala. The amygdala is the central emotional control unit of the brain. The emotion "fear" is located there. The amygdala is mutually connected with cortical and subcortical structures. Sensoric afferences (seeing, hearing and feeling, and also memories of smells, emotions, images and sounds) are connected to the amygdala, which emotionally judges them with joy or fear. The body reacts quickly and unconsciously to its impulses.

It may be helpful to remember the "Three As of Anxiety" (Botto, 2006):

1) Ask how anxious the patient is.
2) Acknowledge what you have heard.
3) Address the patient's fears by offering solutions.

Finally, be honest. Do not make a promise you cannot keep. Once a bond of trust has been established with the child, take care not to break it. If a hurtful procedure has to be undertaken, it is better to announce that there might be some pain than to promise that there will be no pain at all.

Local Anaesthesia

As already mentioned, local anaesthesia in trauma cases rarely poses a problem. Patients may have a fear of injections, for a number of reasons: fear of the needle, fear of the syringe, fear of the pain. Depending on their age, the necessity of using local anaesthetics should be reframed with positive words ("Let's put the gums/teeth to sleep", "We'll gently apply some sleeping drops"). The pain of needle insertion can be minimised by applying a lidocaine gel on to the mucosa. A dry mucosa allows for better diffusion, and the onset of the anaesthetic effect may take 2 minutes. The terminal injection should be performed with a "gentle" thumb, and not hastily. The anaesthetic solution should be allowed to diffuse and take effect in the mucosa before the injection pressure increases. It may sometimes be advisable to ask the patient, especially when they are desperately opening their mouth in a cramped way in expectation of further pain, to loosen the muscles and gently close the mouth a bit. This allows for a gentler diffusion of the anaesthetic solution. Often, when a painless injection can be applied, more than half of the game is won. There are some computerised injection devices on the market that look less like injection needles, and which inject the anaesthetic at slow speed. With these devices, periodontal ligament anaesthesia (PDL), anterior middle superior alveolar block anaesthesia (AMSA) or palatinal anterior superior alveolar block anaesthesia (PASA), for example, can be carried out, which might offer advantages in pain management (Versloot et al., 2005). This is especially true where terminal injections would enter inflamed tissue. The patient and their parents should be reminded upon dismissal that the numbness of some facial regions may last, but not forever, and that biting and nudging of these parts might cause severe wounds (Figure 1.4.5a,b).

In some cases, the compliance of the patient is a priori not sufficient for treatment. It is then advisable to use a sedative regimen. In Switzerland, the two most common methods of conscious sedation are application of nitrous oxide/oxygen inhalation sedation and application of oral midazolam. Both require a healthy lung function without any respiratory obstructions. The patient's paediatrician should be consulted before carrying out either method, and written informed consent should be obtained from the parents. When applying either method in a private dental office, the regulations of the appropriate national dental society should be strictly adhered to.

Nitrous Oxide/Oxygen

The application of nitrous oxide/oxygen is one of the earliest and best studied methods of influencing pain perception and anxiety levels, especially of paediatric patients. Inhalation sedation has an excellent safety record and a proven efficacy in a wide range of patients, both paediatric and adult (IACSD, 2015). Inhalation sedation must not be applied in patients younger than 3 years, in patients with psychic disorders, or in patients with otitis media (SDCEP, 2017). It is also contraindicated when a pregnant woman is in the same room. In dental emergency situations, only mild analgesia and anxiolysis warrant its use.

To achieve the sedation effect, the patient nasally inhales a mixture of nitrous oxide/oxygen up to a concentration of 50% nitrous oxide. In most cases, a lesser nitrous oxide concentration of 65–70% is sufficient. The patient remains conscious during inhalation sedation, and questioning and reframing about their subjective

(a)

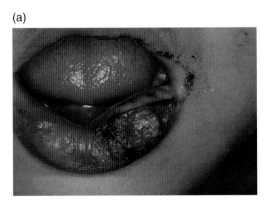

(b)

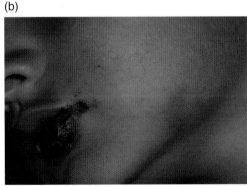

Figure 1.4.5 (a) Serious lip injury 1 day after dental treatment in the lower jaw. (b) Haematoma caused by the injury. It is important to instruct the parents properly following a dental treatment.

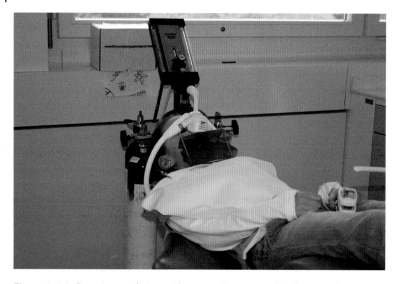

Figure 1.4.6 Conscious sedation with oxygen/nitrous oxide allows perfect treatment conditions. Pulse and oxygen saturation are being monitored (left index finger).

perception of its physical effects (paresthesia of the extremities, cold forehead, warm belly, numb skin) may help deepen them. In order to be able to individually change the ratio of nitrous oxide to oxygen, a delivery device with separate bottles is recommended (Figure 1.4.6). However, this may not be allowed in certain countries, where only prefabricated equimolar 50/50 mixtures are available (e.g. Calinox). The patient is monitored throughout treatment using pulse oximetry. At the end, the patient inhales pure oxygen to prevent a diffusion hypoxia, because they will be exhaling nitrous oxide. Unlike with other sedation methods, after inhalation sedation with nitrous oxide/oxygen the patient is usually fully recovered and has no physical impairments (SDCEP, 2017).

Midazolam

Another possibility for conscious sedation in emergency situations is midazolam. The best way of delivering midazolam is intravenously, but in many clinical settings oral, intranasal or suppository sedation with a concentration of 0.4–0.5 mg/kg body weight is increasingly popular. Ideally, midazolam should be administered titratable intravenously way, but if this cannot be done, an intravenous cannula should be placed in the patient's arm or the back of their hand once the desired sedation effect begins. The effect of midazolam is anxiolytic: the patient becomes drowsy and sometimes experiences a partial retrograde amnesia. However, midazolam has great inter-individual pharmacokinetics and pharmacodynamics; that is, the onset and offset of the effect can vary considerably (usually 20–30 minutes after administration and 30–45 minutes after termination, respectively), and the effect itself can be sufficient or borderline. Still, especially in very young patients, this type of sedation is the method of choice if an operative intervention is mandatory and if general anaesthesia treatment is not an option.

Concomitant pulse oximetry is also mandatory during and after sedation with midazolam (Langhan et al., 2012). The patient must have sufficient respiratory function upon dismissal. Demanding physical activities should be refrained from during the day of sedation, because the reflexes will be subdued, increasing the risk of further accident. If a dentist wants to administer midazolam in the private office setting, local regulative legislation must be followed. In some countries, midazolam may only be administered by anaesthetists or specially trained and certified dentists.

It must be stressed that nitrous oxide/oxygen and midazolam may be combined with local anaesthetics, but not with each other. The combination of midazolam and nitrous oxide by far surpasses the effect of either alone, and once led to the tragic death of a 4-year-old boy (Lee et al., 2017).

Referring the Patient

In some cases, the general state of health of the patient does not permit treatment in a private office. Figure 1.4.7 shows a boy presenting 2 days after a simple extraction of tooth 54. He had swelling, increased mobility of several teeth, pocket probing at depths of 12 mm and more on several teeth, and elevated temperature. Hospitalisation of the patient to receive intravenous antibiotics was the correct treatment. In order to avoid a spreading infection, the prescription of antibiotics and subsequent referral to a clinic or centre that offers treatment in general anaesthesia is recommended in such cases. The aim must always be to help the patient without harming them.

(a)

(b)

(c)

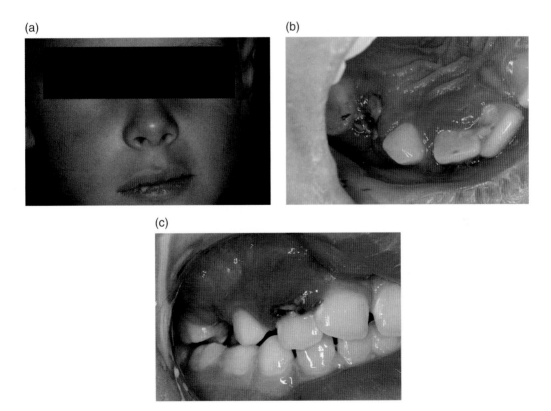

Figure 1.4.7 (a) The facial swelling and the reduced general condition indicate a serious problem. Spreading of the abscess could be seen on the (b) palatal and (c) buccal aspect. The patient had to be hospitalised and received intravenous antibiotic therapy.

References

Agostini, F. G., Flaitz, C. M., Hicks, M. J. 2001. Dental emergencies in a university-based pediatric dentistry postgraduate outpatient clinic: a retrospective study. *ASDC Journal of Dentistry for Children*, **68**, 300–1, 316–21.

Botto, R. W. 2006. Chairside techniques to reduce dental fear. In: Mostofsky, D. I., Forgione, A. G., Giddon, D. B. (eds). *Behavioral Dentistry.* Oxford: Blackwell Munksgaard, pp. 141–52.

Intercollegiate Advisory Committee for Sedation in Dentistry (IACSD). 2015. Standards for conscious sedation in the provision of dental care. Available from https://www.rcseng.ac.uk/-/media/files/rcs/fds/publications/dental-sedation-report-2015-web-v2.pdf (last accessed 30 January 2019).

Gopikrishna, V., Pradeep, G., Venkateshbabu, N. 2009. Assessment of pulp vitality: a review. *International Journal of Paediatric Dentistry*, **19**, 3–15.

Langhan, M. L., Mallory, M., Hertzog, J., Lowrie, L., Cravero, J., Pediatric Sedation Research Consortium. 2012. Physiologic monitoring practices during pediatric procedural sedation: a report from the Pediatric Sedation Research Consortium. *Archives of Pediatric and Adolescent Medicine*, **166**, 990–8.

Lee, H., Milgrom, P., Huebner, C. E., Weinstein, P., Burke, W., Blacksher, E., Lantos, J. D. 2017. Ethics rounds: death after pediatric dental anesthesia: an avoidable tragedy? *Pediatrics*, **140**(6), e20172370.

Scottish Dental Clinical Effectiveness Programme (SDCEP). 2017. Conscious sedation in dentistry. Available from http://www.sdcep.org.uk/wp-content/uploads/2018/07/SDCEP-Conscious-Sedation-Guidance.pdf (last accessed 30 January 2019).

Versloot, J., Veerkamp, J. S., Hoogstraten, J. 2005. Computerized anesthesia delivery system vs. traditional syringe: comparing pain and pain-related behavior in children. *European Journal of Oral Science*, **113**, 488–93.

1.5

Management of Radiographic Needs

Karl Dula[1,2]

[1] Department of Oral Surgery and Stomatology, School for Dental Medicine, Bern, Switzerland
[2] Private dental office, Chiasso, Switzerland

Imaging Procedures in Dentomaxillofacial Radiology

Dentists are using imaging procedures of dentomaxillofacial radiology for diagnostic imaging, some of which have been developed specifically for dentistry. These are all intraoral radiographs (periapical radiographs of various sizes, bitewings and occlusal views) and all extraoral radiographs (panoramic radiographs, cranial and partial cranial views, especially cephalometric radiographs, hand radiographs, conventional tomography (used very rarely today) and cone-beam computed tomography (CBCT)). Other imaging techniques used in medicine are also used in dentistry, such as computed tomography (in particular Dantascan; Schwarz et al., 1987a,b), magnetic resonance imaging and ultrasound. It takes a lot of training to choose from these numerous imaging procedures those that are right for the indication of the individual patient.

Imaging Procedures in Children and Adolescents

In dental medicine, similar emergency situations can generally be experienced by children, adolescents and adults. Almost always, these emergencies are caused by pain or by situations in some way associated with pain. In the age group of children and adolescents, the cause of pain is usually tooth decay, accident or discomfort caused by wisdom teeth.

Dental traumatology is discussed in Chapter 5.2. This chapter will therefore focus on other emergency situations, including tooth decay and discomfort from wisdom teeth, as well as a wide range of pain caused by tooth eruption and inflammation.

Often, therapy differs with regard to the dentition: treatment must be done differently in deciduous teeth than in permanent ones. In deciduous teeth, patient compliance is often poor or absent, making therapy difficult and sometimes impossible. The duration of treatment also plays an important role: especially in children, a longer treatment is often not tolerated – they tire, become restless and react with uncontrolled movements. Most important is patient fear, which sometimes cannot be overcome. Fortunately, with deciduous teeth, a less accurate x-ray examination may often be acceptable, due to their different composition, structure and shape. Obtaining the information necessary for proper treatment is far more important than fulfilling the requirements for good image quality.

In some situations, it may be necessary to prescribe a premedication or to ask the family

Management of Dental Emergencies in Children and Adolescents, First Edition.
Edited by Klaus W. Neuhaus and Adrian Lussi.
© 2019 John Wiley & Sons Ltd. Published 2019 by John Wiley & Sons Ltd.
Companion website: www.wiley.com/go/neuhaus/dental_emergencies

doctor to sedate the young patient. Any therapy involving sedation or even general anaesthesia should be discussed with the anaesthesiologist in advance (see Chapter 1.4).

Biological Risk in Children and Adolescents

As children and adolescents may be affected by orofacial and jaw bone pathologies, x-ray examinations are often required for diagnosis. However, these examinations must be well justified, as this age group is about three times more likely to sustain biological damage from x-rays than adults (UNSCEAR 2013).

One important variable that determines the risk of radiation exposure is the age at exposure. The earlier an organism is irradiated by x-rays, the greater the likelihood of biological damage. This was demonstrated

by BEIR VII, which reviewed the available biological, biophysical and epidemiological literature of recent years (NAS/NCR 2006). The report confirmed that so-called "late" effects, such as cancer, occur many years after initial exposure (Figure 1.5.1).

We now know that the organism of children and adolescents is more sensitive to radiation than that of adults – but why? There are many reasons: the high rate of cell division of the growing tissue – cells in the division phase are much more susceptible to harmful events; the smaller volume of the body – more radiosensitive organs and tissues are irradiated if the aperture is not adapted to the smaller body size and the radiation field thus unnecessarily large; the still immature cell repair mechanisms – cells of a growing body are not yet able to repair radiation damage; the higher radiosensitivity of the immature red bone marrow; the greater water content in the child's body – more

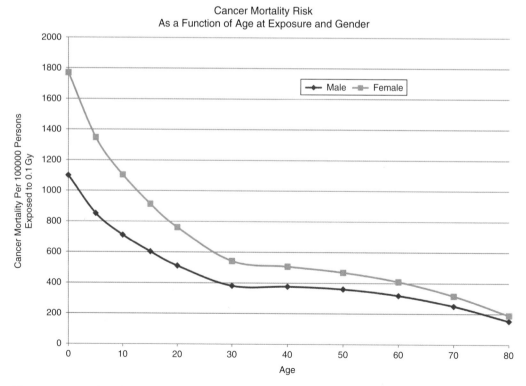

Figure 1.5.1 Number of excess cancer deaths caused by a single radiation exposure of 0.1 Gy as a function of age at the time of exposure and gender. Based on Table 12-D2 in the BEIR VII report (NAS/NCR 2006).

water molecules are available for dissociation and thus for the formation of radicals, which are considered to be cell toxins; and, not least, the longer life expectancy of children, which makes biological harm more likely despite the high latency.

However, the UNSCEAR report (2013) states that the risk from radiation in children appears to be much higher for some organs and tissues, equally high for others and, surprisingly, lower for others still, as compared to adults. This leads to the conclusion that intraoral imaging should be maintained as the standard diagnostic tool in all standard situations (AAPD 2017). Panoramic radiography should be used if a larger overview is required or for radiation protection reasons where more than six intraoral radiographs are needed, since the radiation dose of one panoramic radiograph corresponds to that of six intraoral radiographs (Lübbers et al., 2014). All other imaging techniques in dentomaxillofacial radiology already mentioned are special radiographs that have their own fields of application. Only CBCT need be specifically mentioned here, as there is a risk that it is increasingly being considered some kind of a standard imaging technique. There are several reasons for this. As we live in a three-dimensional world, 3D imaging is a kind of "sympathetic" or "appealing" imaging technique. A drawback of 2D imaging is that superimpositions make interpretation difficult, and sometimes even a game of chance. In intraoral radiography, 2D images offer only a limited field of view. However, since CBCT applies higher doses than almost any other dentomaxillofacial x-ray technology, it may be used with limited indications for special cases, always optimised through the use of the smallest possible field of view (FOV) and after consideration of alternative 2D imaging techniques. The guiding principle, which must be superordinate to any other consideration for justifying 3D imaging, is an honest expectation of additional information relevant to therapy.

If justification has been established, the patient's age should remind the operator to apply the principles of optimisation according to the specific diagnostic needs. It should be mandatory to choose settings for an optimised patient imaging protocol according to age, gender and indication-related parameters. It is not enough to follow the ALARA (As Low As Reasonably Achievable) principle; the clinician should also follow ALADA (As Low As Diagnostically Acceptable), as proposed by Jaju and Jaju (2015), or even ALADAIP (As Low As Diagnostically Acceptable being Indication-oriented and Patient-specific), as discussed in a position statement by the European DIMITRA research group (Oenning et al., 2018).

Because every precaution should be taken to minimise radiation exposure, protective thyroid collars or lead aprons should be used whenever possible, in every imaging technique (AAPD 2012). When CBCT is used, the resulting imaging must be included in the patient records, supplemented with a written report on all findings and interpretations (Dula et al., 2014).

Dental Emergencies in Children and Adolescents

Suspected Caries as a Cause of Pain

Bitewing x-rays are generally accepted for caries detection. Nevertheless, an increasing number of alternative diagnostic procedures without x-rays have been investigated, as they are becoming ever safer and more promising.

It has been found that adjunct methods of caries detection do not significantly improve the detection of primary molar lesions in comparison to visual inspection alone (Mendes et al., 2012). Elhennawy et al. (2018) found that near-infrared digital imaging transillumination (NIDIT) could be used as a radiation-free alternative to x-ray examination to detect carious lesions.

Meta-analyses (Gimenez et al., 2015; Schwendicke et al., 2015) have shown that visual and radiographic examination for the detection of early approximal caries has a very high specificity but low sensitivity. Therefore, Abogazalah and Ando (2017) reviewed the literature regarding the performance of unconventional and novel methods for approximal caries detection, finding that fibre-optic transillumination (FOTI), digital imaging fibre-optic transillumination (DIFOTI), optical coherence tomography (OCT), swept-source optical coherence tomography (SSOCT), laser fluorescence (LF), ultrasound, light-emitting diode (LED) fluorescence, frequency-domain infrared photothermal radiometry and modulated luminescence (PTR/LUM) cannot yet replace conventional methods such as inspection and bitewings for caries detection with any certainty. Therefore, especially in emergency situations in which dental caries is suspected of causing pain, conventional methods should be used for a reliable and stress-free diagnosis.

Wisdom Teeth as a Suspected Cause of Pain

A discrepancy between the size of the jaw and the sum of the mesiodistal crown diameters of all teeth often leads to a lack of space in the area of the last erupting tooth. Therefore, adolescents often suffer from pain in the wisdom tooth area because unerupted or partially erupted wisdom teeth can cause an inflammatory response of the surrounding soft tissues, often accompanied by clinically significant symptoms (increasing swellings in the region of the wisdom tooth, increasing pressure and globus sensation in the throat, increasing trismus, dysphagia with increasingly limited ability to eat and sometimes a sense of illness and rising temperature in advanced stages). In local findings, the mucosa that covers the wisdom tooth is swollen and reddened and hurts when touched or palpated. Lymph nodes begin to swell and become painful as a sign of local defence reaction.

At this stage, the radiological diagnosis of the cause of the pain is important. This should preferably be done with periapical films, provided that the pain, the degree of swelling and the trismus allow the image to be taken. If tooth removal seems to be necessary, it must be decided according to the situation of the wisdom tooth, whether a periapical film provides sufficient information or whether a panoramic radiograph is justified as first admission in order to avoid an insufficient intraoral recording. This can be especially true for more displaced and retained wisdom teeth, where it is important to know the anatomical environment. Only with a panoramic radiograph can full assessment of the anatomical relationship between the wisdom tooth and the mandibular canal be made, since in this image the course of the canal can be fully tracked and determined. This allows signs of an increased risk of nerve damage to be found, as such signs have only been studied, described and validated in the literature for panoramic radiography. In particular, it is important to recognise such signs as the overlapping of the roots with the inferior alveolar canal with obscuration of at least one of the roots, or the diversion or discontinuity of the cortical line of the inferior alveolar canal. These indicate an increased risk of damage to the inferior alveolar nerve (IAN), should the tooth need to be removed (Blaeser et al., 2003).

In acute wisdom tooth inflammation, which must be treated in an emergency, a 3D radiograph (in particular CBCT or computed tomography) is not required. 3D images may never be used as first admission, since they are special radiographic procedures which have to be justified based on the information from 2D images. This implicitly means that 3D images without previously recorded 2D images must not exist, as this precludes a proper justification process! If 3D imaging for surgical removal is subsequently considered necessary, it should be prescribed by the person performing the surgical procedure; otherwise, there is a risk that images will be taken that are not needed (Dula et al., 2001, 2014, 2015). The more experienced the surgeon, the less likely he or she is to require 3D imaging, since the incidence of IAN injuries also decreases as the surgeon's experience increases (Bataineh, 2001; Jerjes et al., 2006).

Other Reasons as a Suspected Cause of Pain

There are a variety of pathological changes in childhood and adolescence that can lead to emergency situations. For the radiological examination of these diseases, it is necessary to select the correct imaging method from amongst all the possible imaging methods already mentioned, whereby the best imaging procedure for a specific task must agree with the best aspects of radiation protection.

Therefore, the radiological diagnosis in children and adolescents should be done whenever possible with intraoral radiographs, as these generally apply a smaller dose than any other dental radiograph (Dula et al., 2001). Here, it is beneficial that the jaw of a child is smaller than that of an adult, which is why the same film format covers a larger area in the child's jaw. Thus, larger areas can be completely seen and interpreted, and no additional panoramic radiograph is required to obtain a larger overview. If it is nevertheless deemed necessary to take a panoramic radiograph, it must be checked whether it is useful to select a child mode, a partial exposure of the jaw (e.g. left/right or anterior region), a sector of the jaw (approximately four teeth) or additional options (e.g. a short scan) to reduce the default exposure values (Svanaes et al., 1985; Esmaeili et al., 2016).

If even the use of CBCT is justified, the operator must have time prior to the exposure to decide on exposure parameters, volume size, resolution, rotation mode (semicircle, three-quarter circle or full circle) and exposure time, taking into account the age and sex of the patient, the objective of the study and the question to be answered.

Case Studies

The following case studies should illustrate which x-ray images are justified for diagnosis in children and adolescents who present to the private practice as emergency patients. An attempt is made to describe the considerations that justify taking images in order to give the reader guidance on what to do in his or her own practice. By selecting these case studies, the author wants to make clear that children and adolescents must have extensive pathological changes in order to justify the application of additional images such as panoramic radiography and CBCT.

Case 1: Pain from Caries in a 7-Year-Old Girl

A 7-year-old girl suffers from pain in her right upper jaw, which is getting progressively worse. Clinically, a deep caries mesial of tooth 53 can already be found in the intraoral examination. To assess the extent of the caries and to examine the other teeth presenting clinically suspicious lesions, bitewings are indicated (Figure 1.5.2). Other lesions can be confirmed and treated.

(a)

(b)

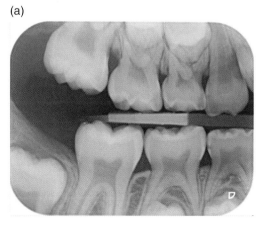
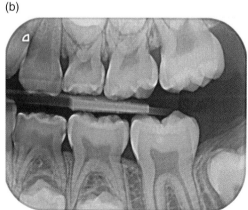

Figure 1.5.2 (a,b) Bitewings for caries detection in children.

Case 2: Pain from Caries in a 17-Year-Old Girl

A 17-year-old girl suffers from sudden, pulsating pain in her right upper jaw. Clinically, intraoral examination reveals a profound caries mesial to tooth 14. Other suspicious lesions are found in the right and left jaws (Figure 1.5.3). Here, taking of bitewings is mandatory, but taking other radiographs would be erroneous.

Case 3: Pain in the Left Lower Jaw

A 17-year old boy feels pain in the left lower jaw and complains of increased restriction of mouth opening and ability to eat. During the examination, the dentist finds a typical situation of complicated wisdom tooth eruption: partial occlusion of the wisdom tooth with gums swollen, reddened and pressure-painful mucosa and soft swollen, painful lymph nodes (Figure 1.5.4a). The dentist manages to take a periapical radiograph (Figure 1.5.4b), which shows the tooth just enough to allow for extraction. (Figure 1.5.4c shows a radiograph of the wisdom tooth of another patient that is not fully visualised. This image is not sufficient for a complete diagnosis, and therefore certainly not sufficient for an extraction.)

Case 4: Pain in the Right Upper Jaw

This case concerns a woman who is still 18 years old at the time of her first admission. She complains about dull pain in her right upper jaw. Her dentist finds all teeth vital and takes two bitewings (Figure 1.5.5a). In the x-ray of the right side, he sees the right upper hypoplastic wisdom tooth. He explains the complaints as pressure from eruption and decides to observe this tooth. One year later, the young woman complains again about pressure in her right upper jaw. The dentist takes two more bitewings (Figure 1.5.5.b), sees that the tooth is slightly erupted and decides to extract it. When the patient continues to complain about the same symptoms three months after extraction, he takes a periapical radiograph (Figure 1.5.5c) and, to his surprise, finds the actual wisdom tooth. He decides to surgically remove it. Since he does not see the root completely represented, he takes a panoramic radiograph (Figure 1.5.5d). This decision is correct, and the panoramic radiograph is justified, since a questionable structure must be represented at least 2–3 mm beyond its borders in order to fully assess it. With this case study, the significance and trueness of this postulation becomes evident – only through the larger overview can the wisdom tooth and a

(a)

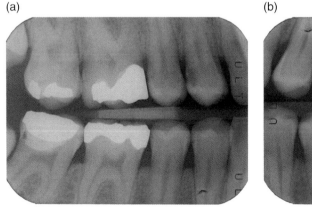

(b)

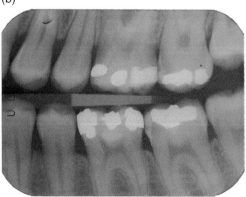

Figure 1.5.3 (a,b) Bitewings for caries detection in adolescents.

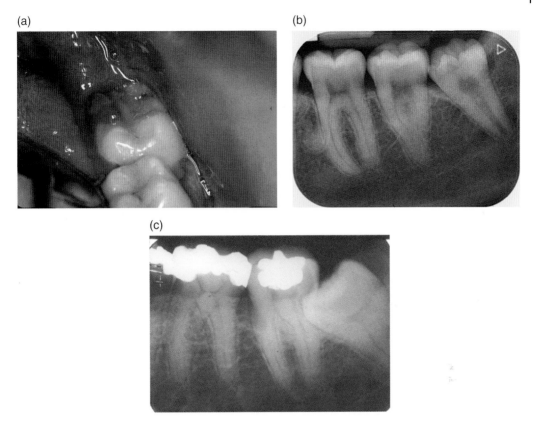

Figure 1.5.4 Complicated wisdom tooth eruption with retromolar swelling. (a) Clinical view. (b) Periapical radiograph. (c) Radiograph of a different patient, showing insufficient visualisation of the third molar. Another radiograph is indicated before extraction.

follicular cyst in antro (border marked by arrows) be found and treated (Figure 1.5.5d).

Case 5: Combined Follicular/Radicular Cysts during Tooth Eruption

The parents of an 8-year-old boy are worried about a slight swelling of his right cheek, which has been increasing for 2 days (Figure 1.5.6a,b). The boy also has pain in the right lower jaw and avoids food intake. Teeth 84 and 85 are slightly mobile and hurt when touched. First, the pulp chamber of tooth 85 is opened, which leads to the outflow of much pus. For reasons of radiation protection, a panoramic radiograph is taken only on the right side, covering the areas that are outside the dimensions of a dental film (Figure 1.5.6c). A greater cystic radiolucency is found, which extends from the roots of the deciduous teeth to the permanent premolars. Radiation transparency surrounds the crowns of the premolars, and the tooth follicle is dissolved. These findings require no further x-ray analysis for diagnosis and therapy: by extracting the deciduous molars, the permanent premolars can erupt, allowing them to "roll up" and dissolve the cystic formation. The clinically visible eruption of the permanent premolars is already a strong sign for the healing of the cystic process. A periapical radiograph is therefore sufficient to confirm the reossification of the cystic lesion (Figure 1.5.6d).

(a)

(b)

(c)

(d)

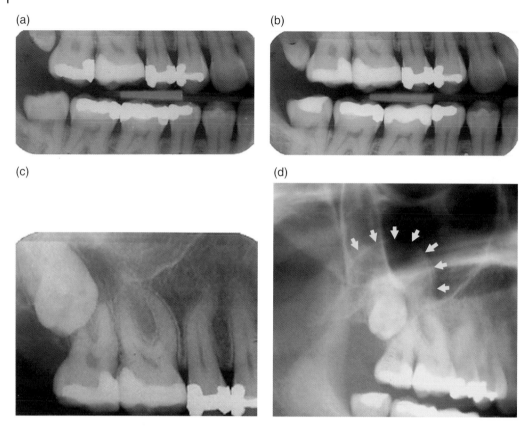

Figure 1.5.5 (a) Initial bitewing radiograph showing a conic tooth 18. (b) The same tooth 1 year later. The tooth is elongated and might be considered a cause for the patient's symptoms. (c) Periapical radiograph of the same patient, showing an impacted wisdom tooth. (d) Cropped part from a panoramic radiograph showing a follicular cyst (arrows).

Case 6: Disturbance of Tooth Eruption due to Malformation

An 8-year-old boy shows a malformation of tooth 32 (Figure 1.5.7a,b). The orthodontist cannot obtain sufficient information about the extent of the malformation with periapical film and panoramic radiography (Figure 1.5.7c–e), and thus transfers him for further clarification. The main question is whether the tooth can momentarily be preserved to gain time for a later implantation. However, as the boy often feels pain in this region, the therapy cannot be postponed. CBCT is justified in order to obtain therapy-relevant additional information.

The CBCT images show the heavily malformed tooth, whose prognosis is unfavourable (Figure 1.5.7f–h). After extraction, these images are fully confirmed by the actual tooth (Figure 1.5.7i–k). Through orthodontic gap closure, a clinically and aesthetically very satisfying long-term solution is achieved (Figure 1.5.7l,m).

Case 7: Invasive Cervical Tooth Resorption

A 9-year-old boy has been teased for a couple of years by his school friends because of a persistent tooth gap (Figure 1.5.8a). He begins to suffer from pain in the upper front tooth region, for which his parents seek help. The orthodontist cannot sufficiently interpret the findings in the standard (panoramic)

(a)

(b)

(c)

(d)

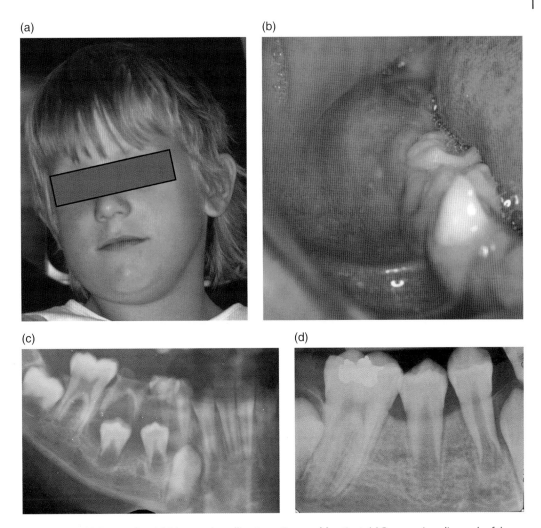

Figure 1.5.6 (a) Extraoral and (b) intraoral swelling in an 8-year-old patient. (c) Panoramic radiograph of the right side only, showing a huge cystic radiolucency. (d) Erupting premolars, proving the reossification of the cystic process after extraction of teeth 84 and 85.

radiograph (Figure 1.5.8b), nor in the occlusal view (Figure 1.5.8c). The boy is referred to an oral surgeon, who decides to use CBCT because he suspects invasive cervical resorption (Figure 1.5.8d,f,h). This decision is correct, because only CBCT shows the extent of the destruction that is the basis for deciding whether the tooth can still be treated conservatively or whether it needs to be extracted.

The CBCT images show a severe destruction of the tooth as a result of invasive cervical resorption. At this stage, tooth preservation by conservative therapy is no longer possible. After extraction, the histological preparation of the tooth confirms this destruction of the dental hard tissues in the crown and root area, the excellent precision of the radiological findings and the value of CBCT in making decisions about therapy (Figure 1.5.8e,g,i).

Case 8: Open Nasopalatine Duct

A 17-year-old boy suddenly experiences increasing pain in the anterior maxilla palatal to the front teeth. His dentist finds a swelling,

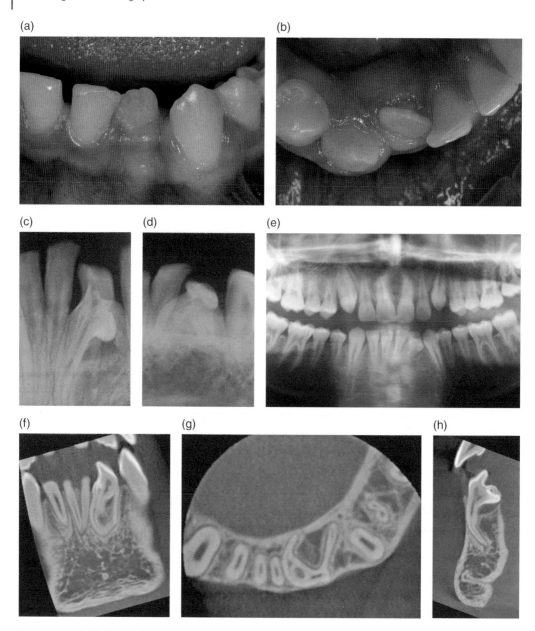

Figure 1.5.7 (a,b) Clinical view of the malformation of tooth 32 in an 8-year-old patient. (c,d) Pariapical radiographs in two different planes, same tooth. (e) A panoramic radiograph rendering insufficient information about the malformation. (f–h) CBCT images of the same situation. (i–k) Clinical view of the extracted tooth. (l,m) Same patient after orthodontic stratification. *Source:* Clinical photoraphs courtesy of Dr U. Picco, Giubiasco, Switzerland.

(i) (j) (k)

(l) (m)

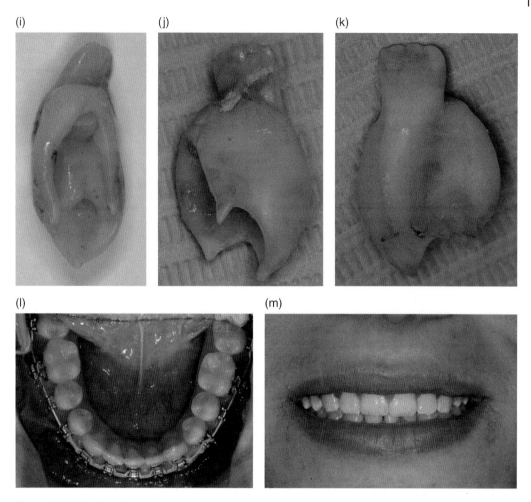

Figure 1.5.7 (Continued)

redness and very severe pain on palpation in the area of the incisive papilla (Figure 1.5.9a). A suspected nasopalatine duct cyst can be excluded by the periapical radiograph (Figure 1.5.9b). All anterior teeth are vital, excluding a palatal abscess by odontogenic inflammation. Upon incision, a slightly yellowish and slightly viscous fluid is discharged. After the swelling has subsided, a fistula-like opening can be seen (Figure 1.5.9c). A gutta-percha point is inserted, which serves as "contrast medium" during the 3D admission (Figure 1.5.9d). CBCT images show the gutta-percha tip in the incisive canal, reaching to the nasal floor, which proves the presence of an open nasopalatine duct (Figure 1.5.9e).

Case 9: Salivary Gland Stone in a 9-Year-Old Boy – A Sialolithiasis of the Submandibular Gland

A 9-year-old boy complains of recurrent swelling in his right lower jaw, which has been painful lately. On the day of admission, a submandibular nodular-humpy induration in the area of the salivary gland is found, which is sensitive to pain. Tooth eruption of the 6-year molar can be detected. All deciduous

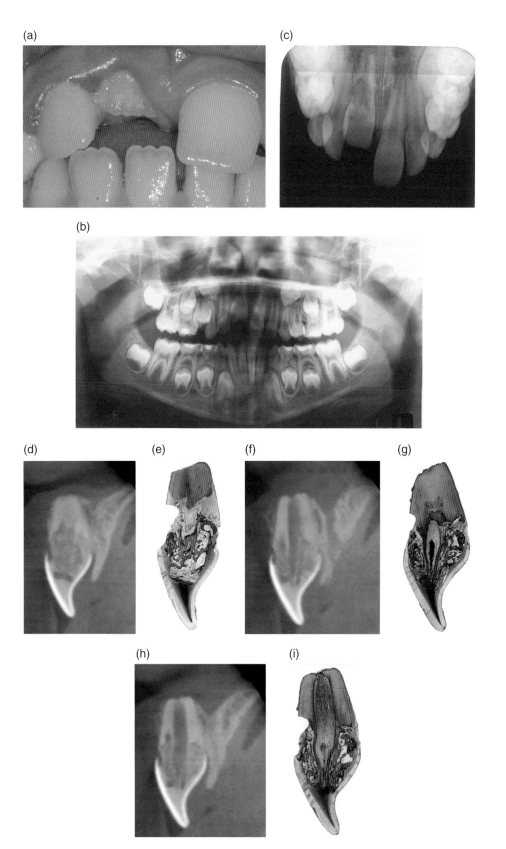

Figure 1.5.8 (a) Clinical view showing incomplete eruption of tooth 11. This situation has persisted for a couple of years. (b) Panoramic radiograph, same patient. (c) Radiograph from the occlusal plane showing a radiolucency in the upper third of the root of tooth 11. (d,f,h) CBCT images of the same tooth indicating the precise extent of the radiolucency and confirming the diagnosis of invasive cervical resorption. (e,g,i) Histology confirming the destruction of the dental hard tissue and plainly showing that any conservative approaches to maintaining such a tooth should be considered hopeless. *Source:* Clinical photograph courtesy of Dr. Samuel Wahlen, Münsingen, Switzerland.

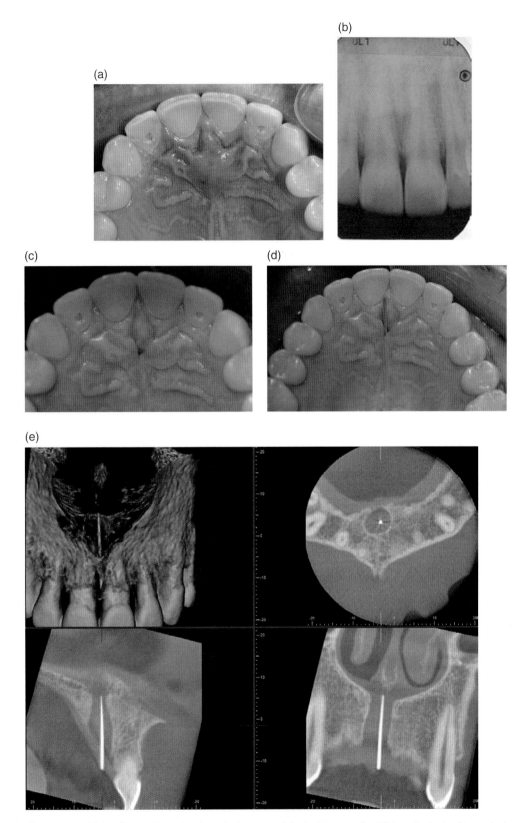

Figure 1.5.9 (a) Swelling, pain and redness in the area of the incisive papilla. (b) A periapical radiograph shows no signs of a nasapalatine duct cyst. (c) After incision and drainage, a fistula-like structure becomes visible. (d) A gutta-percha point is inserted. (e) CBCT confirms an open nasopalatine duct. *Source:* Clinical photographs courtesy of Dr. Andreas Jäggin, Locarno, Switzerland.

teeth are present, and all teeth are free of decay and vital – a clinical situation that justifies not taking a periapical radiograph but immediately ordering a panoramic one, because a larger overview is advisable since the teeth are most likely not the cause of the swelling.

The panoramic radiograph shows a round, approximately pea-sized opaque structure in the posterior mandibular region between the distal root tip of tooth 47 and the basal cortical line (Figure 1.5.10a). The patient's history, the clinical findings and the panoramic radiograph all suggest a salivary gland stone. Therefore, sialography with contrast medium filling of the Wharton duct is performed. A contrast medium recess in the area of the salivary gland stone within the contrast-filled Wharton duct is noted, along with an overall enlargement of the excretory ducts with rarification of the peripheral ducts as a sign of chronic sialadenitis (Figure 1.5.10b). CBCT images show the onion bowl-like structure of the salivary gland stone; the surface-shaded display illustrates the position of the stone within the salivary gland (Figure 1.5.10c–e).

Case 10: Follicular Cyst with Tooth Displacement

A 7-year-old boy has recurrent pain in his left lower jaw. His dentist finds healthy deciduous molars in that region. However, tooth 36 is almost completely retained and buccally displaced, with the distal section appearing distended (Figure 1.5.11a). Since the boy cannot tolerate periapical film inserted in the distal area, a half-side panoramic radiograph is taken (Figure 1.5.11b). This radiograph is justified in such a situation, and shows a slightly displaced tooth 36 and a tooth germ 37 distally displaced by an expanding lesion. Since the lesion superimposes the root area of tooth 36, the situation is indistinct – more information is needed before surgical intervention can be undertaken. Therefore, 3D imaging with CBCT is justified. The CBCT image shows an extensive osteolysis of about 16×22 mm

maximum diameter (Figure 1.5.11c,d,f). The mandibular canal is displaced and therefore not within the area of the expanding lesion. The surface-shaded display impressively illustrates that the lesion has developed vestibularly to tooth 36 and is thus displacing it lingually (Figure 1.5.11e). Histological diagnosis is of a follicular cyst.

Case 11: Initial Osteomyelitis in a Child's Mandible

A 7-year-old girl returns home from school with a swelling of her right cheek. The following night, she has a fever. She has a restless sleep and cries. The next morning, her parents notice a foul smell from the girl's mouth. The dentist finds no tooth decay and all teeth vital, so transfers the child. At the initial examination, the girl complains of pain and is tearful. She has difficulty opening her mouth and shows all symptoms of an infection. Intraoral examination shows a vestibular swelling in the region of the deciduous molars (Figure 1.5.12a) and the permanent first molar, which is not yet completely erupted (Figure 1.5.12b).

The patient's history and the radiographs taken by the private dentist justify the use of panoramic radiography (Figure 1.5.12c). Unfortunately, this only gives a suspicion of inflammatory osteolysis distal to tooth 46, but no definite diagnosis. Therefore, there is an honest expectation that CBCT will provide additional information relevant to therapy. In the surface-shaded CBCT display, a defect in the cortical bone of the lower jaw is visible vestibulo-distally to tooth 46 (Figure 1.5.12d). This is confirmed in the axial and coronal views of the mandible of this region (Figure 1.5.12e). In further views, typical signs of an initial osteomyelitis can be seen: bone sclerosis adjacent to the areas of bone destruction and lifting off of the swollen and slightly sclerosed periosteum by inflammatory processes (Figure 1.5.12f). After initial high-dose antibiosis, the region is surgically revised. The intervention also finds foreign objects reminiscent of leftover food.

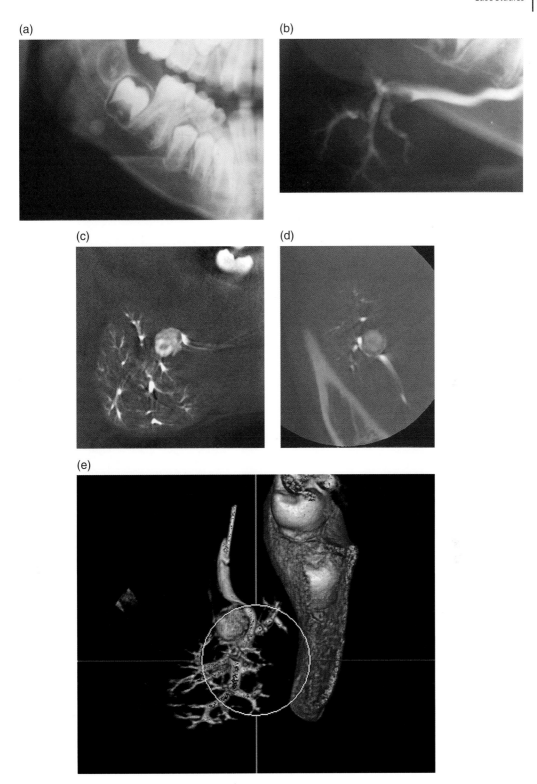

Figure 1.5.10 (a) Panoramic radiograph showing a round opaque structure in the posterior mandibular region between the distal root tip of tooth 47 and the basal cortical line. (b) Sialography with contrast medium filling the Wharton duct, confirming chronic sialadenitis. (c–e) The onion bowl-like structure of the salicary gland stone and its exact location within the salivary gland.

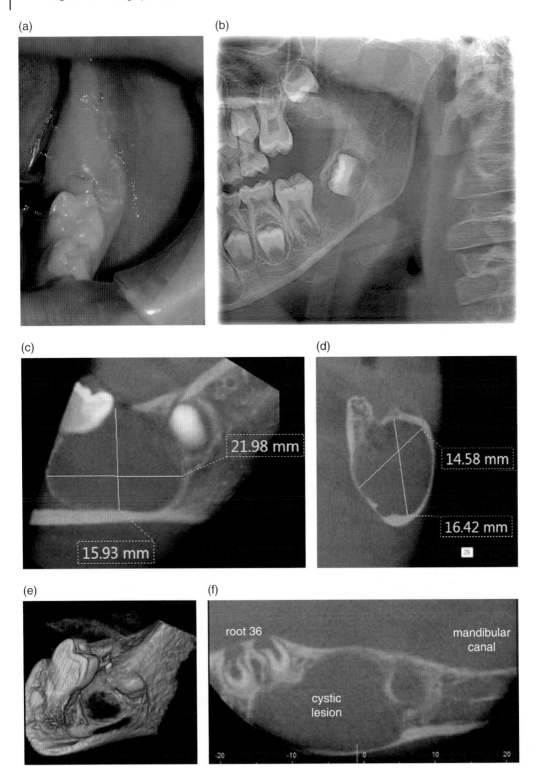

Figure 1.5.11 (a) Clinical view of an incompletely retained tooth 36 in a 7-year-old boy. (b) Because an intraoral radiograph is not tolerated, a half-side panoramic radiograph is taken. The gained intervention is not sufficient for surgical intervention. (c,d,f) The volume of the lesion is measured in CBCT, and the position of the mandibular canal is clearly depicted. (e) The surface-shaded image shows that the lesion has developed buccaly from tooth 36 and is thus displacing it lingually.

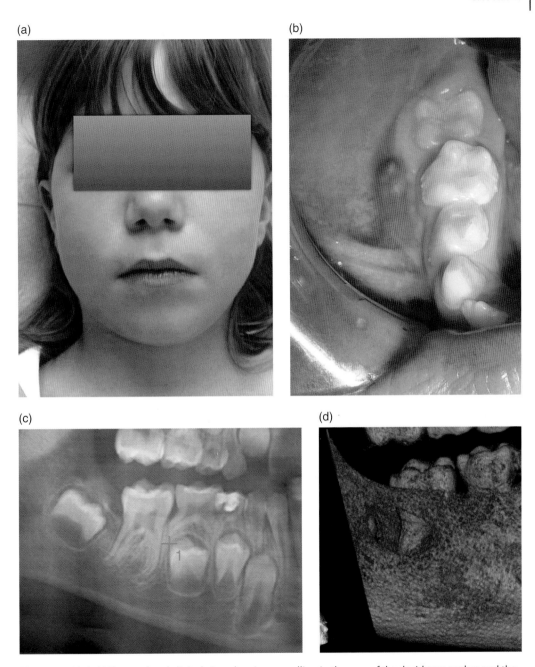

Figure 1.5.12 (a,b) Extraoral and clinical view showing a swelling in the area of the deciduous molars and the first permanent molar of the lower right mandible. All teeth respond to sensitivity test. (c) Panoramic radiograph, giving only a suspicion of inflammatory osteolysis distal to tooth 46. (d) CBCT showing a cortical vestibular defect distal to tooth 46. (e) CBCT images of the same region. (f) CBCT showing bone sclerosis adjacent to the areas of bone destruction and lifting off of the swollen and slightly sclerosed periosteum by inflammatory processes. The diagnosis of osteomyelitis is radiologically confirmed. *Source:* Clinical photograph courtesy of Dr. M. Franscini, Locarno, Switzerland.

(e)

(f)

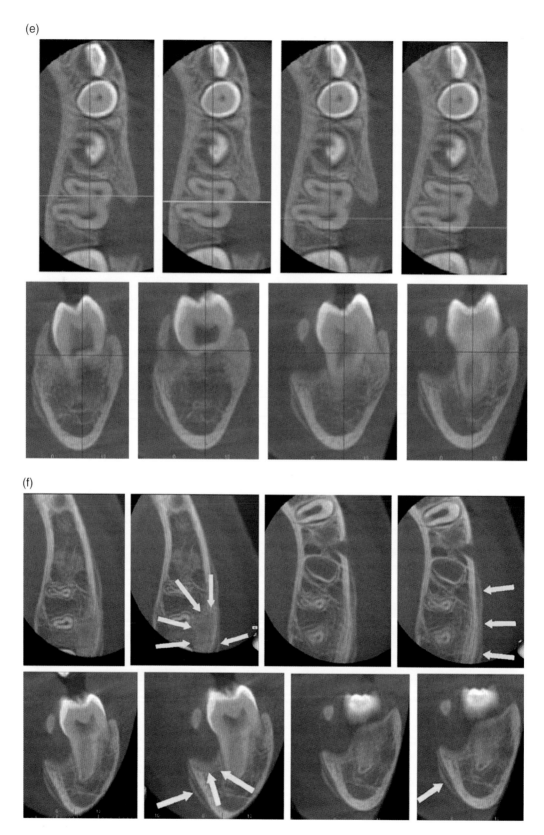

Figure 1.5.12 (Continued)

Conclusion

Children and adolescents are more sensitive to radiation than adults. In emergency situations, they should usually be examined with intraoral dental films.

A meaningful use of CBCT in children and adolescents is limited to specific diseases of particular concern to the general health of the patient, such as serious inflammations, benign and malignant tumours and other very specific pathological changes.

When CBCT is used in children and adolescents, the following issues must be considered:

- Optimisation in radiation protection must be achieved. Patient features like age, size and gender, as well as the specific examination indication, must always be considered and the benefits must be balanced against the possible radiation risk.
- Despite the fact that some CBCT devices offer only standardised, unchangeable exposure values, most allow for custom protocols based on patient size and age.
- ALADAIP (As Low As Diagnostically Acceptable being Indication-oriented and Patient-specific) appears to be the most appropriate current protocol for the use of CBCT in children and adolescents.
- Optimisation in radiation protection is a very challenging task that has to be carried out with great responsibility.

References

Abogazalah, N., Ando, M. 2017. Alternative methods to visual and radiographic examinations for approximal caries detection. *Journal of Oral Science*, **59**(3), 315–22.

American Academy of Pediatric Dentistry (AAPD). 2012. Guideline on prescribing dental radiographs for infants, children, adolescents, and persons with special health care needs. *Pediatric Dentistry*, **34**(5), 319–21.

American Academy of Pediatric Dentistry (AAPD). 2017. Prescribing dental radiographs for infants, children, adolescents, and individuals with special health care needs. *Pediatric Dentistry*, **39**(6), 205–7.

Bataineh, A. B. 2001. Sensory nerve impairment following mandibular third molar surgery. *Journal of Oral Maxillofacial Surgery*, **59**, 1012–17.

Blaeser, B. F., August, M. A., Donoff, R. B., Kaban, L. B., Dodson, T. B. 2003. Panoramic radiographic risk factors for inferior alveolar nerve injury after third molar extraction. *Journal of Oral Maxillofacial Surgery*, **61**, 417–21.

Dula, K., Mini, R., van der Stelt, P. F., Buser, D. 2001. Radiographic assessment of implant patients: decision-making criteria. *International Journal of Oral Maxillofacial Implants*, **16**, 80–9.

Dula, K., Bornstein, M. M., Buser, D., Dagassan-Berndt, D., Ettlin, D. A., Filippi, A., et al. 2014. SADMFR guidelines for the use of cone-beam computed tomography/ digital volume tomography. A consensus workshop organized by the Swiss Association of Dentomaxillofacial Radiology. Part I: Oral and maxillofacial surgery, temporomandibular joint disorders and orthodontics. *Swiss Dental Journal*, **124**, 1170–83.

Dula, K., Benic, G., Bornstein, M. M., Dagassan-Berndt, D., Filippi, A., Hicklin, S., et al. 2015. SADMFR guidelines for the use of cone-beam computed tomography/ digital volume tomography. A consensus workshop organized by the Swiss Association of Dentomaxillofacial Radiology. Part II: Endodontics, periodontology, reconstructive dentistry, pediatric dentistry. *Swiss Dental Journal*, **125**, 945–53.

Elhennawy, K., Askar, H., Jost-Brinkmann, P. G., Reda, S., Al-Abdi, A., Paris, S., Schwendicke, F. 2018. In vitro performance of the DIAGNOcam for detecting proximal carious lesions adjacent to composite restorations. *Journal of Dentistry*, **72**, 39–43.

Esmaeili, E. P., Waltimo-Sirén, J., Laatikainen, T., Haukka, J., Ekholm, M. 2016. Application of segmented dental panoramic tomography among children: positive effect of continuing education in radiation protection. *Dentomaxillofacial Radiology*, **45**, 20160104.

Gimenez, T., Piovesan, C., Braga, M. M., Raggio, D. P., Deery, C., Ricketts, D. N., et al. 2015. Visual inspection for caries detection: a systematic review and meta-analysis. *Journal of Dental Research*, **94**, 895–904.

Jaju, P. P., Jaju, S. P. 2015. Cone-beam computed tomography: time to move from ALARA to ALADA. *Imaging Science in Dentistry*, **45**(4), 263–5.

Jerjes, W., Swinson, B., Moles, D. R., El-Maaytah, M., Banu, B., Upile, T., et al. 2006. Permanent sensory nerve impairment following third molar surgery: a prospective study. *Oral Surgery Oral Medicine Oral Pathology Oral Radiology and Endodontics*, **102**, e1–7.

Lübbers, H. T., Bornstein, M., Dagassan Berndt, D., Filippi, A., Leoncini, S., Suter, V., Dula, K. 2014. Quality guidelines – radiology and radiation protection. SSO. *Swiss Dental Journal*, **124**, 1267–73.

Mendes, F. M., Novaes, T. F., Matos, R., Bittar, D. G., Piovesan, C., Gimenez, T., et al. 2012. Radiographic and laser fluorescence methods have no benefits for detecting caries in primary teeth. *Caries Research*, **46**(6), 536–43.

National Academy of Sciences/National Research Council (NAS/NRC). 2006. *Health Risks from Exposure to Low Levels of Ionizing Radiation, BEIR VII, Phase 2.* Washington, DC: National Academy Press.

Oenning, A. C., Jacobs, R., Pauwels, R., Stratis, A., Hedesiu, M., Salmon, B., DIMITRA Research Group. 2018. Cone-beam CT in paediatric dentistry: DIMITRA project position statement. *Pediatric Radiology*, **48**(3), 308–16.

Schwarz, M., Rothman, S., Rhodes, M., Chafetz, N. 1987a. Computed tomography: Part I. Preoperative assessment of the mandible for endosseous implant surgery. *International Journal of Oral Maxillofacial Implants*, **2**, 137–41.

Schwarz, M., Rothman, S., Rhodes, M., Chafetz, N. 1987b. Computed tomography: Part II. Preoperative assessment of the maxilla for endosseous implant surgery. *International Journal of Oral Maxillofacial Implants*, **2**, 143–8.

Schwendicke, F., Tzschoppe, M., Paris, S. 2015. Radiographic caries detection: a systematic review and meta-analysis. *Journal of Dentistry*, **43**, 924–33.

Svanaes, D., B., Larheim, T. A., Backe, S. 1985. Dose reduction by field size trimming in rotational panoramic radiography. *Scandavian Journal of Dental Research*, **93**, 61–7.

United Nations Scientific Committee on the Effects of Atomic Radiation (UNSCEAR). 2013. *Report: Effects of Radiation Exposure of Children.* Supplement No. 46. New York: United Nations.

Unit 2

Management of Tooth Substance Loss

2.1

Deep Carious Lesions and the Dental Pulp

Falk Schwendicke[1] and Nicola P. Innes[2]

[1] Department of Operative and Preventive Dentistry, Charité Centre for Dental Medicine, Berlin, Germany
[2] Department of Paediatric Dentistry, School of Dentistry, University of Dundee, Dundee, United Kingdom

Introduction

Untreated dental caries affects 2.4 billion people worldwide (Kassebaum et al., 2015). It impacts greatly on children's lives, causing pain and infection; reports on the effect of pain on children (Shepherd et al., 1999; Gilchrist et al., 2015; Pitts et al., 2015; AAPD, 2016) show that it can cause impairment of growth and cognitive development (Alkarimi et al., 2014), affect sleeping, eating and speaking and lead to loss of time at school (Jackson et al., 2011), which may affect attainment (Blumenshine et al., 2008).

Most dentists intervene before it is necessary (Innes and Schwendicke, 2017) to remove all remnants of carious lesions from a cavity, despite evidence showing this is likely to cause more harm than good (Koopaeei et al., 2017). Even in the case of a deep carious lesion that is pain-free or where there is reversible pulpitis, there is still the option of supporting the dental pulp and trying to maintain its health by inactivating or reducing the potency of the carious lesion and allowing the tooth to maintain as much of its integrity as possible. Minimum-intervention approaches are possible for teeth even where there is pain and a deep lesion, provided the diagnosis is correctly established. This relies on a sound understanding of what happens when a deep lesion begins to give pain, whether in a deciduous or a permanent tooth.

Origin of Pulpitis, Pain and Necrosis

Any established carious lesion will obviously directly affect the region of the tooth that is undergoing demineralisation and to which the bacteria are confined. However, there are more distant effects that need to be taken into consideration as well. These occur through stimulation of the pulp–dentinal complex and manifest through reactions in the dental pulp.

Although the dental pulp and dentin are anatomically and histologically separate structures, their tissues are intimately associated and the pulpodentinal complex can be thought of, functionally, as a single structure. Any stimulus to the dentin is detected in the dental pulp and provokes a reaction there through the odontoblasts. It has been shown that even removing dental enamel in a healthy tooth will provoke a response in the dental pulp. The clinical importance of this is that the response can involve reactionary dentin being laid down, but it may also involve pain.

Management of Dental Emergencies in Children and Adolescents, First Edition.
Edited by Klaus W. Neuhaus and Adrian Lussi.
© 2019 John Wiley & Sons Ltd. Published 2019 by John Wiley & Sons Ltd.
Companion website: www.wiley.com/go/neuhaus/dental_emergencies

(a)

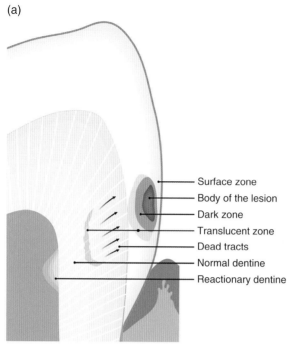

Surface zone
Body of the lesion
Dark zone
Translucent zone
Dead tracts
Normal dentine
Reactionary dentine

Figure 2.1.1 Diagrammatic representation of (a) a noncavitated and (b) a cavitated carious lesion, showing the different components affected by demineralisation and bacteria. (a) Note that even though the lesion has not cavitated, there is reactionary dentin being laid down in the dental pulp. (b) Reactionary dentin is forming, but the lesion is likely to be more aggressive now that cavitation has occurred, as this provides a sheltered environment in which for the lesion to progress. The progress of the lesion may "outrun" the protective reactionary dentin being laid down.

(b)

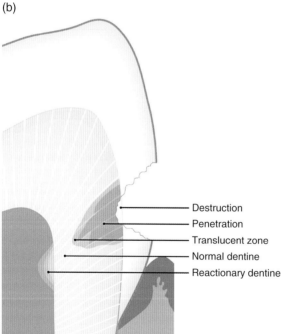

Destruction
Penetration
Translucent zone
Normal dentine
Reactionary dentine

In the case of the deep carious lesion, there isn't just a superficial signal from the enamel, but proteolytic enzymes and bacteria/bacterial byproducts travelling from the biofilm (established in the dentin) down the dentinal tubules and causing a significant stimulus in the dental pulp (see Figure 2.1.1).

This stimulus leads to a response in the pulpodentinal complex, causing reactionary dentin to be laid down. This helps halt the process before the lesion and bacteria reach the dental pulp and cause irreversible inflammation. In effect, there is a race between the dental pulp trying to protect itself as it retreats with a wall of new dentin and the encroaching carious lesion. Through stepwise carious tissue removal, the lesion is sealed in and loses its source of nutrients and hospitable environment. Its progress is slowed or halted, and this allows the pulp to protect itself. Then, when the lesion is opened, further removal of any remaining soft carious tissue is less likely to result in an exposure of the dental pulp.

Pulpitis and Periradicular/Periapical Periodontitis in the Primary and Permanent Dentitions

Dental pain used to be thought to differ between the deciduous and permanent dentition, with deciduous teeth having less innervation and causing less pain than permanent ones. However, over the last few decades, research has shown that there is no difference in innervation between the two (Rodd and Boissonade, 2001). There are, however, differences beyond the teeth themselves that make treating the deciduous and permanent teeth slightly different. One factor is that the permanent teeth have a much longer lifespan; others relate to the age of the child and their ability to communicate and to cope with treatment. Young children do not find it as easy to describe and report pain as older children and young adults. Cognitively, the ability to understand pain and differentiate a chronic pain from the absence of pain is a complex phenomenon. Young children who grow up with pain from an early age may not realise that this is not normal. When they do realise they have pain, it can be difficult for them to describe it precisely in order to help reach an accurate diagnosis.

The Spectrum of Pain

Dental pain resulting from carious lesions can be thought of as a spectrum rather than three distinct states. When a lesion is left untreated and reaches a stage of causing pain, this stretches from reversible pulpitis, through irreversible pulpitis to periradicular/periapical periodontitis. This spectrum, however, is not a straightforward progression from one stage to the next, and neither is it inevitable that the progression will continue. Pulpitis is defined by the American Association of Endodontists (AAE) as "a clinical and histologic term denoting inflammation of the dental pulp; clinically described as reversible or irreversible and histologically described as acute, chronic or hyperplastic" (AAE, 2015).

Reversible Pulpitis

Reversible pulpitis is defined as "a clinical diagnosis based on subjective and objective findings indicating that the inflammation should resolve and the pulp return to normal" (AAE, 2015). As the carious lesion becomes established in the dentin, pathophysiologically an inflammatory response is stimulated in the dentition and odontoblasts are stimulated to lay down reactionary dentin. Histopathologically, the pulp will show inflammatory cells close to the site of the reaction, but this will resolve if the stimulus (the carious lesion) is removed or made impotent.

The patient's symptoms will be intermittent. Classically, the patient will describe the pain as coming and going, usually provoked by a stimulus such as something sweet or cold. This pain will not outlast the provoking stimulus and will not tend to awaken the patient at night.

Irreversible Pulpitis

Irreversible pulpitis can be either asymptomatic or symptomatic, where the symptoms are "lingering thermal pain, spontaneous pain, [and] referred pain" (AAE, 2015). It is "a clinical diagnosis based on subjective and objective findings indicating that the vital inflamed pulp is incapable of healing" (AAE, 2015). This happens when the lesion continues to progress, having affected the dental pulp to the extent that it has overwhelmed the protective mechanisms. The inflammatory response increases in an attempt to lay down adequate reactionary dentin, but as the disease continues, the pulp can fail to provide enough reactionary dentin, and quickly enough, to protect itself. The inflammation becomes so great that it no longer provides protection and actually becomes the problem for the tooth. The inflamed tissue, in a confined space without the ability to resolve the inflammation, increases pressure, and pain is acute and unresolving. The pulp will show more inflammatory signs than it did with reversible pulpitis. The patient's symptoms will have progressed to be more continuous. Pain will start spontaneously. It may also waken them from sleep and keep them awake.

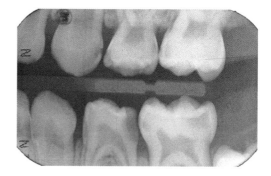

Figure 2.1.2 Radiograph of tooth 74 (lower left first primary molar) showing a deep occluso-distal lesion encroaching on the pulp. There is some evidence of a radiolucent area in the furcal area, indicating periradicular pathology and pulp necrosis.

Pulp Necrosis with or without Periradicular Periodontitis

Pulp necrosis is "a clinical diagnosi[s] … indicating death of the dental pulp. The pulp is usually nonresponsive to pulp testing" (AAE, 2015). At some stage, the pulp will not be able to withstand the bacterial toxins and the persistent damage caused by the inflammation. The bacteria will have travelled through the tooth as the mineral was destroyed and then through any remaining dentinal tubules to reach the dental pulp. At this stage, there is liquefaction inflammation and necrosis of the cells, with bacteria present within the pulp cavity and, eventually, the root canals. This will not necessarily cause symptoms/pain. However, bacterial byproducts or the bacteria themselves will stimulate an inflammatory reaction in the periradicular or periapical bone. In many cases, this can be seen radiographically as a radiolucency in the furcal area between the roots (in deciduous teeth) (Figure 2.1.2) or around the apices (in permanent teeth). This chronic inflammation may stay asymptomatic in the long term, but it can also show acute exacerbation (secondary acute inflammation). In some

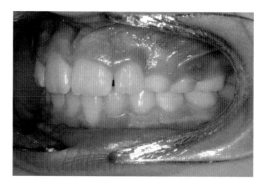

Figure 2.1.3 Abscess at the mucogingival junction of the buccal mucosa of tooth 64 (upper left first primary molar). The tooth is pain-free except occasionally when the patient bites on it. It is tender to percussion.

cases, an acute reaction can happen without the chronic phase (primary acute inflammation). In this case, there are usually signs visible within the bone on a radiograph. In both types of acute inflammation, patients will experience the tooth as very painful; they will be unable to bite on it without pain, as the inflammation has extended to the root canal system and out into the periradicular tissues. This means that the tooth is being pushed out of its socket, in some places, by the inflammation. There may be a visible sinus, abscess or pus extruding from a pocket of the tooth (Figure 2.1.3).

Managing Deep Lesions: Treat the Carious Lesion or Treat the Pulp?

Diagnosis of the extent of the lesion and the inflammation of the dental pulp is not always easy, and because the treatment very much depends on getting the diagnosis correct, the factors involved in making this assessment have to be understood.

The disease has been described in terms of progression, but it is very important to re-emphasise that there is not necessarily a straightforward progression through these symptoms, and a number of influencing factors will change the course of the disease, its speed and the extent to which the patient experiences symptoms. For example, teeth, especially deciduous teeth, have multiple root canals and accessory canals, making them complex systems. The different parts can have different responses to an inflammatory stimulus, including remaining unaffected, depending on where the stimulus is. The carious lesion may undergo a change in its ecosystem whereby it becomes less cariogenic, progression slows and reparative dentin is able to shield the dental pulp and reduce inflammation. The same patient can experience and express pain differently at different times. A common definition of pain is "whatever the experiencing person says it is, existing whenever the experiencing person says it does" (McCaffery, 1968), which is often shortened to, "Pain is what the patient says it is".

Despite these many and complicating factors, to treat the disease well, an accurate diagnosis has to be established based on the patient's history, a thorough clinical assessment, a radiographic assessment and possibly (for permanent teeth) vitality testing.

Strategies for Dealing with Carious Lesions

The options for management mean that when the pulp is reversibly inflamed, it is possible to resolve the pain simply by managing the carious lesion. By removing it, inactivating it or slowing its progress, the reactionary dentin laid down by the dental pulp can provide enough of a barrier for the pulp to stop the stimulus that is causing it to be inflamed. However, if the pulp has reached a stage where it is irreversibly inflamed, the only possibilities are to remove the pulp and carry out a root canal treatment or to extract the tooth. In the deciduous dentition, the root treatment might be a pulpotomy or a pulpectomy, again depending on the level of inflammation of the pulp.

A diagnosis of reversible pulpitis means that the tooth can be managed by removing the lesion or reducing its potency. A number of options are available:

- Nonselective removal of the carious lesion.
- Stepwise removal of the carious lesion.
- Selective removal of the carious lesion.
- Sealing of the carious lesion, without removing it.
- A nonrestorative cavity-control approach (appropriate mainly for deciduous teeth).

Previously, the only treatment for a carious lesion was to completely remove it – this is now known as nonselective removal of carious tissue (Innes et al., 2016). However, it has been shown that a carious lesion does not need to be completely removed (Ricketts et al., 2013, Schwendicke et al., 2013). In fact, doing so in deep lesions means that there is a much higher chance of causing pulp exposure and iatrogenic damage to the tooth, leading to unnecessary pulp treatment.

Stepwise carious tissue removal offers the chance to carry out nonselective removal of carious tissue over two visits, around 6–9 months apart (Bjørndal et al., 2017). The first part of the removal makes the cavity appropriate to keep the restoration in place, by clearing the walls of carious tissue and ensuring there is good adhesion and a good seal. This allows the remaining carious tissue on the floor of the cavity to arrest as it is sealed and gives the dental pulp time to lay down reparative dentin. This means that in the second stage, any remaining soft dentin can be removed with much less chance of exposing the dental pulp.

Selective carious tissue removal has the same first stage but no re-entry to the cavity. The success of the treatment relies on the lesion being sealed and arresting.

There are two treatments that are particular to deciduous teeth. The first is where no removal of the deep lesion takes place and it is sealed into the tooth. This can be done in two ways. The Hall Technique uses a preformed metal or stainless steel crown to seal the lesion into the tooth without any caries or tooth tissue removal and with no need to use local anaesthesia. Deep lesions on occlusal surfaces can also be sealed in using restorative materials, but this relies on there being sufficient depth for the material and on the walls providing a solid adhesive surface.

Removing Deep Lesions: Nonselective, Stepwise or Selective?

As already briefly described, one strategy for the treatment of the painful pulp is to remove some or all of the contaminated dentin from the cavity, along with the bacteria and bacterial toxins causing the pulpal inflammation. As well as reducing inflammation, this reduces pain. Again, however, it should be noted that removing carious dentin is not a suitable treatment for irreversibly inflamed or necrotic pulp; in these cases, endodontic treatments are needed (see Chapter 3.3).

Removal of carious tissues (also known as "caries excavation") traditionally aimed to remove all contaminated (or "infected") and all demineralised (or "affected") dentin (Fusayama and Kurosaki, 1972). The logic behind this goal was to remove all bacteria, as caries was thought to be an infectious disease. Treating caries was synonymous with preventing infection, or – where infection had occurred – removing all causative agents from the mouth (and the affected teeth). This understanding of caries, however, is not supported by current evidence. Instead, the presence of cariogenic bacteria in the dental biofilm is most likely to be a normal status in most individuals. The harmful effects of these bacteria are only fully seen when

fermentable carbohydrates (mainly low-molecular sugars) are frequently consumed: cariogenic bacteria are all acidogenic, which means they lower the pH in their local environment by metabolising sugar to acid. They are also aciduric, which means they can tolerate this lower pH. Notably, and most relevantly, many other (noncariogenic) bacteria aren't, leading to a shift in the composition of the biofilm towards cariogenic species, and thus a change in the biofilm activity towards intense and long-lasting acidity. The result is mineral loss from dental hard tissues (Marsh, 2006). Following this logic, caries management and the management of carious lesions (the symptoms of caries) should aim not to remove all bacteria, but rather to control biofilm composition and activity. Given this established pathogenesis, one main strategy of control is to isolate the bacteria from carbohydrates.

Bacteria left beneath intact restorations are largely isolated from the mouth, and thus from their carbohydrate nutrition. Most cariogenic bacteria are dependent on this nutrition; they die when sealed (and deprived from nutrition) for long periods (Oong et al., 2008). Clinically, understanding this has driven a paradigm shift towards less removal of carious tissues, especially in deep lesions.

Traditional removal of "all" carious dentin used a number of criteria to establish when this aim had been achieved: hardness (all remaining dentin is "hard" (i.e. resistant against probing) everywhere in the cavity), moisture (all dentin is dry), colour (all dentin is yellow, like sound dentin), and stainability (all dentin can no longer be stained, as measured using a caries-detector dye). This carious removal strategy – nonselective excavation – had significant disadvantages when treating deep lesions (Schwendicke et al., 2015a). The greatest was the high risk of pulp exposure: 30–40% in deep or very deep carious lesions (those in close proximity to the pulp, radiographically often defined as reaching the inner third or quarter of dentin) (Figure 2.1.4). Given that exposed pulps are usually managed using direct pulp capping,

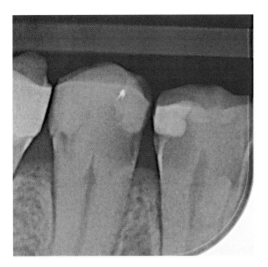

Figure 2.1.4 Deep carious lesions on the lower right first and second premolar. In the first premolar, only a thin band of sound dentin remains above the pulp; the carious lesion reaches into the inner quarter of the dentin. On the second premolar, the lesion reaches into the inner third and the sound dentin band is thicker. Both teeth were clinically asymptomatic, with vital pulps.

which shows highly unsatisfactorily success rates (at least when performed conventionally; further details are beyond the scope of this chapter), or root-canal treatment, exposing the pulp has grave consequences for the tooth and should be avoided (Aguilar and Linsuwanont, 2011; Schwendicke and Stolpe, 2014; Schwendicke et al., 2013, 2014b, 2015b). Similarly, nonselective removal can irritate the pulp and increases the risks of post-operative pulp complications in the teeth where the pulp is not exposed. In summary, nonselective removal does not seem to be the best strategy for managing (reversibly inflamed) painful pulp or preventing pain (and pulp inflammation).

For over 80 years, one established alternative has been stepwise removal, where, first, carious dentin is sealed beneath a temporary restoration and, second, nonselective removal of carious tissue is carried out. Between these two steps, reactionary dentin is laid down (reducing the risk of pulp exposure during the second step), the lesion is inactivated and the bacteria are killed by depriving them from carbohydrates and demineralised dentin is (partially) remineralised and rehardened (Bjørndal et al., 2017). One often stated advantage of this technique is that the carious lesion can be re-inspected prior to restoration. For painful teeth, there is also the advantage of being able to gauge the pulp's clinical reaction to the removal of most of the bacteria and bacterial toxins: if the pain persists during the temporary sealing phase, this is usually an indicator for an irreversible pulp inflammation, which requires endodontic therapy (as described). This means that stepwise removal can be helpful in reaching a definitive diagnosis regarding the status of the pulp. Another advantage is that the definitive restoration is carried out on dentin that is hard and similar to sound dentin after the second removal step. This is relevant, as the quality of the dentin (sound, demineralised or bacterially contaminated) has been found to significantly affect the bond strengths of dental adhesives (reducing them) and the mechanical support of the overlying restoration against masticatory forces. Placing a restoration onto soft dentin may produce a "trampoline" effect, with the restoration fracturing "into" the lesion during chewing. This is avoided in stepwise removal. However, stepwise removal has its disadvantages, too: the risk of pulp exposure is lower than in nonselective removal, but remains significant at around 10% for deep lesions. In addition, the second step generates costs, is burdensome for patients and may, especially in children, induce unnecessary anxiety, with long-term consequences. For this reason, stepwise removal is no longer commonly recommended, at least in children (Schwendicke et al., 2016).

Instead, the third strategy – selective carious tissue removal – is increasingly being recommended. In selective removal, different dentin is left in proximity to the pulp than to the periphery. Peripherally, the aim is to prepare the dentin (and the enamel) for a strong-sealing and supportive, long-lasting restoration. Thus, only sound enamel and hard dentin is left there. In proximity to the pulp (usually the deepest part of the cavity), on the other hand, avoiding pulp exposure (and not restoration survival) is the priority. Soft or leathery dentin is left and sealed under the restoration. According to Innes et al. (2016), "Soft dentin will deform when a hard instrument is pressed onto it, and can be easily scooped up (e.g. with a sharp hand excavator) with little force being required", while "leathery dentin can still be easily lifted without much force being required", but "does not deform when an instrument is pressed onto it". Selective removal (Figure 2.1.5) dramatically reduces the risk of pulp exposure. If the indication is correct and the pulp is truly only reversibly inflamed, the carious lesion itself is only seldom extended right up to the pulp; instead, a band of sound dentin usually separates the pulp from the

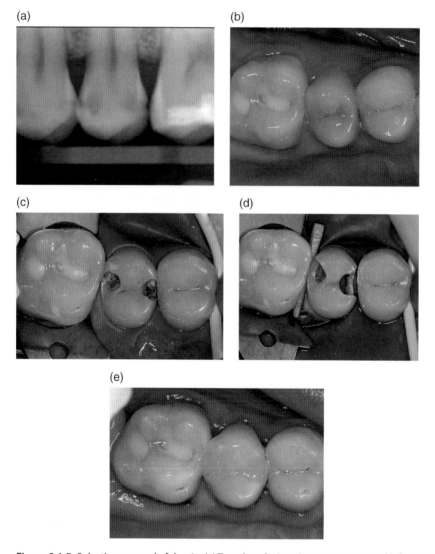

Figure 2.1.5 Selective removal of dentin. (a) Two deep lesions in an upper second left premolar. The patient complains only of intermittent pain on cold stimulus. (b) Clinically, a dentin shadow is detected (ICDAS score 4). (c) After opening the lesion. Soft and wet dentin is found. (d) After cleaning the enamel and initially scooping out the soft dentin. Leathery dentin remains. (e) After restoration.

lesion (this band can be seen as radiopacity on most radiographs) (see Figure 2.1.4). When not aiming to remove firm or hard dentin close to the pulp, but actively restricting the carious tissue removal until soft or leathery dentin remains, it is highly unlikely that pulp exposure occurs at all (Ricketts et al., 2013; Schwendicke et al., 2013). If the pulp is nevertheless exposed when applying these criteria, it is very likely that the pulp diagnosis was incorrect: if the carious lesion is so obviously extended to the pulp, an irreversible inflammation or pulp necrosis is far more likely than a reversible inflammation (in such cases, endodontic therapy is the suitable choice). Selective removal can thus also be recommended for painful teeth – if the pulp is not exposed during excavation and a strong-sealing, long-lasting restoration can be placed, pulp survival is often possible. However, in line with the arguments for stepwise removal, painful teeth treated this way should be monitored regularly for signs of pathology. In summary, selective removal is a promising strategy for dealing with reversibly inflamed pulps and their associated pain, or for preventing any pain in teeth which have deep lesions. Given the restoration mechanical support and bond strength issues already discussed, however, selective removal may have disadvantages when it comes to placing definitive restorative materials. These are discussed in the next section.

Restoring Deep Lesions

Restoring deep lesions usually means restoring extensive lesions, and restoration survival is known to be closely associated with the number of surfaces involved (Demarco et al., 2012). There are additional factors that might affect restoration survival in teeth with deep lesions and irreversible pulpitis (or in teeth without pain). Selective removal is the recommended strategy for managing or preventing pain (see last section), but residual carious (soft, leathery) dentin reduces restoration bond strength in this area, and therefore local mechanical support

of the restoration. However, this seems to depend on (i) the lesion extent and (ii) the lesion location. Clinical studies where only minimal amounts of carious dentin were left beneath restorations did not find the restoration survival to be significantly inferior to that in teeth where nonselective excavation was carried out (note that pulp exposure and complications were usually reduced in the selective excavation group) (Schwendicke et al., 2013). In contrast, leaving large amounts of carious dentin does seem to significantly impact restoration longevity. This indicates that if selective removal is performed, only pulpoproximal carious dentin should remain (Bakhshandeh et al., 2012; Hesse et al., 2014). The second aspect, lesion location, is relevant because masticatory force mainly comes from a coronal direction (admittedly, there are also some lateral forces). While no clinical studies are available to support this, in vitro research points towards residual carious dentin on occlusal cavity walls being potentially more disadvantageous than that on axial walls. This is because of biomechanical forces; as the masticatory forces act on the lesion in occlusal walls, and the restoration is loaded but not fully supported, if large amounts of carious dentin are left, the restoration may not withstand these "bending" stresses (flexure) and may fracture into the (soft) lesion. In cavities where carious dentin is left on axial walls, forces are directed not onto, but along, the lesion; the restoration itself is supported by hard dentin in the occlusal and proximal box floors. In this case, leaving even more extensive amounts of carious dentin has been found to not significantly disadvantage the restoration (Hevinga et al., 2010; Schwendicke et al., 2014a).

The restoration of any deep (and extensive) lesion in children is challenging. First, restoration survival is significantly worse in children (especially in deciduous teeth) than in adults. The choice of material and strategy is especially relevant. Similarly, for painful teeth with deep lesions (or those without pain, where pain prevention is paramount), selective removal should be performed: here, a strong-sealing restoration is a requirement for clinical success! Finally, given that deep lesions are – as already discussed – located close to the pulp, the risk of irritating the pulp during the restoration process or via an inadequate restoration is high.

We will start by discussing adhesive composite or compomer restorations. Current adhesives are usually either etch-and-rinse or self-etch types. The etch-and-rinse adhesives have superior enamel bond strengths given effective conditioning of the enamel using phosphoric acid. However, in dentin, they can cause over-etching and over-drying after rinsing. Careful adherence to timing for the etchant (usually, 15–20 seconds) and cavity re-wetting after drying (before applying the adhesive) are recommended. For re-wetting (not only in deep cavities), water can be used. Alternatively, chlorhexidine has been recommended, for two reasons. First, it inhibits matrix metalloproteinases (MMPs): dentin enzymes activated under acidic condition (e.g. an active carious lesion, but also when applying an acidic etchant) and thought to cleave the collagen within the hybrid layer, degrading it and thus limiting the longevity of the restoration (Mazzoni et al., 2015). To date, however, this is mainly a theoretical construct; clinical data supporting the use of anti-MMP rinses or MMP-inhibiting adhesives are not convincing (Göstemeyer and Schwendicke, 2016). Given that re-wetting is needed anyway, however, chlorhexidine can be recommended for this purpose. The second rationale might underpin this recommendation: chlorhexidine is antibacterial. However, the relevance of such antibacterial cavity pretreatment is questionable, too: studies show that placing a sealing restoration that isolates bacteria from carbohydrate nutrients is the best antibacterial treatment possible.

Given the additional steps involved in the use of etch-and-rinse adhesives and these challenges, self-etch or universal adhesives have been increasingly recommended for deep lesions. They avoid over-etching and the need for re-wetting, and do not remove the smear layer, reducing the risk of methacrylate penetration into the pulp via the tubules. To overcome the lower bond strengths of such self-etch or universal adhesives to enamel, a selective etching step is recommended for enamel, which is technically easy to perform. The phosphoric acid gel can then be rinsed off and the whole cavity treated using (mainly) universal adhesives (Figure 2.1.6).

When dealing with deep lesions, traditionally a lining material was placed over the pulpal floor of the cavity (this is also known as indirect pulp capping, although the exact definition of the term is very opaque). The liner, conventionally calcium hydroxide, was thought to isolate the pulp from thermal and chemical damage, kill any remaining dentin bacteria and induce reactionary dentin. As an alternative to calcium hydroxide, nowadays calcium silicates like mineral trioxide aggregate or biodentine are recommended.

(a)   (b)   (c)   (d)   (e)

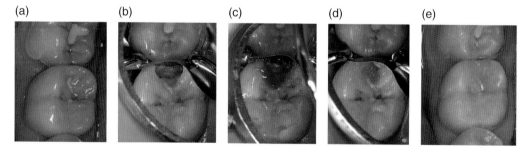

Figure 2.1.6 Selective enamel etching. (a) Initial situation. A dentin shadow is detectable. (b) After carious tissue removal. (c) Selective enamel etching using phosphoric acid. A universal self-etch adhesive was used afterwards on both enamel and dentin. (d) Following restoration of the cavity using a hybrid composite. (e) Final restoration.

However, again, clinical studies do not support using a liner: in deciduous teeth, the benefits of this treatment are doubtful, while in permanent teeth, these linings might even be disadvantageous (as they weaken the restoration) (Schwendicke et al., 2015c). This latter aspect might be overcome when using mineral trioxide aggregate (MTA) or Biodentine, as they are mechanically stronger than calcium hydroxide. However, this still involves an additional treatment step. Also, in teeth with pain due to reversible pulpitis or with deep lesions where pain should be prevented, there is no case for requiring the use of liners prior to restoration placement.

With regards to the material choice, further detail is beyond the scope of this chapter, but it needs highlighting that – as previously mentioned – all direct plastic restoration materials (e.g. composites, compomers, glass ionomer cements) perform worse in deciduous teeth than in permanent ones (Hickel et al., 2005). There are a number of reasons for this, including the different anatomies of the two teeth types, but also the difficulties in operating in a child's mouth. In particular, moisture control, a prerequisite for many direct materials, can be challenging. Often, glass ionomer cements are recommended where this is an issue. However, it should be highlighted that their survival is limited in comparison to the other materials when a proximal surface is involved (Chadwick and Evans, 2007; Klinke et al., 2016), due to the lower flexural strength of glass ionomer cements compared with composites or compomers.

As a result of the poor performance of most direct plastic materials, alternatives have been sought for decades. One is the stainless steel crown, in use since the 1950s (see Chapter 4.2). Stainless steel crowns come with much better survival rates than all other materials in deciduous teeth (they are almost never placed in permanent teeth, partially because the alloy is not wear-resistant over decades). They can be used to restore teeth with deep lesions (with or without reversible pain) following selective removal. They can also be used when managing deep lesions without removing any carious dentin, as discussed in the next section.

Sealing Deep Lesions without Removal

Sealing allows control of carious lesions and bacteria. Given the risks associated with and the effort required in carious tissue removal, this raises an important question: Why remove at all? In theory, arresting a lesion and inactivating bacteria does not require any carious tissue removal; sealing the lesion alone is sufficient. However, there are two issues with this approach. Firstly, as already discussed, in deep lesions, a large number of bacteria and bacterial toxins are present within the carious dentin. Concern has been expressed that if all these bacteria and toxins are sealed beneath a sealant without any attempt at removal, the pulp might be harmed. So far, however, no clinical study has supported this theoretical concern. Secondly, sealing deep lesions carries the same inherent mechanical issues already discussed; the sealing restoration sits on soft, nonsupportive dentin, and on dentin and enamel where dental adhesives show low, or even no, bond strength at all, detrimentally affecting sealant survival. Sealing cavitated lesions that are subject to masticatory forces using plastic materials is therefore not possible at present.

A restoration that circumvents this problem is the Hall Technique. Briefly, the Hall Technique is carried out by pushing a stainless steel crown (also known as a preformed metal crown) onto a deciduous molar tooth without removing any carious tissue or carrying out any tooth removal. A crown the right size to cover the tooth is chosen and is cemented with glass ionomer cement by pushing it on (or asking the child to bite down on) the tooth. More information and a manual on how to carry out the technique can be found at https://en.wikipedia.org/wiki/Hall_Technique. These have been clinically shown to have a high success rate for sealing cavitated lesions. Trials, either completed (Innes et al., 2011; Santamaria et al., 2017) or underway (Narbutaite et al.,

2014; Tonmukayakul et al., 2015; Hesse et al., 2016), have found the technique to be more acceptable to children, parents and dentists, with clinical success rates (no pain or infection) of 99% (UK trial) (Innes et al., 2007) and 100% (Germany) at 1 year (Santamaria et al., 2014), 98% (UK) and 93% (Germany) over 2 years (Innes et al., 2007; Santamaria et al., 2017) and 97% (UK) over 5 years (Innes et al., 2011). In one study, around two-thirds of lesions were over halfway into dentin radiographically (Innes et al., 2011), and the technique can therefore be recommended for teeth that are cavitated or have deep lesions. Using the diagnostic sign of a bridge of dentin being visible radiographically between the lesion and the pulp gives a 97% chance of success in treatment over an average of 3 years. There have, however, been no studies involving teeth with pain (reversible pulpitis), and whilst the Hall Technique is used by some for this indication, it has no evidence to support.

Conclusion

Deep carious lesions can often be managed with minimal intervention approaches, even when they are associated with pain. This depends on the correct diagnosis (reversible pulpitis, irreversible pulpitis, pulp necrosis with or without periradicular periodontitis) being established, which allows for choice of the correct treatment. For teeth without pain and deep lesions, or those with possibly reversible inflammation and pain, dentists should not aim to remove all carious dentin, but should manage the carious lesion biologically. This can involve stepwise, selective or no removal (in the latter case, it is necessary to seal the lesion, e.g. with a crown placed using the Hall Technique). Teeth should be followed up regularly, as there remains the risk of having misdiagnosed the pulp status, which would necessitate endodontic therapy later on.

References

Aguilar, P., Linsuwanont, P. 2011. Vital pulp therapy in vital permanent teeth with cariously exposed pulp: a systematic review. *Journal of Endodontics*, **37**, 581–7.

Alkarimi, H. A., Watt, R. G., Pikhart, H., Sheiham, A., Tsakos, G. 2014. Dental caries and growth in school-age children. *Pediatrics*, **133**, e616–23.

American Academy Of Pediatric Dentistry (AAPD). 2016. Policy on early childhood caries (ECC): classifications, consequences, and preventive strategies. *Pediatric Dentistry*, **38**, 52–4.

American Association of Endodontists (AAE). 2015. *Glossary of Endodotic Terms*. Chicago, IL: American Association of Endodontists.

Bakhshandeh, A., Qvist, V., Ekstrand, K. 2012. Sealing occlusal caries lesions in adults referred for restorative treatment: 2–3 years of follow-up. *Clinical Oral Investigations*, **16**, 521–19.

Bjørndal, L., Fransson, H., Bruun, G., Markvart, M., Kjaeldgaard, M., Näsman, P., et al. 2017. Randomized clinical trials on deep carious lesions: 5-year follow-up. *Journal of Dental Research*, **96**, 747–53.

Blumenshine, S. L., Vann, W. F., Gizlice, Z., Lee, J. Y. 2008. Children's school performance: impact of general and oral health. *Journal of Public Health Dentistry*, **68**, 82.

Chadwick, B. L., Evans, D. J. 2007. Restoration of class II cavities in primary molar teeth with conventional and resin modified glass ionomer cements: a systematic review of the literature. *European Archives of Paediatric Dentistry*, **8**, 14–21.

Demarco, F. F., Correa, M. B., Cenci, M. S., Moraes, R. R., Opdam, N. J. 2012. Longevity of posterior composite restorations: not only a matter of materials. *Dental Materials*, **28**, 87–101.

Fusayama, T., Kurosaki, N. 1972. Structure and removal of carious dentin. *International Dental Journal*, **22**, 401–11.

Gilchrist, F., Marshman, Z., Deery, C., Rodd, H. D. 2015. The impact of dental caries on children and young people: what they have to say? *International Journal of Paediatric Dentistry*, **25**, 327–38.

Göstemeyer, G., Schwendicke, F. 2016. Inhibition of hybrid layer degradation by cavity pretreatment: meta- and trial sequential analysis. *Journal of Dentistry*, **49**, 14–21.

Hesse, D., Bonifacio, C. C., Mendes, F. M., Braga, M. M., Imparato, J. C., Raggio, D. P. 2014. Sealing versus partial caries removal in primary molars: a randomized clinical trial. *BMC Oral Health*, **14**, 58.

Hesse, D., De Araujo, M. P., Olegário, I. C., Innes, N. P., Raggio, D. P., Bonifácio, C. C. 2016. Atraumatic restorative treatment compared to the Hall Technique for occluso-proximal cavities in primary molars: study protocol for a randomized controlled trial. *Trials*, **17**, 169.

Hevinga, M. A., Opdam, N. J., Frencken, J. E., Truin, G. J., Huysmans, M. C. 2010. Does incomplete caries removal reduce strength of restored teeth? *Journal of Dental Research*, **89**, 1270–5.

Hickel, R., Kaaden, C., Paschos, E., Buerkle, V., García-Godoy, F., Manhart, J. 2005. Longevity of occlusally-stressed restorations in posterior primary teeth. *American Journal Dentistry*, **18**, 198–211.

Innes, N. P. T., Schwendicke, F. 2017. Restorative thresholds for carious lesions: systematic review and meta-analysis. *Journal of Dental Research*, **96**, 501–8.

Innes, N. P., Evans, D. J., Stirrups, D. R. 2007. The Hall Technique; a randomized controlled clinical trial of a novel method of managing carious primary molars in general dental practice: acceptability of the technique and outcomes at 23 months. *BMC Oral Health*, **7**, 18.

Innes, N. P., Evans, D. J., Stirrups, D. R. 2011. Sealing caries in primary molars: randomized control trial, 5-year results. *Journal of Dental Research*, **90**, 1405–10.

Innes, N. P., Frencken, J. E., Bjorndal, L., Maltz, M., Manton, D. J., Ricketts, D., et al. 2016. Managing carious lesions: consensus recommendations on terminology. *Advances in Dental Research*, **28**, 49–57.

Jackson, S. L., Vann, W. F. Jr., Kotch, J. B., Pahel, B. T., Lee, J. Y. 2011. Impact of poor oral health on children's school attendance and performance. *American Journal of Public Health*, **101**, 1900–6.

Kassebaum, N., Bernabe, E., Dahiya, M., Bhandari, B., Murray, C., Marcenes, W. 2015. Global burden of untreated caries: a systematic review and metaregression. *Journal of Dental Research*, **94**(5), 650–8.

Klinke, T., Daboul, A., Turek, A., Frankenberger, R., Hickel, R., Biffar, R. 2016. Clinical performance during 48 months of two current glass ionomer restorative systems with coatings: a randomized clinical trial in the field. *Trials*, **17**, 239.

Koopaeei, M. M., Inglehart, M. R., McDonald, N., Fontana, M. 2017. General dentists', pediatric dentists', and endodontists' diagnostic assessment and treatment strategies for deep carious lesions: a comparative analysis. *Journal of the American Dental Association*, **148**, 64–74.

Marsh, P. D. 2006. Dental plaque as a biofilm and a microbial community – implications for health and disease. *BMC Oral Health*, **6**, S14.

Mazzoni, A., Tjaderhane, L., Checchi, V., Di Lenarda, R., Salo, T., Tay, F. R., et al. 2015. Role of dentin MMPs in caries progression and bond stability. *Journal of Dental Research*, **94**, 241–51.

McCaffery, M. 1968. *Nursing Practice Theories Related to Cognition, Bodily Pain, and Man–Environment Interactions*. Los Angeles, CA: University of California at Los Angeles Students' Store.

Narbutaite, J., Maciulskiene, V., Splieth, C., Innes, N. P., Santamaria, R. M. 2014. Acceptability of three different caries treatment methods for primary molars among Lithuanian children. 12th Congress of the European Academy of Paediatric Dentistry: "A Passion for Paediatric Dentistry", 5–8 June 2014. Sopot, Poland.

Oong, E. M., Griffin, S. O., Kohn, W. G., Gooch, B. F., Caufield, P. W. 2008. The effect of dental sealants on bacteria levels in caries lesions. *Journal of the American Dental Association*, **139**, 271–8.

Pitts, N., Chadwick, B., Anderson, T. 2015. *Children's Dental Health Survey Report 2: Dental Disease and Damage in Children: England, Wales and Northern Ireland*. London: Health and Social Care Information Centre.

Ricketts, D., Lamont, T., Innes, N. P., Kidd, E., Clarkson, J. E. 2013. Operative caries management in adults and children. *Cochrane Database of Systematic Reviews*, CD003808.

Rodd, H. D., Boissonade, F. M. 2001. Innervation of human tooth pulp in relation to caries and dentition type. *Journal of Dental Research*, **80**, 389–93.

Santamaria, R. M., Innes, N. P., Machiulskiene, V., Evans, D. J., Splieth, C. H. 2014. Caries management strategies for primary molars: 1-yr randomized control trial results. *Journal of Dental Research*, **93**, 1062–9.

Santamaria, R. M., Innes, N. P., Machiulskiene, V., Schmoeckel, J., Alkilzy, M., Splieth, C. 2017. Alternative caries management options for primary molars: 2.5-yr outcomes of a randomised clinical trial. *Caries Research*, **51**(6), 605–14.

Schwendicke, F., Stolpe, M. 2014. Direct pulp capping following a carious exposure versus root canal treatment: a cost-effectiveness analysis. *Journal of Endodontics*, **40**(11), 1764–70.

Schwendicke, F., Dörfer, C. E., Paris, S. 2013. Incomplete caries removal: a systematic review and meta-analysis. *Journal of Dental Research*, **92**, 306–14.

Schwendicke, F., Kern, M., Meyer-Lueckel, H., Boels, A., Doerfer, C., Paris, S. 2014a. Fracture resistance and cuspal deflection of incompletely excavated teeth. *Journal of Dentistry*, **42**, 107–13.

Schwendicke, F., Paris, S., Stolpe, M. 2014b. Cost-effectiveness of caries excavations in different risk groups – a micro-simulation study. *BMC Oral Health*, **14**, 153.

Schwendicke, F., Paris, S., Tu, Y. 2015a. Effects of using different criteria and methods for caries removal: a systematic review and network meta-analysis. *Journal of Dentistry*, **43**(1), 1–15.

Schwendicke, F., Stolpe, M., Innes, N. 2015b. Conventional treatment, Hall Technique or immediate pulpotomy for carious primary molars: a cost-effectiveness analysis. *International Endodontic Journal*, **49**(9), 817–26.

Schwendicke, F., Tu, Y. K., Hsu, L. Y., Göstemeyer, G. 2015c. Antibacterial effects of cavity lining: a systematic review and network meta-analysis. *Journl of Dentistry*, **43**, 1298–307.

Schwendicke, F., Frencken, J. E., Bjorndal, L., Maltz, M., Manton, D. J., Ricketts, D. N. J., et al. 2016. Managing carious lesions: consensus recommendations on carious tissue removal. *Advances in Dental Research*, **28**(2), 58–67.

Shepherd, M. A., Nadanovsky, P., Sheiham, A. 1999. Dental public health: the prevalence and impact of dental pain in 8-year-old school children in Harrow, England. *British Dental Journal*, **187**, 38–41.

Tonmukayakul, U., Martin, R., Clark, R., Brownbill, J., Manton, D., Hall, M. 2015. Protocol for the Hall Technique study: a trial to measure clinical effectiveness and cost-effectiveness of stainless steel crowns for dental caries restoration in primary molars in young children. *Contemporary Clinical Trials*, **44**, 36–41.

2.2

Management of Crown Fractures and Crown-Root Fractures

Gabriel Krastl[1] and Julia Amato[2]

[1] *Department of Conservative Dentistry and Periodontology and Center of Dental Traumatology, University Hospital of Würzburg, Würzburg, Germany*
[2] *Department of Periodontology, Endodontology and Cariology, University Center for Dental Medicine Basel, University of Basel, Basel, Switzerland*

Epidemiological Data

Fractures of the tooth crown are amongst the most common injuries to the permanent teeth, accounting for up to 50% of injuries sustained. These fractures mainly affect the enamel and the dentin. The pulp is exposed in approximately 25% of all crown fractures. Crown-root fractures represent less than 5% of traumatic dental injuries (TDIs).

The teeth most frequently affected are the upper central incisors, followed by the laterals. More than 40% of all injuries to the permanent dentition occur before the age of 14, and nearly one-quarter of these occur before the age of 9 (Borum and Andreasen, 2001). In young children, the roots of the affected teeth are not yet fully developed. Thus, preserving pulp vitality and avoiding conventional root canal treatment must be the goal of every restorative treatment in this age group.

Enamel Infractions

Infractions are incomplete fractures of a tooth which remains morphologically intact (Figure 2.2.1). In most cases, solely enamel is involved, but the crack line may extend into the

dentin as well. Various patterns of infraction lines may be seen. The crack lines are hard to visualise and frequently overlooked. Illuminating the tooth with different light sources from various directions makes the fine discontinuities in the enamel visible and may help to estimate the extent of the infraction. An exact assessment of the depth of the crack and crack propagation prediction is not feasible, however. Although in vitro studies have identified enamel cracks as potential portals of entry for microorganisms, an infection of the endodontic system is unlikely if the pulp is healthy. The risk of pulp necrosis in teeth with infraction as the only damage is 3.5% (Ravn, 1981).

Infractions do not generally require treatment. In severe cases, sealing with adhesive resin may be recommended. However, there is no evidence whether sealing increases the fracture resistance of the crown or prevents pulp necrosis or discolouration of the crack lines.

Crown Fractures

Crown fractures may be restricted to the enamel or may involve the dentine and the pulp. Enamel fractures are frequently

Management of Dental Emergencies in Children and Adolescents, First Edition.
Edited by Klaus W. Neuhaus and Adrian Lussi.
© 2019 John Wiley & Sons Ltd. Published 2019 by John Wiley & Sons Ltd.
Companion website: www.wiley.com/go/neuhaus/dental_emergencies

localised in the incisal region, leaving behind a rough, sharp-edged surface (Figures 2.2.2 and 2.2.3a,b). Clinical symptoms are rather unlikely if there is no concomitant luxation injury. Crown fractures affecting the dentine

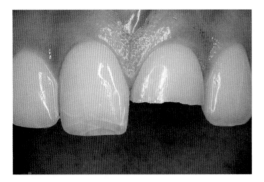

Figure 2.2.1 Enamel cracks of the upper right central incisor and crown fracture of the upper left central incisor.

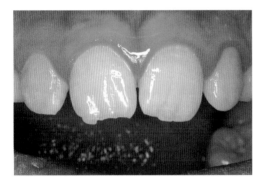

Figure 2.2.2 Small enamel fractures of both upper central incisors.

or even the pulp are usually accompanied by hypersensitivity. Restorative treatment of crown fractures confined to the enamel is not essential in every case. Smoothening and polishing of the sharp edges may be sufficient. For aesthetic reasons, small direct composite restorations can be performed (Olsburgh et al., 2002).

Most crown fractures expose dentine. In children, 80% of the total cross-sectional area in the proximity of the pulp consists of the lumina of the dentinal tubules. Thus, infection of the pulp tissue may occur. The risk of pulp necrosis is further increased in cases of concomitant luxation injury (Robertson et al., 2000).

A definitive bacteria-tight restoration should be performed as soon as possible after the accident. If this is not feasible during emergency treatment, placement of the restoration can be postponed if the dentinal wound is sealed properly to avoid pulp infection. Immediate dentin sealing can be carried out using a recent dentin adhesive and a layer of flowable composite. Dentin protection with a calcium hydroxide cement or a glass ionomer cement is less effective and should only be applied if subsequent treatment is to take place within the next few days.

When the pulp of a previously intact tooth is traumatically exposed, it can generally be assumed that it is healthy and is capable of regeneration. The conditions for maintaining vitality are favourable if the blood supply to

(a)

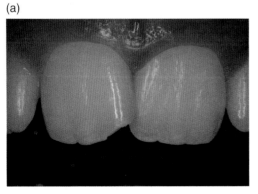

(b)

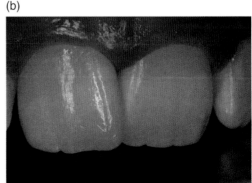

Figure 2.2.3 (a) Enamel fracture of the upper right central incisor. Dentin is not exposed. (b) Restoration of the tooth with a universal composite, for aesthetic purposes.

the pulp is intact. This can be expected in young patients without pre-existing pulpal damage caused by carious lesions or earlier TDIs. The longer the pulp is exposed to the oral cavity, the greater the probability that the pulpal tissue will become infected. In addition, concomitant dislocation injuries substantially reduce the pulp's regenerative capacity, because of the compromised pulpal blood supply. Crown fractures with exposed pulps normally require prompt treatment. Provided that the indication is correct, vital pulp therapy methods after TDIs have a high success rate, particularly in partial pulpotomy, which has a prognosis of over 90% (Krastl and Weiger, 2014) (for details, see Chapter 3.1).

Reattachment Restoration

The adhesive reattachment of the coronal fragment is a simple and conservative approach to reestablishing function and aesthetics. If the fragment was stored under moist conditions after the accident, reattachment should ideally be performed immediately during the emergency treatment (Figure 2.2.4a–c). However, if the fragment is dehydrated due to dry storage for an extended period (>1 hour), both the aesthetic result and the bond strength may be compromised. Storage in saline or water for 1 day is recommended in such cases to allow for rehydration of the fragment (Figure 2.2.5a–d) (Farik et al., 1999); in the meantime, the dentine should be covered with a temporary material that is easy to remove (e.g. calcium hydroxide cements). Rehydration time may be shortened by wet storage of the fragment in a pressure vessel. According to our clinical experience, effective rehydration in terms of a resolved colour disharmony between fragment and tooth seems to occur within 30–60 minutes with this technique.

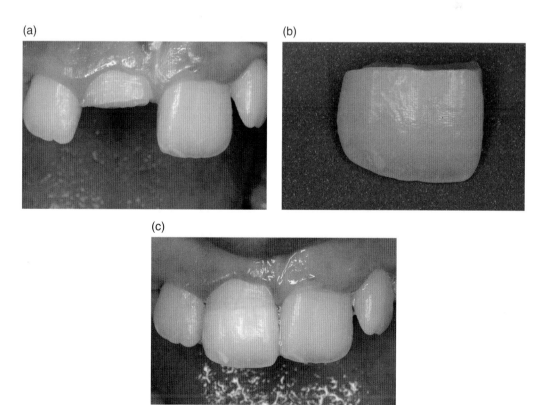

(a)

(b)

(c)

Figure 2.2.4 (a) Crown fracture. (b) Tooth fragment kept under moist conditions following the accident. (c) Same tooth following immediate adhesive reattachment of the fragment.

(a) (b) (c) (d)

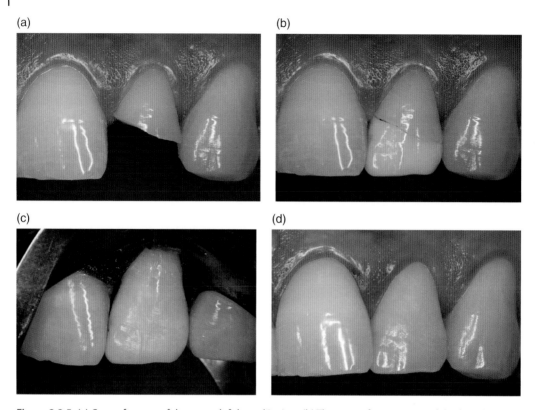

Figure 2.2.5 (a) Crown fracture of the upper left lateral incisor. (b) The crown fragment was dehydrated and could not be reattached immediately. (c) Adhesive reattachment of the crown fragment 1 day later. The fragment was kept in water, to provide rehydration. (d) Clinical situation 9 months after reattachment.

Further, the use of multimode adhesives may compensate for shorter rehydration times, as recently demonstrated by Poubel et al. (2017). Rehydration of crown fragments in a special cell culture medium (tooth rescue box) is not necessary, since no vital cells need to be kept alive. (If such a medium was chosen for storage at the place of the accident, no negative impact on bond strength is expected.) Further alternative rewetting media, such as milk, egg white or hypertonic solutions, have been proposed, but evidence on their benefit compared to saline or water is scarce and partly contradictory (Yilmaz et al., 2010; Sharmin and Thomas, 2013; Shirani et al., 2013).

Before fragment bonding, both fragment and tooth should be cleaned thoroughly. Sandblasting might be a good option to remove any remnant of provisional material

placed to seal dentin during the emergency treatment. However, careful consideration is necessary in areas with a reduced dentin thickness.

Additional preparation, such as chamfering the enamel margins or placement of an internal groove, will lead to an improved bond strength but impede the exact repositioning of the fragment. Tooth surface and fragment should be pretreated with an adhesive system, whereby previous enamel etching with phosphoric acid is highly recommended. Precuring the bonding agent will impair the fit and should therefore be avoided. A flowable resin composite should be applied to the fracture surfaces of both parts and thoroughly spread over the surface. After repositioning the fragment, excess material can be removed and the fracture line cured from the labial and the palatal side. High-power curing lights and a longer irradiation time are recommended to ensure enough energy is delivered through the tooth structure to the entire bonding surface. Cooling the tooth with compressed air helps reduce the temperature rise during photopolymerisation and may prevent heat-induced pulp damage.

Direct Composite Restoration

If repositioning of a coronal fragment is difficult or even impossible in cases of multiple or missing fragments, current composites are used on a routine basis for the restoration of fractured teeth. Smaller defects in particular can be easily built up "freehand" with a universal composite (Figure 2.2.3a,b). If extended parts of the crown have to be restored, more sophisticated polychromatic, multiple-layer techniques using aesthetic composites provide excellent results (Vanini and Mangani, 2001; Dietschi et al., 2006). Whenever possible, isolation with a rubber dam should be attempted. However, in a mixed dentition with partially erupted teeth or in partly subgingivally located defects, the application of a rubber dam is not always feasible (Figure 2.2.6a–i). In these cases, alternative methods of isolation utilising cotton rolls in combination with efficient saliva suction may be implemented. To facilitate a predictable outcome, a mock-up is fabricated directly in the patient's mouth and a silicone key is created. After shade selection, the margins are bevelled. In the labial area, a much wider bevel of 1–2 mm is established to mask the transition between the composite and the tooth. With the help of the silicone key, the palatal wall can be easily constructed with enamel composite material. The resulting artificial enamel frame should precisely reproduce the palatal and incisal outline of the reconstruction, but should not yet be in contact with the adjacent teeth. Various matrix techniques can be used to build the proximal walls. The dentine core is built up with an opaque dentin mass. The core makes up the largest part of the restoration,

leaving only a small space of approximately 0.5 mm for the buccal enamel layer. In young teeth, replication of the optical properties of the incisal area can be challenging. Thus, enough space should be provided in this region for the characterisation of mamelons with translucent and opalescent resin materials.

After application and light-curing of the last artificial enamel layer, excess bonding or composite can be removed at the restoration margins with a curved scalpel. With appropriate finishing and polishing techniques, surface lustre and micromorphology can be adapted almost perfectly to the rest of the dentition (Figure 2.2.7a–c).

Indirect Ceramic Restorations

All-ceramic restorations (veneers or crowns) are a feasible alternative to the direct composite technique. Tooth preparation, however, is more invasive and entails additional damage to the pulp, especially in immature teeth with extended coronal pulps. Thus, the indication for indirect restorations should be restricted to extensive defects in adult patients.

Crown-Root Fractures

In upper anterior permanent teeth, crown-root fractures have a typical fracture line: on the facial side, the fracture is localised paragingivally or supragingivally, whilst palatally the defect often extends far into the root region (Figure 2.2.8a–c). Although the coronal fragment reveals increased mobility, it is still retained palatally by the intact periodontal fibre attachment. Usually, only one fracture line is diagnosed in the periapical radiographs, which corresponds to the buccal fracture line. The palatally situated fracture is usually not visible because of an overlap with the alveolar bone and the absence of diastasis between the fragments in this region. The pulp is frequently, but not always, involved.

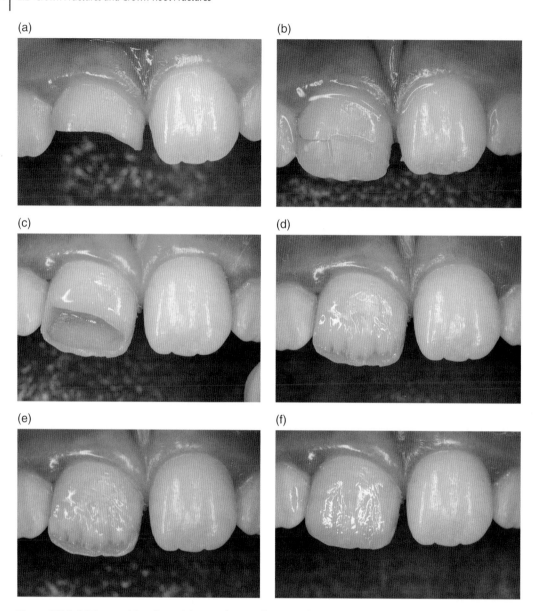

Figure 2.2.6 (a) 7-year-old patient with typical crown fracture of the upper right central incisor. Placement of rubber dam is difficult, because the teeth are not fully erupted. (b) Direct mock-up with composite. (c) The artificial enamel frame is build first using a silicone key. Cotton rolls are used in combination with efficient saliva suction for isolation. (d) The dentin core is reconstructed, leaving only limited space for the buccal enamel. (e) White tints are used for characterisation. (f) Completed restoration before finishing. (g) Restoration after finishing and polishing. (h) Patient's smile. (i) Clinical situation after 1.5 years.

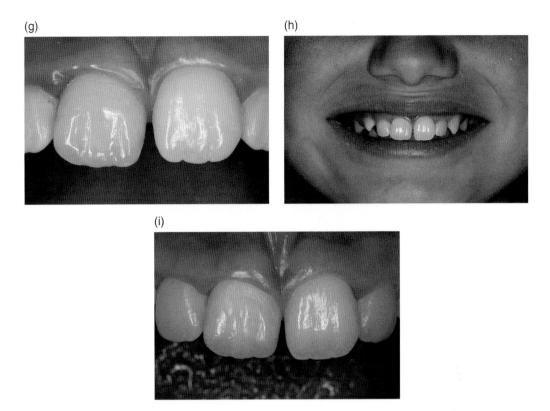

Figure 2.2.6 (Continued)

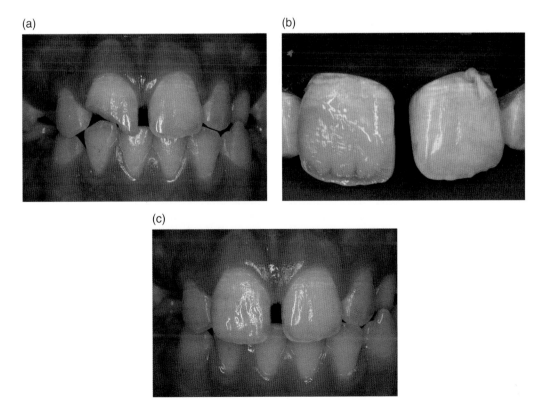

Figure 2.2.7 (a) Crown fracture. (b) Direct composite restoration under optimal conditions. (c) Aesthetic result.

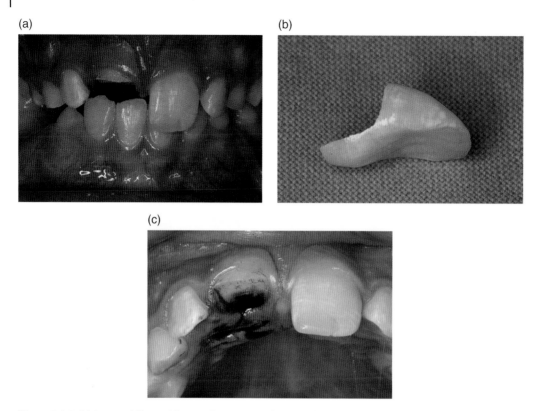

Figure 2.2.8 (a) 9-year-old boy with typical crown-root fracture of the upper right central incisor after removal of the mobile coronal tooth fragment. (b) Coronal fragment. (c) Incisal view of the palatally subgingival defect. The pulp is exposed.

Emergency Treatment for Crown-Root Fractures

To assess the extent of the fracture and identify additional fractures which are often located at the palatal side of the root, it is necessary to remove the mobile coronal fragment. All fragments must be removed in order to assess the situation and properly initiate treatment. This will induce bleeding and makes the sealing of the dentin or the pulp–dentin wound more demanding than in supragingival crown fractures. Astringent haemostatic agents with or without retraction cords may be used to control sulcus bleeding and reduce the flow of sulcular exudates. However, the clinician should be aware that bond strength to astringent-contaminated dentin is considerably reduced, particularly when self-etch adhesives are used (Bernades Kde et al., 2014).

Adhesive reattachment of the crown fragment is a very conservative but technique-sensitive approach to the restoration of crown-root fractures. Ideal conditions for adhesive procedures often require the preparation of a mucoperiostal access flap. Thus, fragment reattachment under less than ideal conditions during emergency treatment is not recommended.

A very simple emergency treatment for crown-root fractures with a mobile but still attached coronal fragment is adhesive sealing of the accessible (usually labial) part of the fracture with overcontoured composite. This approach cannot prevent pulp infection, but eliminates pain and discomfort for the patient. Further treatment can be postponed for a few days.

Table 2.2.1 Treatment options for crown-root fractures (modified after Weiger et al., 2014).

Clinical situation	Options for restorative treatment
Only slightly subgingival defect, with reasonable access after placement of retraction cords, gingivectomy or surgical flap	**OPTION 1:** Restoration with reattachment of the coronal fragment, direct composite restoration or indirect restoration
Inaccessible defect due to deep subgingival/subosseous extension	**OPTION 2:** Restorative treatment of the accessible regions (mostly supragingival)
	OPTION 3: Surgical crown lengthening + restoration
	OPTION 4: Orthodontic extrusion of the apical fragment (forced eruption) + restoration
	OPTION 5: Surgical extrusion (intra-alveolar transplantation) + restoration
Unrestorable tooth due to deep subosseous extension or additional fractures of the root	**OPTION 6:** Extraction

Definite Treatment for Crown-Root Fractures

The definite treatment for crown-root fractures is difficult, requiring consideration of periodontal, endodontic and, in particular, restorative aspects. Treatment options for different clinical situations are presented in Table 2.2.1.

If the subgingival defect margins can be accessed after placement of retraction cords, gingivectomy or fracture-site exposure by the preparation of a surgical flap, the restoration is comparable to the restoration of supragingival crown fractures and includes fragment reattachment, direct composite restoration and indirect restoration.

For fragment reattachments performed meticulously after preparation of a mucoperiostal access flap, excellent results during the first 2 years have been reported (Eichelsbacher et al., 2009). However, long-term results are still needed.

If a composite restoration is the treatment of choice, a two-step procedure with elevation of the margin in the first step can combine good marginal adaptation with an optimal anatomic reconstruction of the crown (Frese et al., 2014).

If the defect margin is very difficult to access and the fractured surface shows a steep inclination, a supragingival restoration that covers only the accessible regions may be a reasonable compromise over more invasive methods. However, some fractured subgingival dentine areas remain unsealed with this approach.

In most cases, adequate treatment depends on good access to the defect site. This can be achieved by performing surgical crown lengthening, provided that aesthetics are not compromised. Selective reduction of the alveolar bone on the palatal site makes the defect accessible for restorative treatment and reestablishes the biological width. However, the benefits should be balanced against the drawbacks. In particular, the bone loss associated with this approach may result in a more unfavourable situation for any future implant placement if the treatment fails.

Extrusion of the remaining root is another alternative; one which can be carried out either orthodontically (forced eruption) (Faria et al., 2015) or surgically (intra-alveolar transplantation) (Das and Muthu, 2013). With surgical extrusion, the root is extracted, replanted after 180° rotation and splinted in a position sited farther coronally (Figure 2.2.9a–d) (Krastl et al., 2011). A significant advantage of this method is that the

(a) (b) (c) (d)

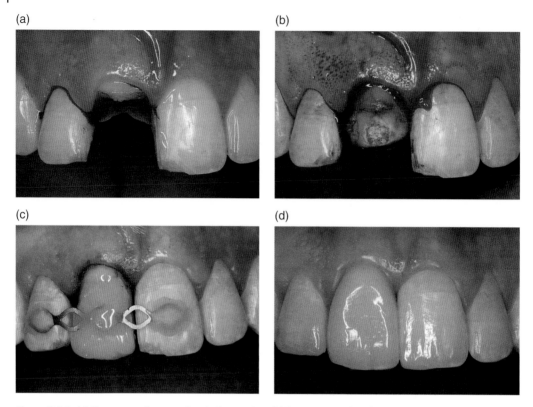

Figure 2.2.9 (a) Crown-root fracture. Surgical extrusion: (b) Extraction and replanting of the root after 180° rotation. (c) Splinting and provisional restoration. (d) Restoration with direct composite after periodontal healing for 2 months following extrusion.

inspection of the whole root surface can easily be performed, so that additional fractures are not overlooked. Provided that an atraumatic extraction technique is employed, there is little mechanical damage to the root cement layer. Periodontal healing (without ankylosis) can therefore be expected (Kelly et al., 2016). Clinical studies confirm the favourable prognosis of this method, with minimal adverse events (Elkhadem et al., 2014). Aesthetic rehabilitation includes all methods of restorative treatment from composite build-ups to the placement of crowns, depending on the residual tooth substance.

Although the treatment of crown-root fractures is one of the most technically demanding procedures in dental traumatology, and in many cases is considered a long-term temporary restoration, even tooth conservation up to the age at which implants can be placed is accepted as success.

Management of Crown and Crown-Root Fractures of Deciduous Teeth

In deciduous teeth, fractures occur less often compared to dislocation injuries. In cases of minor crown fracture, sharp edges are smoothened. If the dentine is involved, restorations with resin composites can be performed (Figure 2.2.10). In cases of crown-root fracture, restorative treatment may be considered if only a small part of the root is involved. In most clinical situations, however, deciduous teeth with crown-root fracture are deemed nonretainable and should be extracted (Figure 2.2.11) (Malmgren et al., 2012).

Besides all medical considerations, in young children the therapy mainly depends on the amenability of the child to dental treatment.

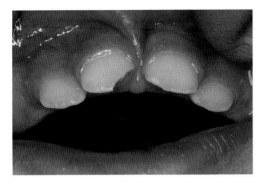

Figure 2.2.10 Crown fractures of upper central primary incisors in a 1.5-year-old boy

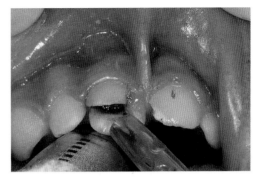

Figure 2.2.11 Crown-root fracture of a primary incisor. Extraction is necessary.

References

Bernades Kde, O., Hilgert, L. A., Ribeiro, A. P., Garcia, F. C., Pereira, P. N. 2014. The influence of hemostatic agents on dentin and enamel surfaces and dental bonding: a systematic review. *Journal of the American Dental Association*, **145**(11), 1120–8.

Borum, M. K., Andreasen, J. O. 2001. Therapeutic and economic implications of traumatic dental injuries in denmark: an estimate based on 7549 patients treated at a major trauma centre. *International Journal of Paediatric Dentistry*, **11**(4), 249–58.

Das, B., Muthu, M. S. 2013. Surgical extrusion as a treatment option for crown-root fracture in permanent anterior teeth: a systematic review. *Dental Traumatology*, **29**(6), 423–31.

Dietschi, D., Ardu, S., Krejci, I. 2006. A new shading concept based on natural tooth color applied to direct composite restorations. *Quintessence International*, **37**(2), 91–102.

Eichelsbacher, F., Denner, W., Klaiber, B., Schlagenhauf, U. 2009. Periodontal status of teeth with crown-root fractures: results two years after adhesive fragment reattachment. *Journal of Clinical Periodontology*, **36**(10), 905–11.

Elkhadem, A., Mickan, S., Richards, D. 2014. Adverse events of surgical extrusion in treatment for crown-root and cervical root fractures: a systematic review of case series/reports. *Dental Traumatology*, **30**(1), 1–14.

Faria, L. P., Almeida, M. M., Amaral, M. F., Pellizzer, E. P., Okamoto, R., Mendonca, M. R. 2015. Orthodontic extrusion as treatment option for crown-root fracture: literature review with systematic criteria. *Journal of Contemporary Dental Practice*, **16**(9), 758–62.

Farik, B., Munksgaard, E. C., Andreasen, J. O., Kreiborg, S. 1999. Drying and rewetting anterior crown fragments prior to bonding. *Endodontics & Dental Traumatology*, **15**(3), 113–16.

Frese, C., Wolff, D., Staehle, H. J. 2014. Proximal box elevation with resin composite and the dogma of biological width: clinical r2-technique and critical review. *Operative Dentistry*, **39**(1), 22–31.

Kelly, R. D., Addison, O., Tomson, P. L., Krastl, G., Dietrich, T. 2016. Atraumatic surgical extrusion to improve tooth restorability: a clinical report. *Journal of Prosthetic Dentistry*, **115**(6), 649–53.

Krastl, G., Weiger, R. 2014. Vital pulp therapy after trauma. *Endodontic Practice Today*, **8**(4), 293–300.

Krastl, G., Filippi, A., Zitzmann, N. U., Walter, C., Weiger, R. 2011. Current aspects of restoring traumatically fractured teeth. *European Journal of Esthetic Dentistry*, **6**(2), 124–41.

Malmgren, B., Andreasen, J. O., Flores, M.T., Robertson, A., DiAngelis, A. J., Andersson, L., et al. 2012. International association of dental traumatology guidelines for the management of traumatic dental injuries: 3. Injuries in the primary dentition. *Dental Traumatology*, **28**(3), 174–82.

Olsburgh, S., Jacoby, T., Krejci, I. 2002. Crown fractures in the permanent dentition: pulpal and restorative considerations. *Dental Traumatology*, **18**(3), 103–15.

Poubel, D. L. N., Almeida, J. C. F., Dias Ribeiro, A. P., Maia, G. B., Martinez, J. M. G., Garcia, F. C. P. 2017. Effect of dehydration and rehydration intervals on fracture resistance of reattached tooth fragments using a multimode adhesive. *Dental Traumatology*, **33**(6), 451–7.

Ravn, J. J. 1981. Follow-up study of permanent incisors with enamel cracks as result of an acute trauma. *Scandinavian Journal of Dental Research*, **89**(2), 117–23.

Robertson, A., Andreasen, F. M., Andreasen, J. O., Noren, J. G. 2000. Long-term prognosis of crown-fractured permanent incisors. The effect of stage of root development and associated luxation injury. *International Journal of Paediatric Dentistry*, **10**(3), 191–9.

Sharmin, D. D., Thomas, E. 2013. Evaluation of the effect of storage medium on fragment reattachment. *Dental Traumatology*, **29**(2), 99–102.

Shirani, F., Sakhaei Manesh, V., Malekipour, M. R. 2013. Preservation of coronal tooth fragments prior to reattachment. *Australian Dental Journal*, **58**(3), 321–5.

Vanini, L., Mangani, F. M. 2001. Determination and communication of color using the five color dimensions of teeth. *Practical Procedures & Aesthetic Dentistry*, **13**(1), 19–26, quiz 28.

Weiger R, Krastl G, Filippi A, Lienert N. 2014. AcciDent (App for iOS and Android).

Yilmaz, Y., Guler, C., Sahin, H., Eyuboglu, O. 2010. Evaluation of tooth-fragment reattachment: a clinical and laboratory study. *Dental Traumatology*, **26**(4), 308–14.

2.3

Management of Root Fractures

Dan-Krister Rechenberg

Clinic of Preventive Dentistry, Periodontology and Cariology, Center of Dental Medicine, University of Zurich, Zurich, Switzerland

Introduction

Traumatic dental injury (TDI) describes injury to teeth and other tissues of the oral cavity (such as the gums, periodontium and alveolar bone) and their adjacent soft tissues (lips, tongue and cheek). The main reasons for TDI are accidents happening at sports or play or in traffic, which by definition occur unexpectedly (Skaare and Jacobsen, 2003). They are prevalent in all age groups and constitute approximately 5% of all (non-oral) injuries (Petersson et al., 1997), although they occur most frequently during childhood and adolescence (Bücher et al., 2013a). Depending on the impact (force, vector) and the stage of tooth/root development, TDIs can cause different forms of injury, including crown fractures, luxation, avulsion and root fractures. Root fractures, however, are rare, being present in only 8% of TDI cases (Andreasen et al., 2004a, 2007). Because of the protrusion and therefore exposed position, maxillary permanent incisors are most often involved (Andreasen, 1970). In contrast, deciduous teeth and teeth without finished root development are rarely affected (Majorana et al., 2002). The sponge-like bone structure surrounding deciduous teeth is known to be pliable and provides reduced periodontal support, much like permanent teeth without finished root development (see Chapter 1.1). Hence, such teeth tend to luxate or avulse during TDI (Andreasen and Hjorting-Hansen, 1967; McTigue, 2009). The biological principles of a root fracture in deciduous teeth are not very different from those in permanent teeth. Consequently, they will be dealt with together in this chapter, whilst relevant differences will be presented separately.

Biological Considerations

If an injured tooth suffers a root fracture, different tissues are involved: the root itself, the supporting periodontium (periodontal ligament (PDL), cementum and alveolar bone), the pulp and gingival soft tissues (Figure 2.3.1). A TDI may produce an incomplete root fracture, complete root fracture or multiple complete root fractures. The root fracture itself can extend in different angulations and may be located at any level of the root. However, root fractures occur most commonly at the mid-root level and are less common at the cervical and apical levels (Hovland, 1992; Calişkan and Pehlivan, 1996; Andreasen et al., 2012b). The biological conditions and the treatment of supracrestal root fracture are comparable to those of crown-root fractures (Heithersay

Management of Dental Emergencies in Children and Adolescents, First Edition.
Edited by Klaus W. Neuhaus and Adrian Lussi.
© 2019 John Wiley & Sons Ltd. Published 2019 by John Wiley & Sons Ltd.
Companion website: www.wiley.com/go/neuhaus/dental_emergencies

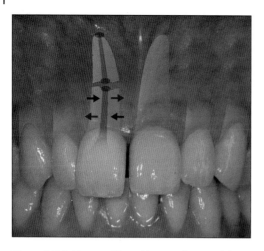

Figure 2.3.1 Tissues affected by root fracture injury: pulp (purple) and periodontium (green). Periodontal tearing is indicated by blue arrows, whilst the compression site is indicated by red arrows.

and Moule, 1982) (see Chapter 2.2). A complete root fracture separates the root into two fragments: an apical and a coronal. Whilst the apical fragment commonly remains uninjured and in its natural position, the coronal fragment is frequently displaced from its alveolar bone socket and is therefore comparable to a (lateral) luxation injury. The impact provokes stretching/tearing of the periodontium on some parts of the coronal root surface, and compression at the opposing parts (Figure 2.3.1). The tissue damage will inevitably result in local inflammation. However, if the coronal fragment is repositioned close to its natural position in a timely fashion and kept in place, the inflammation will ultimately lead towards periodontal repair. During reorganisation, the periodontal tissues may undergo different forms of resorption. Histologically and radiographically, external and internal surface resorption have been described, as well as internal tunneling resorption and transient apical breakdown (Andreasen and Andreasen, 1988). External and internal surface resorption refers to the resorptive blunting of the external (proximal) or internal (central) root fracture edges. Internal tunnelling resorption is described as a burrowing behind the pre-dentin layer along the root canal walls affecting

the coronal fragment, and transient apical breakdown as a temporary resorption of the periodontium from the apical fragment (Andreasen, 2003). Collectively, these processes aim to remove damaged periodontal tissue and replace it through mineralisation. They occur predominantly in the first 2 years after root fracture and can eventually be detected radiographically (Andreasen and Andreasen, 1988). Clinically, they are of low concern (for more detail, see Andreasen and Andreasen, 1988 and Andreasen, 2003). However, they should not be confused with pathological events such as external replacement resorption, inflammatory root resorption or periodontitis caused by root canal infection (Andreasen et al., 2007).

The pulp is another important tissue affected by root fracture (Figure 2.3.1). It must be remembered that TDIs are most prevalent in children and adolescents, and maxillary incisors represent the teeth most affected (Andreasen, 1970; Bücher et al., 2013a). These are mostly free of caries and restorations (Steiner et al., 2010). Consequently, in most cases of root fracture, the pulp is in a perfectly healthy, immunocompetent condition when the injury occurs. The pulpal trauma can range from stretching and tearing of the neurovascular bundle to a total rupture of the nerve-vessel bundle. Even if the pulp ruptures because of a severely dislocated coronal root fragment, the apical fragment usually maintains its vitality since it is not affected by displacement and receives an unimpeded neurovascular supply (Andreasen et al., 2004a, 2004b). The neurovascular supply of the coronal fragment, on the other hand, may be either compromised or entirely interrupted. In the latter case, the coronal aspect of the pulp initially becomes ischaemic and ultimately develops a coagulation necrosis (Andreasen, 1988). If the displaced coronal fragment receives appropriate treatment, including repositioning and flexible splinting, the chances for pulpal revascularisation – and consequently the maintenance of pulpal vitality – are fairly good (Andreasen et al., 1989). Preserving pulpal vitality is desired, since a vital pulp provides immunocompetence and facilitates continuing root development/ hard tissue formation.

Depending on the periodontal and pulpal damage, as well as patient- and treatment-related factors, a root fracture may heal in either a desirable or an undesirable fashion (Heithersay and Kahler, 2013). One factor of utmost importance to the outcome is the potential access of microorganisms to the injury site. Microorganisms from the oral environment may gain direct access through a breach in the tissues (Figure 2.3.2). If the root fracture is located more towards the cervical root level, the risk of microbial infection increases significantly (Welbury et al., 2002; Andreasen et al., 2012b). In case of concomitant coagulation necrosis of the coronal fragment, the pulpal space may become infected and cause (apical) perio-dontitis (Nair, 1997). If there is no access for microorganisms (i.e. aseptic trauma), heal-ing may occur unaffected by infection, even if the pulp of the coronal fragment has become necrotic (Bender and Freedland, 1983). However, over time, the chances increase that microorganisms will access the necrotic pulp space through cracks in the enamel and dentin, or possibly through anachoresis (Figure 2.3.2) (Grossman, 1967;

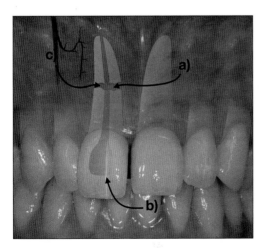

Figure 2.3.2 Routes for microbial infection of the root fracture injury site: (a) through a trauma-caused breach in the tissues, connecting the injury site with the oral environment; (b) through enamel/dentin cracks; (c) through anachoresis, i.e. via bloodborne microbial infection.

Love, 1996). (The latter route is mentioned here for the sake of completeness, and is not supported by much evidence.)

Regardless of the presence of microor-ganisms, pulpal and periodontal healing at the root fracture site may be synergistic or competitive. Depending on which of the tissues dominates the healing process, differ-ent outcomes are described histologically (Kronfeld, 1935; Hammer, 1939; Schindler, 1941; Andreasen and Hjorting-Hansen, 1967; Andreasen and Andreasen, 1988):

1) **Hard tissue healing.** This occurs when the fracture space between the apical and the coronal fragments is solidly bridged by hard tissue deposition. Pulpal odonto-blasts and periodontal cells serve as the source for a mixed pulpoperiodontal tis-sue (dentin, osteodentin and cementum). Remaining pulpal vitality is a prerequisite for this most favourable type of healing.

2) **Connective tissue healing.** Periodontally derived connective tissue occupies the fracture gap between the fragments. It is assumed that the pulp must have suffered moderate damage in order to develop this healing pattern, so periodontal (instead of pulpal) cells dominate the healing process. Ultimately, this results in an organised, cementum-covered PDL, separating the two fragments.

3) **Interposition of granulation tissue.** If microorganisms have access to the root fracture, infection of the coronal and api-cal aspect of the pulp may occur. This sit-uation can be viewed as an (ordinary) necrotic root canal infection. Proteolytic enzymes and bacterial byproducts cause soft tissue breakdown and bone resorp-tion between the fragments. Finally, inflamed granulation tissue interposes the root fracture gap. Consequently, this third outcome is not healing, but can still represent a steady-state situation without clinical signs or symptoms.

Having understood the biological foundation of the tissues involved, the diagnosis and therapy of teeth affected by root fracture become apparent: treatment should aim to create an environment that (i) enables undisturbed periodontal healing and (ii) facilitates the maintenance of pulpal vitality.

Diagnostics of Root Fractures

The primary diagnostic goal is to recognise and distinguish a root fracture from other TDIs (e.g. crown-root fracture, intrusion, luxation injuries). All diagnostic test results should be compared to those obtained with non-affected adjacent or contralateral teeth. In order to avoid missing any potentially relevant diagnostic information, a systematic approach is recommended; this has been shown to be beneficial in the management of TDI (Bücher et al., 2013b).

Inspection

In contrast to crown fracture and crown-root fracture, root fracture cannot be confirmed by direct visual inspection. The position of a root-fractured coronal fragment may be unaltered, intruded, extruded or laterally luxated. Patients may complain about occlusal interference. A coronal fragment that is slightly extruded and displaced towards the lingual or palatal aspect is most common (Feiglin, 1995). However, based on clinical examination alone, it is not possible to differentiate a root fracture from a (lateral) luxation injury. Discolouration of the tooth crown after root fracture injury is infrequent (Malmgren and Hubel, 2012). Nevertheless, a reddish discolouration may rarely evolve over the short term (2–3 days) – a so-called transient coronal discolouration – caused by extravasation of blood into the dentinal tubules (Kronfeld, 1935). As the name indicates, this is a temporary phenomenon that in most cases disappears within weeks or months (Malmgren and Hubel, 2012).

Mobility

The coronal fragment may show increased mobility due to periodontal compression. This can be tested by gentle palpation of the tooth crown. An increased mobility of multiple teeth in unison may be suggestive of alveolar process fracture. Sometimes, the coronal fragment shows no mobility at all during palpation. This is indicative of intrusion and may be confirmed by percussion (see later).

Probing Depth

Forceful periodontal probing of traumatised teeth (e.g. to confirm a potential fracture line) is not advisable, since it may cause additional trauma to the periodontium.

Percussion

Gentle tapping and percussion on the tooth crown may elicit some form of pain or periodontal discomfort. This suggests periodontal involvement in the injury. A nonmobile, intruded tooth fragment may provoke a characteristic high-pitched, metallic sound during percussion, similar to that of an ankylotic tooth.

Pulpal Sensitivity Tests

Pulpal sensitivity tests are highly subjective (i.e. depending on the patient's response), and in general are not a perfect measure (Dummer et al., 1980). The most common sensitivity tests involve the application of a thermal stimulus (cold test) or electric current (electric pulp test, EPT) to the tooth. These tests aim to evoke a neurogenic response by direct (EPT) or indirect (thermal) stimulation of pulpal nerve fibres. Hence, a positive test response indirectly suggests neurogenic activity and is highly indicative of vital pulpal conditions (Seltzer et al., 1965; Villa-Chavez et al., 2013). In contrast, the significance of a negative test result is limited (Seltzer et al., 1965; Gazelius et al., 1988; Andreasen et al., 1989). However, a nonresponsive pulp is a common finding after traumatic root fracture, perhaps due to some form of injury-related, temporary neuronal degeneration (Andreasen, 1989; Ozcelik et al., 2000). It is known that the neurovascular supply needs time to recover, and that it can take the pulp several months to regain sensory excitability (Gazelius et al.,

1988). Furthermore, it should be noted that EPT in permanent but developing teeth with wide-open apices may lack a positive response (Fulling and Andreasen, 1976). This observation is attributed to incomplete innervation until the final stages of root development (Bernick, 1964). For these reasons, a negative pulpal sensitivity response in teeth with root fracture must be interpreted with care. With respect to pulpal sensitivity tests in deciduous teeth, it must be mentioned that they are known to be difficult to perform and even more difficult to interpret (Gopikrishna et al., 2009).

Radiographic Imaging

The presence of a root fracture can only be confirmed (or excluded) radiographically (Wilson, 1995). The radiographic appearance on a periapical radiograph is described as a radiolucent line separating the coronal from the apical fragment, or even separating multiple fragments, and as a discontinuity of the PDL space (Figure 2.3.3a) (Whaites and

Drage, 2013). If the radiolucent line continues in the same direction through several tooth roots, this is suggestive of an alveolar process fracture. Both the plane of the root fracture (i.e. angulation) and the direction of the central beam have an influence on the radiographic projection. If the central beam does not project in parallel through the fracture plane, the root fracture may remain covered on a radiograph due to superimposition. To compensate for this shortcoming, it is advisable to use multiple radiographs at different vertical and horizontal angulations (Kullman and Al Sane, 2012). Currently, there is no final agreement on the number of radiographs that are needed to confirm or exclude a root fracture. However, four (one orthogonal exposure, one steep occlusal exposure and one mesial and one distal eccentric exposure) are recommended by a panel of experts, and have shown to be more reliable than one, two or three (Wenzel and Kirkevang, 2005; Flores et al., 2007; Diangelis et al. 2012).

(a)

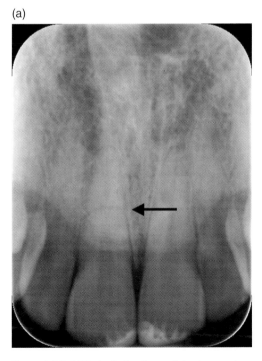

(b)

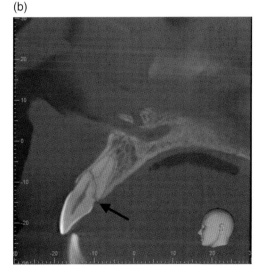

Figure 2.3.3 (a) Periapical radiograph (orthogonal exposure) suggesting a complete root fracture at the mid-root level of the right permanent central incisor (black arrow). (b) More accurate depiction of the fracture plane in the same right central incisor by CBCT revealing cervical involvement (black arrow). Note: neither the periapical radiograph (a), nor the CBCT (b) reveal radiographic signs for inflammation. Hence treatment is not indicated.

Cone-beam computed tomography (CBCT) is superior to conventional radiography in the detection of root fracture (Cohenca et al., 2007), and is recommended by dental societies for this indication (Figure 2.3.3b) (Special Committee, 2015). For deciduous teeth in particular, it might be the imaging modality of choice, because their roots are often masked by permanent teeth (Flores, 2002). However, CBCT imaging requires a significantly higher radiation dose compared to conventional radiography (Pauwels et al., 2012). Therefore, especially in children and adolescents, an individual dose risk assessment must be made (for further information, see Chapter 1.5).

Treatment and Prognosis of Root Fractures

Emergency treatment of a root fracture may require acute priority; that is, treatment should be performed within a few hours after injury (Andreasen et al., 2002). Delayed treatment can lead to impaired periodontal healing and therefore undesired outcomes. With respect to injured pulpal and periodontal tissues, the coronal and apical fragment of a fractured root can be viewed as separate entities from a treatment perspective. In the majority of cases, treatment is only necessary for the coronal fragment. The most common therapy involves repositioning and temporary immobilisation of the displaced coronal fragment. It is important to understand that all manipulations subsequent to a root fracture represent some form of additional trauma to the tissues involved. Consequently, it is of ultimate importance to perform these procedures as gently as possible (Andreasen et al., 2006).

General Treatment Considerations

Rinsing the soft-tissue wound with water to remove debris is advocated (Valente et al., 2003).

Table 2.3.1 Factors related to favourable pulpal (PU) and periodontal (PE) healing after root fracture injury.

Patient-related factors	Selected studies demonstrating a favourable effect
Incomplete root development with open apical foramen (PU/PE)	Zachrisson and Jacobsen (1975), Cvek et al. (2001), Andreasen et al. (2004b)
No communication with oral environment (PU/PE)	Welbury et al. (2002)
Positive pulpal sensitivity on testing immediately after root fracture injury (PU)	Andreasen et al. (1989), Cvek et al. (2002)
Root fracture line located more towards the apical than the cervical root level (PU/PE)	Cvek et al. (2008), Welbury et al. (2002), Andreasen et al. (2012b)
Small distance between fragments (PU)	Andreasen et al. (2004b), Cvek et al. (2001)
Physiologic mobility of the coronal fragment (PE)	Andreasen et al. (1989, 2004b)
No or slight displacement of the coronal fragment (PE)	Zachrisson and Jacobsen (1975), Andreasen et al. (1989), Cvek et al. (2001)
Treatment-related factors	
Gentle application of a semi-rigid splint for a (short) period of approx. 4 weeks (PE)[a]	Andreasen et al. (1989, 2004a)
Repositioning of the coronal fragment close to the natural position (PU/PE)	Andreasen et al. (2004a), Cvek et al. (2002)
Root canal treatment confined to the pulp-necrotic coronal fragment only (PU)	Jacobsen and Kerekes (1980), Cvek et al. (2004)
Use of MTA for an apexification procedure, rather than calcium hydroxide (PU)	Damle et al. (2012)

[a] Alveolar process fracture, or root fractures located towards the cervical root aspect with the coronal fragment exhibiting increased mobility, may require prolonged splinting (see text).
MTA, mineral trioxide aggregate.

Moreover, it may be necessary to remove dislodged objects from the soft tissue to prevent local inflammation and to suture the wound. If pain is present, it should be managed by reasonable medication (see Chapter 1.4). If the patient's general condition does not require antibiotic prophylaxis, a routine prescription for inflammatory prophylaxis after root fracture injury is not supported by evidence and therefore not recommended (Andreasen et al., 1989, 2004b). For further reading, see Chapter 1.3.

Treatment of Periodontium

Root Fractures *Without Displacement* of the Coronal Fragment

In root fractures without displacement of the coronal fragment (i.e. a concussed or subluxated fragment), the fracture line is usually located at the apical level, or towards the mid-root. Hence, the periodontium provides sufficient support for the coronal fragment, showing almost normal tooth mobility. In case of mild to moderate injury, such fractures may even remain unnoticed by the patient and the clinician (Molina et al., 2008). Later, they can accidentally become evident during routine radiographic examination. Fortunately, root fractures without displacement and increased mobility rarely require any form of therapy (Oztan and Sonat, 2001; Cvek et al., 2002). In the case of slight occlusal interference, minor adjustment to the antagonist and a soft diet for up to 2 weeks are advisable (Andreasen et al., 2007).

As indicated in Table 2.3.1, the overall prognosis of root fractures depends upon certain patient- and treatment-related factors. The prognosis of those without displacement of the coronal fragment is most favourable: the majority of cases develop hard-tissue healing and maintain pulpal vitality (Andreasen et al., 1989, 2004a; Welbury et al., 2002).

Root Fractures *With Displacement* of the Coronal Fragment

A fractured and displaced coronal fragment may be intruded, extruded or laterally luxated. Moreover, the fragment may be clocked in its position or may show increased mobility on palpation. The fracture line is usually located at the mid-root level, or towards the cervical aspect of the root (Hovland, 1992; Calişkan and Pehlivan, 1996; Welbury et al., 2002). Whatever the displacement, the treatment of a displaced coronal fragment always aims to reposition it to relieve periodontal and pulpal compression/stretching (Figure 2.3.1). Unless there is an alveolar process involvement, the repositioning of a root fracture rarely requires the injection of a local anaesthetic. Subsequently, the coronal fragment should be stabilised using a semi-rigid splint. Semi-rigid orthodontic wires and fibre composites are appropriate materials, and can be bonded to the coronal fragment and the adjacent teeth. Splinting for 4 weeks has been shown to provide sufficient time for the periodontium to heal (Cvek et al., 2001). However, if the fracture line is located towards the cervical aspect of the root, and the fragment exhibits great mobility, a prolonged splinting time of up to 4 months may be necessary to enable stability (Cvek et al., 2002). Treatment alternatives, including the removal of the coronal fragment, should also be considered (see also Chapter 2.2) (Heithersay, 1973; Heithersay and Moule, 1982). In any case of splinting, the patient should receive appropriate oral hygiene instructions. If there is no microbial infection, the majority of root fractures with displaced crowns develop connective tissue healing at the fracture site (Cvek et al., 2001; Andreasen et al., 2004a). This healing pattern is less ideal, but should be considered as acceptable.

Treatment of the Pulp

Revascularisation of the Coronal Fragment

The pulp of a coronal fragment survives root fracture injury in the vast majority (about 60–80%) of cases (Zachrisson and Jacobsen, 1975; Andreasen, 1989; Calişkan and Pehlivan, 1996). It must be reiterated that a negative response to pulpal sensitivity tests immediately after root fracture injury is a common finding and does not represent an indication for root canal treatment without further evidence of pulpal necrosis. No treatment (i.e. watchful waiting) is still a form of treatment. In case of doubt, it is more advisable to monitor the situation closely than to initiate treatment (Jacobsen and Kerekes, 1980). A frequently observed reaction of a traumatised but vital pulp indicates pulp canal obliteration (Lundberg and Cvek, 1980). The pulp continuously deposes hard tissue (dentin) along the pulp canal walls, leading to a narrowing of the entire pulpal space (Andreasen, 1989). In case of root fracture, pulp canal obliteration is usually confined to the apical fragment, but in rare cases the coronal fragment may be affected too (Saroglu and Sonmez, 2008). Pulp canal obliteration should be considered a vital pulp's reaction to trauma (Andreasen, 1989). Affected teeth rarely develop pulpal necrosis (Robertson et al., 1996). Positive prognostic predictors for pulpal survival are given in Table 2.3.1.

Pulpal Necrosis of the Coronal Fragment

Signs and symptoms for pulpal necrosis after root fracture are an enduring negative response to pulpal sensitivity testing, presence of (pulpal) pain, pain on percussion, oedema, sinus tract, progressive blackish discolouration of the tooth crown, radiographic evidence for bone resorption and arrested root development. Mostly, only the coronal fragment develops pulpal necrosis (Andreasen and Hjorting-Hansen, 1967). In these cases *root canal treatment should be confined to this fragment only*. It should be noted that the apical terminus of a root-fractured coronal fragment is wide open. Therefore, an apexification procedure should be performed before obturation to avoid excessive overfill. Traditionally, this was done by long-term medication with calcium hydroxide (Cvek, 1974; Cvek et al., 2004), but this should be considered as outdated (Duggal et al., 2017) Because of their favourable characteristics and ease of use (e.g. reduced number of visits), hydraulic calcium silicate cements such as mineral trioxide aggregate (MTA), are advocated for use in apexification procedures (Damle et al., 2012; Duggal et al., 2017). However, it must be borne in mind that some

(but not all) MTA formulations are known to irreversibly stain teeth (Jacobovitz and De Pontes Lima, 2009). After sufficient root canal treatment of the necrotic coronal fragment, the prognosis of root-fractured teeth may be considered promising (Cvek et al., 2008).

Pulpal Necrosis of the Apical Fragment

In extremely rare cases of root fracture, the apical fragment may develop pulpal necrosis (Cvek et al., 2002). The tentative diagnosis can only be confirmed radiographically, since pulpal sensitivity tests are not possible there. It has been shown that conventional root canal treatment cannot adequately seal off the root canal of the apical fragment (Cvek et al., 2004). Hence, combining endodontic treatment of the coronal fragment with the surgical removal of the infected apical fragment is indicated in these rare cases (Cvek et al., 2004).

Treatment of Root Fractures in Deciduous Teeth

Root fracture in deciduous teeth is rare (Majorana et al., 2002). The aim of treatment is similar to that in permanent teeth: to facilitate periodontal and pulpal healing. However, intervention should be reduced to the minimum. Moreover, therapeutic options may be limited in deciduous teeth due to noncompliant behaviour (Veire et al., 2012). If the coronal fragment is merely slightly displaced, it may be left untreated and will eventually realign spontaneously. The apical fragment will then resorb physiologically. Because of the anterior open bite, occlusive disturbances are rare. More severely displaced coronal fragments may be actively repositioned; however, extra care must be taken not to damage the succeeding tooth germ (Andreasen et al., 1971; Lenzi et al., 2015). The application of a bonded splint is usually not necessary. An exception occurs with an accompanying alveolar process fracture, which should be splinted for 2–3 weeks (Malmgren et al., 2012). If the coronal fragment displays signs and symptoms of pulpal necrosis, it should be removed instantly to avoid potential damage to the permanent successor. Again, the apical fragment does not require therapy and will resorb physiologically. Unless there are additional complicating factors (e.g. a recurring trauma), the prognosis of root fractures in the deciduous dentition is comparable to that in permanent teeth (Wilson, 1995).

Recall

The patient should be recalled for clinical and radiographic examination at 1-, 1.5-, 4-, 6- and 12-month intervals, and again after 5 years (Diangelis et al., 2012). If possible, the splint should be removed after 4 weeks. The examinations should include the diagnostic procedures previously described and should aim to exclude periodontal inflammation and pulpal necrosis. Typically, signs of pulpal necrosis appear within the first 3 months after injury

(Jacobsen and Kerekes, 1980; Andreasen, 1989). In addition, the emerging outcome may be evaluated. Hard-tissue healing may be assessed radiographically by a vanishing fracture gap and a positive response to pulpal sensitivity testing along with physiologic tooth mobility. In case of connective tissue healing, the fracture gap persists radiographically and blunting of the peripheral fracture edges can be observed (Andreasen and Andreasen, 1988). Frequently, increased tooth mobility may persist for these teeth (Zachrisson and Jacobsen, 1975; Cvek et al., 2002). However, over time, this effect has been shown to decline (Andreasen et al., 2012a). In contrast, interposition with granulation tissue is characterised by radiographic loss of the lamina dura, advancing rarefaction and widening of the fracture line, along with clinical signs and symptoms of pulpal necrosis.

References

Special Committee to Revise the Joint AAE/ AAOMR Position Statement on Use of CBCT in Endodontics. 2015. AAE and AAOMR Joint Position Statement: use of cone beam computed tomography in endodontics 2015 update. *Journal of Endodontics*, **41**(9), 1393–6.

Andreasen, J. O. 1970. Etiology and pathogenesis of traumatic dental injuries. A clinical study of 1298 cases. *Scandinavian Journal of Dental Research*, **78**(4), 329–42.

Andreasen, F. M. 1988. Histological and bacteriological study of pulps extirpated after luxation injuries. *Endodontics & Dental Traumatology*, **4**, 170–81.

Andreasen, F. M. 1989. Pulpal healing after luxation injuries and root fracture in the permanent dentition. *Endodontics & Dental Traumatology*, **5**(3), 111–31.

Andreasen, F. M. 2003. Transient root resorption after dental trauma: the clinician's dilemma. *Journal of Esthetics and Restorative Dentistry*, **15**(2), 80–92.

Andreasen, F. M., Andreasen, J. O. 1988. Resorption and mineralization processes

following root fracture of permanent incisors. *Endodontics & Dental Traumatology*, **4**(5), 202–14.

Andreasen, J. O., Hjorting-Hansen, E. 1967. Intraalveolar root fractures: radiographic and histologic study of 50 cases. *Journal of Oral Surgery*, **25**(5), 414–26.

Andreasen, J. O., Sundstrom, B., Ravn, J. J. 1971. The effect of traumatic injuries to primary teeth on their permanent successors. I. A clinical and histologic study of 117 injured permanent teeth. *Scandinavian Journal of Dental Research*, **79**(4), 219–83.

Andreasen, F. M., Andreasen, J. O., Bayer, T. 1989. Prognosis of root-fractured permanent incisors – prediction of healing modalities. *Endodontics & Dental Traumatology*, **5**(1), 11–22.

Andreasen, J. O., Andreasen, F. M., Skeie, A., Hjorting-Hansen, E., Schwartz, O. 2002. Effect of treatment delay upon pulp and periodontal healing of traumatic dental injuries – a review article. *Dental Traumatology*, **18**(3), 116–28.

Andreasen, J. O., Andreasen, F. M., Mejàre, I., Cvek, M. 2004a. Healing of 400 intra-alveolar root fractures. 1. Effect of pre-injury and injury factors such as sex, age, stage of root development, fracture type, location of fracture and severity of dislocation. *Dental Traumatology*, **20**(4), 192–202.

Andreasen, J. O., Andreasen, F. M., Mejàre, I., Cvek, M. 2004b. Healing of 400 intra-alveolar root fractures. 2. Effect of treatment factors such as treatment delay, repositioning, splinting type and period and antibiotics. *Dental Traumatology*, **20**(4), 203–11.

Andreasen, J. O., Bakland, L., Andreasen, F. M. 2006. Traumatic intrusion of permanent teeth. Part 3. A clinical study of the effect of treatment variables such as treatment delay, method of repositioning, type of splint, length of splinting and antibiotics on 140 teeth. *Dental Traumatology*, **22**(2), 99–111.

Andreasen, J. O., Andreasen, F. M., Andersson, L. 2007. Root fractures. In: Andreasen, J. O., Andreasen, F. M., Andersson, L. (eds). *Textbook and Color Atlas of Traumatic Injuries to the Teeth*. Oxford: Blackwell Munksgaard.

Andreasen, J. O., Ahrensburg, S., Tsilingaridis, G. 2012a. Tooth mobility changes subsequent to root fractures: a longitudinal clinical study of 44 permanent teeth. *Dental Traumatology*, **28**(5), 410–14.

Andreasen, J. O., Ahrensburg, S. S., Tsilingaridis, G. 2012b. Root fractures: the influence of type of healing and location of fracture on tooth survival rates – an analysis of 492 cases. *Dental Traumatology*, **28**(5), 404–9.

Bender, I. B., Freedland, J. B. 1983. Clinical considerations in the diagnosis and treatment of intra-alveolar root fractures. *Journal of the American Dental Association*, **107**(4), 595–600.

Bernick, S. 1964. Differences in nerve distribution between erupted and non-erupted human teeth. *Journal of Dental Research*, **43**, 406–11.

Bücher, K., Neumann, C., Hickel, R., Kühnisch, J. 2013a. Traumatic dental injuries at a German university clinic 2004–2008. *Dental Traumatology*, **29**(2), 127–33.

Bücher, K., Neumann, C., Thiering, E., Hickel, R., Kühnisch, J., International Association of

Dental Traumatology. 2013b. Complications and survival rates of teeth after dental trauma over a 5-year period. *Clinical Oral Investigations*, **17**(5), 1311–18.

Calişkan, M., Pehlivan, Y. 1996. Prognosis of root-fractured permanent incisors. *Endodontics and Dental Traumatology*, **12**(3), 129–36.

Cohenca, N., Simon, J. H., Roges, R., Morag, Y., Malfaz, J. M. 2007. Clinical indications for digital imaging in dento-alveolar trauma. Part 1: Traumatic injuries. *Dental Traumatology*, **23**(2), 95–104.

Cvek, M. 1974. Treatment of non-vital permanent incisors with calcium hydroxide. IV. Periodontal healing and closure of the root canal in the coronal fragment of teeth with intra-alveolar fracture and vital apical fragment. A follow-up. *Odontologisk Revy*, **25**(3), 239–46.

Cvek, M., Andreasen, J. O., Borum, M. 2001. Healing of 208 intra-alveolar root fractures in patients aged 7–17 years. *Dental Traumatology*, **17**(2), 53–62.

Cvek, M., Mejàre, I., Andreasen, J. O. 2002. Healing and prognosis of teeth with intra-alveolar fractures involving the cervical part of the root. *Dental Traumatology*, **18**(2), 57–65.

Cvek, M., Mejàre, I., Andreasen, J. O. 2004. Conservative endodontic treatment of teeth fractured in the middle or apical part of the root. *Dental Traumatology*, **20**(5), 261–9.

Cvek, M., Tsilingaridis, G., Andreasen, J. O. 2008. Survival of 534 incisors after intra-alveolar root fracture in patients aged 7-17 years. *Dental Traumatology*, **24**(4), 379–87.

Damle, S. G., Bhattal, H., Loomba, A. 2012. Apexification of anterior teeth: a comparative evaluation of mineral trioxide aggregate and calcium hydroxide paste. *Journal of Clinical Pediatric Dentistry*, **36**(3), 263–8.

Diangelis, A., Andreasen, J. O., Ebeleseder, K., Kenny, D., Trope, M., Sigurdsson, A., et al. 2012. International Association of Dental Traumatology guidelines for the management of traumatic dental injuries: 1. Fractures and luxations of permanent teeth. *Dental Traumatology*, **28**(1), 2–12.

Duggal, M., Tong, H. J., Al-Ansary, M., Twati, W., Day, P. F., Nazzal, H. 2017. Interventions for the endodontic management of non-vital traumatised immature permanent anterior teeth in children and adolescents: a systematic review of the evidence and guidelines of the European Academy of Paediatric Dentistry. *European Archives of Paediatric Dentistry*, **18**(3), 139–51.

Dummer, P. M., Hicks, R., Huws, D. 1980. Clinical signs and symptoms in pulp disease. *International Endodontic Journal*, **13**(1), 27–35.

Feiglin, B. 1995. Clinical management of transverse root fractures. *Dental Clinics of North America*, **39**(1), 53–78.

Flores, M. T. 2002. Traumatic injuries in the primary dentition. *Dental Traumatology*, **18**(6), 287–98.

Flores, M., Andersson, L., Andreasen, J. O., Bakland, L., Malmgren, B., Barnett, F., et al. 2007. Guidelines for the management of traumatic dental injuries. *I. Fractures and luxations of permanent teeth. Dental Traumatology*, **23**(2), 66–71.

Fulling, H. J., Andreasen, J. O. 1976. Influence of splints and temporary crowns upon electric and thermal pulp-testing procedures. *Scandinavian Journal of Dental Research*, **84**(5), 291–6.

Gazelius, B., Olgart, L., Edwall, B. 1988. Restored vitality in luxated teeth assessed by laser doppler flowmeter. *Endodontics & Dental Traumatology*, **4**(6), 265–8.

Gopikrishna, V., Pradeep, G., Venkateshbabu, N. 2009. Assessment of pulp vitality: a review. *International Journal of Paediatric Dentistry*, **19**(1), 3–15.

Grossman, L. I. 1967. Origin of microorganisms in traumatized, pulpless, sound teeth. *Journal of Dental Research*, **46**(3), 551–3.

Hammer, H. 1939. Die Heilungsvorgänge bei Wurzelbrücken. *Deutsche Zahn-, Mund- und Kieferheilkunde*, **6**, 273–87.

Heithersay, G. S. 1973. Combined endodontic-orthodontic treatment of transverse root fractures in the region of the alveolar crest. *Oral Surgery Oral Medicine Oral Pathology*, **36**(3), 404–15.

Heithersay, G. S., Kahler, B. 2013. Healing responses following transverse root fracture: a historical review and case reports showing

healing with (a) calcified tissue and (b) dense fibrous connective tissue. *Dental Traumatology*, **29**(4), 253–65.

Heithersay, G. S., Moule, A. J. 1982. Anterior subgingival fractures: a review of treatment alternatives. *Australian Dental Journal*, **27**(6), 368–76.

Hovland, E. J. 1992. Horizontal root fractures. Treatment and repair. *Dental Clinics of North America*, **36**(2), 509–25.

Jacobovitz, M., De Pontes Lima, R. K. 2009. The use of calcium hydroxide and mineral trioxide aggregate on apexification of a replanted tooth: a case report. *Dental Traumatology*, **25**(3), e32–6.

Jacobsen, I., Kerekes, K. 1980. Diagnosis and treatment of pulp necrosis in permanent anterior teeth with root fracture. *Scandinavian Journal of Dental Research*, **88**(5), 370–6.

Kronfeld, R. 1935. A case of tooth fracture, with special emphasis on tissue repair and adaptation following traumatic injury. *Journal of Dental Research*, **15**, 429–45.

Kullman, L., Al Sane, M. 2012. Guidelines for dental radiography immediately after a dento-alveolar trauma, a systematic literature review. *Dental Traumatology*, **28**(3), 193–9.

Lenzi, M., Alexandria, A., Ferreira, D., Maia, L. 2015. Does trauma in the primary dentition cause sequelae in permanent successors? A systematic review. *Dent Traumatol*, **31**(2), 79–88.

Love, R. M. 1996. Bacterial penetration of the root canal of intact incisor teeth after a simulated traumatic injury. *Endodontics & Dental Traumatology*, **12**(6), 289–93.

Lundberg, M., Cvek, M. 1980. A light microscopy study of pulps from traumatized permanent incisors with reduced pulpal lumen. *Acta Odontologica Scandinavica*, **38**(2), 89–94.

Majorana, A., Pasini, S., Bardellini, E., Keller, E. 2002. Clinical and epidemiological study of traumatic root fractures. *Dental Traumatology*, **18**(2), 77–80.

Malmgren B, Andreasen J. O., Flores M. T., Robertson A, DiAngelis A. J., Andersson L., et al. 2012. International Association of Dental Traumatology guidelines for the management of traumaticdental injuries: 3.

Injuries in the primary dentition. *Dent Traumatol*, **28**(3), 174–182.

Malmgren, B., Hubel, S. 2012. Transient discoloration of the coronal fragment in intra-alveolar root fractures. *Dental Traumatology*, **28**(3), 200–4.

McTigue, D. 2009. Managing injuries to the primary dentition. *Dental Clinics of North America*, **53**(4), 627–38, v.

Molina, J., Vann, W., McIntyre, J., Trope, M., Lee, J. 2008. Root fractures in children and adolescents: diagnostic considerations. *Dental Traumatology*, **24**(5), 503–9.

Nair, P. N. 1997. Apical periodontitis: a dynamic encounter between root canal infection and host response. *Periodontology 2000*, **13**, 121–48.

Ozcelik, B., Kuraner, T., Kendir, B., Asan, E. 2000. Histopathological evaluation of the dental pulps in crown-fractured teeth. *Journal of Endodontics*, **26**(5), 271–3.

Oztan, M., Sonat, B. 2001. Repair of untreated horizontal root fractures: two case reports. *Dental Traumatology*, **17**(5), 240–3.

Pauwels, R., Beinsberger, J., Collaert, B., Theodorakou, C., Rogers, J., Walker, A., et al. 2012. Effective dose range for dental cone beam computed tomography scanners. *European Journal of Radiology*, **81**(2), 267–71.

Petersson, E. E., Andersson, L., Sorensen, S. 1997. Traumatic oral vs non-oral injuries. *Swedish Dental Journal*, **21**(1–2), 55–68.

Robertson, A., Andreasen, F. M., Bergenholtz, G., Andreasen, J. O., Noren, J. G. 1996. Incidence of pulp necrosis subsequent to pulp canal obliteration from trauma of permanent incisors. *Journal of Endodontics*, **22**(10), 557–60.

Saroglu, I., Sonmez, H. 2008. Horizontal root fracture followed for 6 years. *Dental Traumatology*, **24**(1), 117–19.

Schindler, J. 1941. Kasuistischer Beitrag zum Problem der Heilung von Zahnwurzelfrakturen mit Erhaltung der Vitalität der Pulpa. *Schweizerische Monatsschrift für Zahnheilkunde*, **51**, 474–86.

Seltzer, S., Bender, I. B., Nazimov, H. 1965. Differential diagnosis of pulp conditions. *Oral Surgery Oral Medicine Oral Pathology*, **19**, 383–91.

Skaare, A. B., Jacobsen, I. 2003. Etiological factors related to dental injuries in Norwegians aged 7–18 years. *Dental Traumatology*, **19**(6), 304–8.

Steiner, M., Menghini, G., Marthaler, T. M., Imfeld, T. 2010. Changes in dental caries in Zurich school-children over a period of 45 years. *Schweizerische Monatsschrift für Zahnmedizin*, **120**(12), 1084–104.

Valente, J. H., Forti, R. J., Freundlich, L. F., Zandieh, S. O., Crain, E. F. 2003. Wound irrigation in children: saline solution or tap water? *Annals of Emergency Medicine*, **41**(5), 609–16.

Veire, A., Nichols, W., Urquiola, R., Oueis, H. 2012. Dental trauma: review of common dental injuries and their management in primary and permanent dentitions. *Journal of the Michigan Dental Association*, **94**(1), 41–5.

Villa-Chavez, C. E., Patino-Marin, N., Loyola-Rodriguez, J. P., Zavala-Alonso, N. V., Martinez-Castanon, G. A., Medina-Solis, C. E. 2013. Predictive values of thermal and electrical dental pulp tests: a clinical study. *Journal of Endodontics*, **39**(8), 965–9.

Welbury, R., Kinirons, M. J., Day, P., Humphreys, K., Gregg, T. A. 2002. Outcomes for root-fractured permanent incisors: a retrospective study. *Pediatric Dentistry*, **24**(2), 98–102.

Wenzel, A., Kirkevang, L. L. 2005. High resolution charge-coupled device sensor vs. medium resolution photostimulable phosphor plate digital receptors for detection of root fractures in vitro. *Dental Traumatology*, **21**(1), 32–6.

Whaites, E., Drage, N. 2013. Trauma to teeth and facial sceleton. In: Whaites, E., Drage, N. (eds). *Dental Radiography and Radiology*, 5th edn. London: Churchill Livingston.

Wilson, C. F. 1995. Management of trauma to primary and developing teeth. *Dental Clinics of North America*, **39**(1), 133–67.

Zachrisson, B., Jacobsen, I. 1975. Long-term prognosis of 66 permanent anterior teeth with root fracture. *Scandinavian Journal of Dental Research*, **83**(6), 345–54.

Unit 3

Management of Open Pulp in Permanent Teeth

3.1

Pulpotomy after Trauma

Hrvoje Jurić

Department of Paediatric and Preventive Dentistry, School of Dental Medicine, University of Zagreb, Zagreb, Croatia

Introduction

Dental trauma refers to trauma or injury to the teeth or periodontium (gums, periodontal ligament (PDL), alveolar bone), as well as nearby soft tissues such as the lips and tongue. The study of dental trauma is called dental traumatology (Andreasen and Andreasen, 2007). Dental trauma by definition is always a result of acute energy transmission directly or indirectly to the tooth and surrounding tissues, which can result in crown-root fracture, alveolar bone injuries and injuries of the soft tissue of the oral cavity. Children are prone to dental trauma, especially in young permanent dentition, mostly because of their excessive physical activity. There are numerous epidemiological studies in dental traumatology which confirm this (Škaričić et al., 2014).

From epidemiological studies, we know that around two-thirds of all cases of hard dental tissue injury involve central and lateral maxillary incisors (Škaričić et al., 2016). Data from these studies show that around 20% of all children aged up to 18 suffer from some kind of dental trauma in the permanent dentition. Furthermore, most dental traumas occur between the ages of 7 and 15. At this stage, especially between 7 and 10 years, apexogenesis of permanent incisors has not finished, which greatly affects treatment planning and long-term prognosis for every injured tooth. Therefore, our treatment plan is always focused on how to preserve dental pulp vitality in order to promote finishing of the physiological growth and development of the root (apexogenesis). For this reason, in these cases, one of the most favourable clinical procedures is pulpotomy.

Pulpotomy involves treating the exposed vital pulp in the coronal portion of the pulp chamber. The desired outcome of our therapy in young permanent teeth is preservation of pulp vitality. Normal pulpal circulation is the key to success, because circulation will ensure future root maturation. Pulpotomy is highly appropriate for young permanent teeth, in which apexogenesis is often an ongoing process; only a vital dental pulp with its own undamaged circulation can ensure an increase in the quality and quantity of the root. Pulpotomy is especially indicated in cases of traumatic injury of young permanent teeth with an incomplete root, where we try to create favourable conditions in order to complete apexogenesis, because any other endodontic treatment which completely eliminates the dental pulp tissue from the pulp chamber threatens our treatment and long-term prognosis for the tooth.

Management of Dental Emergencies in Children and Adolescents, First Edition.
Edited by Klaus W. Neuhaus and Adrian Lussi.
© 2019 John Wiley & Sons Ltd. Published 2019 by John Wiley & Sons Ltd.
Companion website: www.wiley.com/go/neuhaus/dental_emergencies

Dental Trauma

In this chapter, the focus will be on hard dental tissue injuries, especially crown fractures. There are many different classification systems for dental trauma (Garcia-Godoy, 1984; Spinas and Altana, 2002; Flores et al., 2007; Pagadala and Tadikonda, 2015). For clinical work, in our opinion, the most important one is based on the severity of the injury. Crown fractures can be divided as shown in Figure 3.1.1.

Different diagnoses strongly affect the treatment plan, which should aim to ensure the best final outcome for the patient and the best long-term prognosis for the injured tooth. Crown fracture with pulp involvement is always a very difficult diagnosis for young permanent teeth, and a lot of different cofactors can influence decision-making and the treatment plan; the most important are the size of the pulpal wound, the time from injury to treatment, any concomitant luxation injury and the stage of root maturation. Each of these cofactors has a different influence on the treatment outcome. A smaller pulpal wound is preferable to a big pulp exposure. A shorter time from injury to treatment has a better influence on treatment outcome; for this reason, crown fracture should always be treated as soon as possible. Additional luxation injury strongly influences long-term prognosis and decreases pulp survival rate. Incomplete root development of the injured

tooth with pulpal involvement is very often a double-edged sword: on the one hand, the pulpal circulation is more abundant in such teeth and the capability for recovery from the pulp injury is much higher than in teeth with complete root development; on the other, complications are more serious when root development is incomplete and are associated with loss of pulp vitality. The result of such a clinical situation is stagnation of apexogenesis, with all its associated problems. In these cases, much more complex and time-consuming treatments (e.g. apexification, regenerative endodontic treatments (revascularisation)) must be provided, with unpredictable results. Some experts claim that clinical judgement and the presence of cofactors are not as important to clinical decision-making as is often assumed, because of the strong self-protective abilities of dental pulp. Recently, the International Association of Dental Traumatology (IADT) published guidelines recommending well-known procedures like pulp capping and partial/coronal pulpotomy for the treatment of complicated crown fracture, but the rationale for the choice of treatment remains unclear (Diangelis et al., 2012).

Proper diagnostics and clinician experience should lead to the correct treatment plan through evidence-based dentistry. Thus, superficial pulp infection and degradation of the pulp tissue can be successful controlled by the pulp itself for a period of up to

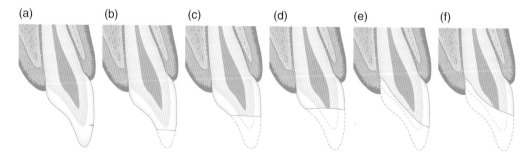

Figure 3.1.1 Illustration of different crown fractures according to our suggested classification: (a) enamel infraction; (b) enamel fracture; (c) enamel-dentine fracture without dental pulp involvement; (d) enamel-dentine fracture with dental pulp involvement; (e) complete crown fracture (enamel-dentine-root) without dental pulp involvement; (f) complete crown fracture (enamel-dentine-root) with dental pulp involvement.

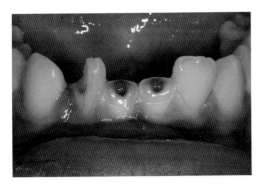

Figure 3.1.2 Strong proliferative pulp reaction following complicated crown fracture 48 hours after trauma and without any treatment.

48 hours. After that, we can expect an infection deeper in the pulp tissue and our treatment should be more radical in an apical direction (Figure 3.1.2). In those circumstances, the size of the pulpal wound also plays a role, where smaller equals better (Ozçelik et al., 2000). From the clinician's perspective, the most important point is to make a precise diagnosis which leads to the treatment plan with the best possible outcome.

In the remainder of this chapter, we will present some different clinical situations from everyday practice and suggest the treatment possibilities in crown fractures with an exposed pulp.

Pulp Histology

The dental pulp is a specific soft dental tissue of mesenchymal origin, situated inside the tooth and surrounded by hard dentin walls. It is also a highly innervated tissue which contains sensory trigeminal afferent axons (Byers, 1984; Byers and Närhi, 1999). Dentin and pulp are strongly connected, each influencing the other. For that reason, we often refer to the "dentin–pulp complex." This complex, and its positive regenerative reaction in cases of traumatic injury, is the cornerstone of successful therapy.

Pulp is actually a single neurovascular bundle made up different cell types and blood vessels. From the nerve supply in the dentin–pulp complex, we have two types of fibre, A and C. These fibres have different diameters and are responsible for the transition of different kinds of sensation from the pulp (Abd-Elmeguid and Yu, 2009). The A fibres are myelinated and are subdivided into two further types, A-delta and A-beta; 90% are of the delta type. They are mainly located at the coronal dentin–pulp border and are concentrated in the pulpal horns. The C fibres are unmyelinated and are located in the pulp core, with an extension into the cell-free zone and under the odontoblastic layer (Byers and Dong, 1983; Bender, 2000). In young permanent teeth with incomplete roots, the ratio of myelinated to unmyelinated fibres is very unpredictable, because the myelin sheath develops later during tooth maturation (Johnsen et al., 1983). The A-delta fibres are smaller in diameter but have a better conduction capacity than the C fibres, especially when they are transmitting pain directly to the thalamus. From the location and conduction velocity of A fibres, it is clear that they transmit the sharp and fast pain produced by such stimulations as drilling, probing and the hydrodynamic effect. The hydrodynamic effect is caused by rapid movement of dentin fluid and produces a fast, sharp pain transmitted by A fibres in the case of dentin desiccation (extensive drying) or hot/cold stimulation. It is very easy for patients to localise this kind of pain. The C fibres are mostly located in the pulp core, and their transmission velocity is lower than that of A fibres. Because of this, the C fibres are responsible for the kind of dull, diffuse pain which is very often difficult to localise. This is because C fibres innervate more than one tooth (Närhi et al., 1992; Andrew and Matthews, 2000). Another important point that should be kept in mind when treating patients with pulp injury is that C fibres can survive in a hypoxic environment. This explains situations where patients feel pain during root canal treatment even when the pulp is necrotic (Mullaney et al., 1970).

It must be stressed, in case of crown fracture with pulp involvement, that with increasing time from injury, increasing neural degradation occurs in pulp tissue. Degradation of the myelin sheath can already be seen 17 hours after traumatic injury (Ozçelik et al., 2000). In this situation, activation of the repair processes by neural signalling occurs – so-called neurogenic inflammation. During this degenerative process, afferent nerve fibres respond to bacterial antigens by releasing neuropeptides, which activate the immune cell system due to the presence of neuropeptide receptors on their cell surfaces, leading to activation of the repair processes (Haug and Heyeraas, 2006).

Pulp Vascularisation

In a traumatised young permanent tooth with a crown fracture, the most important factor for a successful treatment outcome is the positive vascular reaction of the pulp. The question is, what do clinicians consider a positive vascular reaction? From a clinical perspective, we expect successful bleeding control from the pulp after treatments such as partial or cervical pulpotomy, without the use of any bleeding-control agents like astringents or hydrogen peroxide. This indicates good control of local pulp tissue inflammation and indicates improved healing of the dentin–pulp complex, with the formation of a dentin bridge and preservation of pulp vitality. From a histological perspective, on the other hand, the most important thing is normal vascularisation close to the pulp injury. Good vascularisation ensures an adequate anti-inflammatory response limiting the infection and the degradation process close to the pulpal wound, which as a consequence imparts a better regenerative potential to the injured tooth. In that case, it is clear that a tooth with an incomplete apex and without periodontal (luxation) injury has a much better chance of healing with a maintained vital pulp (Josell, 1995; Andreasen and Kahler, 2015).

In one study, a rapid increase of vascularisation was observed 1.5 hours after the injury, which is important to a positive long-term prognosis for the injured tooth (Ozçelik et al., 2000). There was extensive neovascularisation 4 days after the injury, and the newly formed blood vessels were filled with plasma and blood cells (Ozçelik et al., 2000). From another study, we know that the most important driving force behind angiogenesis of the injured dental pulp is hypoxia (Aranha et al., 2010). Under hypoxic conditions, dental pulp cells start expressing different molecules, such as vascular endothelial growth factor (VEGF), angiopoietins or fibroblast growth factor 2 (FGF-2), which kickstart the intensive process of angiogenesis (Tran-Hung et al., 2008; Zimna and Kurpisz, 2015). Angiogenesis is an important step in the efficient defensive reaction of the vital dental pulp. New blood vessels with an appropriate circulation enhance wound cleaning, maintain an adequate local anti-inflammatory reaction and ensure the soft pulp tissue is well oxygenated. Under these conditions, pulp wound healing is more predictable for a positive final outcome.

One more important point should be made. With a complicated crown fracture, the surface of the fracture line after trauma is usually straight, some larger parts of the dentin can be found in the pulp tissue and a healthy vital pulp reacts strongly against contamination from the oral cavity. This reaction is macroscopically visible as pulpal outgrowth from the dentin wound (Figure 3.1.3). When the pulp is exposed during caries excavation, the pulpal wound looks very different compared to the traumatised tooth, with some necrotic parts of the pulp close to the dentin, different amounts of residual dentin in the pulp tissue and the surface of the trepanation site much more irregular. In these cases, after caries excavation, we have a much less favourable situation for pulpal wound healing, which is very important in decision-making and treatment planning (Mjör, 2002).

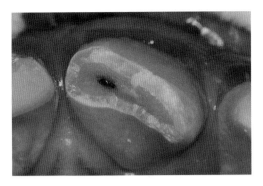

Figure 3.1.3 Fast pulpal reaction with overgrowth of the pulp soft tissue through the dentin 12 hours after injury.

Pulpotomy

Pulpotomy is a therapeutic procedure targeting vital pulp, in which the coronal portion of the pulp, or even a part of it, is surgically removed and the remaining pulp is preserved intact. After removal, a suitable material is used to replace it, in order to protect the remaining pulp against further insult. Furthermore, pulpotomy tends to initiate healing and repair of the injured hard and soft dental tissue (Eghbal et al., 2009). The two main forms are partial (Cvek) pulpotomy (Cvek, 1978) and cervical (full) pulpotomy (Corbman, 1947). In some cases, especially where there is an incomplete, wide apex, the intention of therapy is to maintain apexogenesis in order to complete root formation.

In special cases, such as where there is huge pulp exposure (≥3 mm), delayed intervention or uncontrollable pulpal bleeding following Cvek or cervical pulpotomy, a more radical procedure can be performed, termed extended pulpotomy.

Partial (Cvek) Pulpotomy

Partial pulpotomy was invented and suggested as a clinical procedure by Dr Miomir Cvek in the late 1970s. The main idea was to remove the coronal pulp tissue to the level of the healthy portion of the pulp in order to preserve pulp vitality and maintain normal function (Cvek, 1978).

Indications

The primary indication for Cvek pulpotomy is a crown fracture with pulp involvement in a case where direct pulp capping is not indicated. Today, direct pulp capping indications are limited to cases where we have pinpoint exposure of the pulp and the injured tooth is treated within a few hours after the accident (Dean, 2016). This means that further indications for Cvek pulpotomy are delayed intervention and pulp exposure ≥1 mm. Results from different studies indicate that Cvek pulpotomy up to 30 hours after injury has a success rate of around 90%; the same is true for pulp exposure in the range 1–4 mm (Bimstein and Rotstein, 2016; Wang et al., 2017). Other very important factors for good long-term prognosis are an additional luxation injury and the stage of root maturation, where a luxation injury decreases the success rate and an incomplete root increases it (Fong and Davis, 2002; Lauridsen et al., 2012). Finally, the most important reason for promoting Cvek pulpotomy as the first choice of therapy in a crown fracture with pulp involvement, instead of cervical pulpotomy, is that a cell-rich coronal pulp has a greater potential to facilitate the healing process than radicular pulp. Radicular pulp is a more fibrous and unicellular tissue with less capacity to respond to the healing process (de Blanco, 1996).

Clinical Procedure

The first step in treatment is a quick clinical examination, taking a short dental and medical history, collecting important information about the accident and making a few clinical pictures (Figure 3.1.4). Radiographic examination is also very important and should never be omitted. Following this, a final decision can be made and a treatment plan can be drawn up.

The next important step is successful pain control. For a good local analgesia, the amide group of local anaesthetics (e.g. lidocaine 2%, articaine 4% or mepivacaine 3%) should be used. One important issue when choosing a local anaesthetic for partial pulpotomy is the concentration of vasoconstrictor (epinephrine)

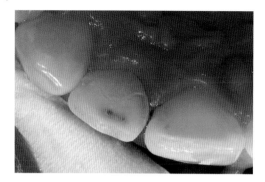

Figure 3.1.4 Diagnostic procedure in complicated crown fracture – clinical pictures.

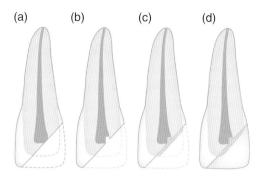

Figure 3.1.5 (a) Complicated crown fracture. (b) Surgical removal of the injured pulp. (c) Final restoration with pulp capping material. (d) Final restoration with dentin bridge formation.

in the solution, which should be either low ($1:200\,000/1:400\,000$) or zero. This is mainly to avoid periapical vasoconstriction, which can compromise treatment success by giving a false-positive clinical sign of good pulpal bleeding control and causing amputation to end too early, in the coronal pulp. Further, when the vasoconstrictor is washed out from the periapical region, blood clot formation starts below the capping material, which can initiate a degenerative process in the pulp tissue that often leads to pulp necrosis.

After analgesia, the working field should be isolated. The best option is a rubber dam, but where this cannot be applied (e.g. in traumatised children), cotton rolls should be used instead (Wang et al., 2017).

Once good pain control has been achieved and the working field has been isolated, pulp amputation can be performed (Figure 3.1.5). For pulpotomy, it is recommended to use a high-speed handpiece cooled under water spray and a round diamond bur (1.0–1.2 mm diameter) (Figure 3.1.6a,b). The approach with the bur should be direct to the exposed pulp to 1–3 mm depth, without widening the access cavity. The pulpal wound should be rinsed with saline solution and compressed with a cotton pellet (moistened with saline to avoid desiccation of the superficial pulp tissue and contamination of the wound with cotton fibres) (Figure 3.1.6c). Use of aggressive solutions such as NaOCl, CHX or H_2O_2 for wound cleaning or bleeding control should be avoided. The most important clin-

ical sign that enough pulpal tissue has been removed and the underlying remaining pulp is healthy is successful bleeding control within 2–3 minutes. After that, the pulp should be capped with a biostimulating agent and restored with a definitive restoration to prevent coronal microleakage, which is one of the main reasons for Cvek pulpotomy failure (Fong and Davis, 2002).

There are many suggestions and recommendations for pulp capping materials in the literature, but the most common are calcium hydroxide ($Ca(OH)_2$), mineral trioxide aggregate (MTA) and a cement based on di- and tricalcium silicate. All of these are successfully used in everyday clinical practice, according to their different advantages and disadvantages.

$Ca(OH)_2$ has been in common clinical use for more than 35 years, indicating how effective it can be, but it still its disadvantages (Cvek, 1978). First, it loses its antibacterial capacity (high pH) very rapidly when it comes in contact with pulp tissue fluid due to the decrease in pH. It also does not seal the pulpal wound against bacterial penetration very well, and because of that it depends on the overlying restorative material to prevent bacterial coronal microleakage. Ultimately, its high pH causes the necrotic zone on the pulp surface to become a hotbed of bacterial growth, which can later penetrate through the rather permeable dentinal bridge and

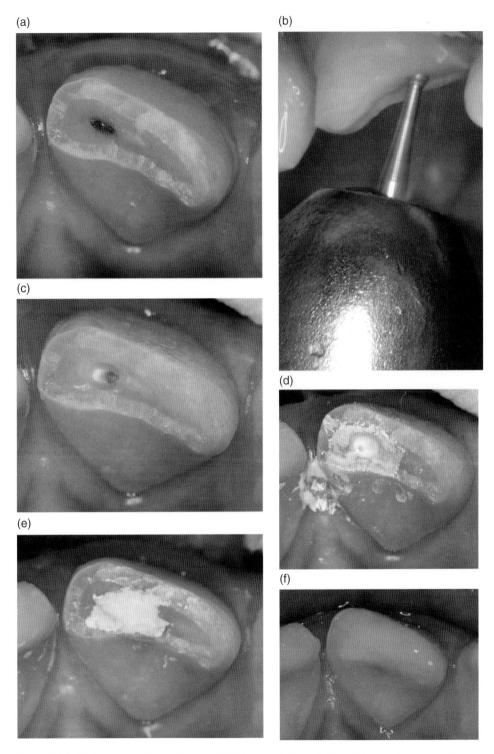

Figure 3.1.6 (a) Complicated crown fracture. (b) Pulp amputation – fast handpiece, water spray and round diamond bur. (c) Good bleeding control after pulpotomy (rinsing with saline). (d) Application of single-component $Ca(OH)_2$ and cleaning of the remaining paste with a dry cotton pellet. (e) Application of two-component $Ca(OH)_2$ cement over the paste. The remaining enamel cement should be thoroughly cleaned to achieve good marginal adaptation of the composite resin restoration. (f) Final restoration with composite material.

cause delayed pulpal damage (Bakland, 2009). Despite these drawbacks, $Ca(OH)_2$ is still the first choice of capping material in our clinical practice because of its long history of proven effectiveness and relatively low cost. To improve its clinical performance, we suggest some modifications when applying $Ca(OH)_2$ in Cvek pulpotomy. The single-component $Ca(OH)_2$ paste (Calcipulpe, UltraCal XS) should be placed directly on the pulp and compressed with a dry sterile cotton pellet (Figure 3.1.6d). With this technique, an intimate contact is achieved between the capping material and the pulp, making application of a two-component $Ca(OH)_2$ cement (Dycal, Kerr Life) much easier and more precise (Figure 3.1.6e). The most challenging aspect of $Ca(OH)_2$ cement application is how rapidly it sets when it touches the moist surface of the pulp tissue. Our "two consistencies" technique avoids this problem and provides a better prognosis for the final outcome. It also greatly reduces the material's porosity. Finally, a composite resin restoration should be placed (Figure 3.1.6f).

When MTA was introduced as a material of choice for pulpotomy, promising clinical results were reported from a number of studies and case reports, with a success rate of more than 90% (even better than for $Ca(OH)_2$; da Rosa et al., 2018). Apart from its difficult handling, long setting time and high price, the biggest disadvantage of MTA is the greyish discolouration it produces in the tooth, even when white MTA is used (Belobrov and Parashos, 2011). Thus, since maxillary incisors are the most commonly injured teeth, we cannot recommend it as the first choice for pulp capping after pulpotomy.

Recently introduced medical cements based on di- and tricalcium silicate (Biodentine, Septodont) show very good results in partial pulpotomy in a number of different studies, comparable with those for $Ca(OH)_2$ and MTA (Nowicka et al., 2013; Martens et al., 2015). Their consistency ensures much better handling than MTA, they have very good sealing properties, their pulpal response is favourable (with compact dentin-like hard dental tissue formation) and no discolouration is reported. Thus, these silicate-based cements look very promising, but results from long-term clinical studies are needed before their use can definitely be recommended.

Finally, pulp vitality should be tested at least 4 weeks after pulpotomy, and x-ray should be taken after 3 months (Figure 3.1.7). Subsequent x-rays are required for the next 2–3 years, in order to monitor treatment success and to recognize any complications at an early stage.

Cervical (Full) Pulpotomy

Cervical pulpotomy was first suggested as a clinical procedure for the treatment of traumatised young permanent teeth more than 70 years ago (Corbman, 1947). Today, it is indicated only in special cases where the crown is severely injured, with a big loss of hard dental tissue and large pulp exposure, or where control of pulpal bleeding has been unsuccessful following Cvek pulpotomy in teeth with incomplete root formation.

Clinical Procedure

Many of the clinical steps are the same as for Cvek pulpotomy (Figures 3.1.8 and 3.1.9). When good pain control (anaesthesia) and isolation of the working filed are achieved, pulp tissue should be removed more apically than in Cvek pulpotomy, to the root canal orifices. After that, the pulpal wound should be rinsed with saline and compressed with a moistened cotton pellet. When the bleeding is stopped, biostimulating capping material should be placed on the remaining root pulp. When using $Ca(OH)_2$, the same "two consistencies" technique as described for Cvek pulpotomy is recommended. Definitive restoration should be done using composite resin. The schedule for control visits is the same as described for Cvek pulpotomy.

Extended Pulpotpmy

As already mentioned, the aim of extended pulpotomy is to ensure a suitable environment

(a) (b)

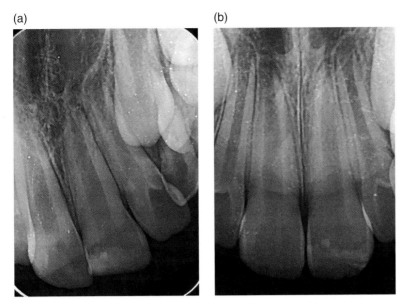

Figure 3.1.7 (a) x-ray taken immediately after Cvek pulpotomy. (b) x-ray taken 3 months after Cvek pulpotomy, showing dentin bridge formation.

Figure 3.1.8 (a) Complicated crown fracture. (b) Surgical removal of the pulp tissue to the root canal orifice. (c) Final restoration with pulp capping material below the restoration. (d) Positive outcome with dentin bridge formation and definitive composite resin restoration of the fractured crown.

(a) (b) (c) (d)

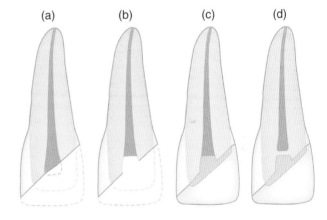

for the physiological root development of traumatised young permanent teeth. Under growing skeletal conditions, maintaining a root symptomless in the jaw can only be advantageous. The main goal of the procedure is to avoid the need for apexification or regenerative endodontics if these are not an option due to compliance, technical issues or time constraints while performing root canal treatment in young permanent teeth (Kahler et al., 2017). Extended pulpotomy is not a standard clinical procedure, but in some clinical cases it can give us alternative possibilities when treating very complicated traumatic injuries.

The following clinical case will describe an attempt to prolong apexogenesis in a very severe crown fracture of a right central maxillary incisor under unusual clinical circumstances. An 8-year-old patient presented at the dental office 3 days after sustaining this injury. He was without any pain and had

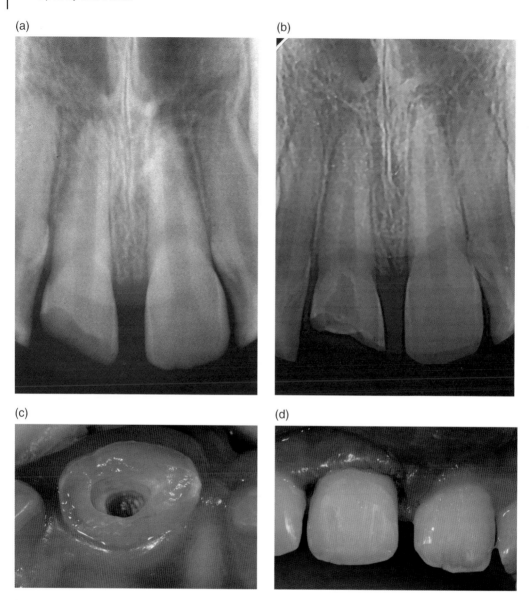

Figure 3.1.9 (a) x-ray taken 30 hours after injury. A large pulpal wound and incomplete root formation is visible. Cervical pulpotomy was performed using the "two consistencies" Ca(OH)$_2$ technique. (b) Control x-ray taken 12 months after the first intervention. Loss of composite restoration after repeated trauma and dentin bridge formation with normal root development without periapical pathology can be seen. (c) Dentin bridge. (d) New definitive restoration with composite resin immediately after treatment.

previously been treated in an emergency care setting, where a cotton pellet moistened with sodium hypochlorite was placed directly on the pulp tissue and covered with a temporary restoration (Cavit). After taking x-rays and administering a local anaesthesic (plain 3% mepivacaine), a rubber dam was used to isolate the site and treatment started with a plan to perform a cervical pulpotomy. Following cervical pulpotomy, bleeding could not be effectively controlled, but the idea was to avoid pulpectomy because of the

(a)   (b)   (c)

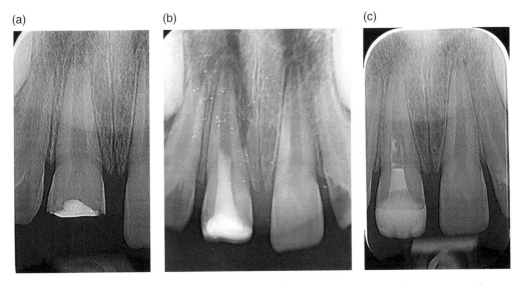

Figure 3.1.10 (a) x-ray taken before extended pulpotpmy. (b) x-ray taken 5 months after treatment with Ca(OH)$_2$ in the root canal. Normal root development can be observed, as in the adjacent, non-injured tooth. (c) Dentin bridge formation and root development 10 months after injury. Final restoration over Ca(OH)$_2$ was done using GIC and composite resin.

very immature root. Therefore, the clinical decision was to extend the pulp tissue amputation more apically. Removal of the pulp was performed with a fast handpiece and a long-neck round diamond bur under water spray cooling. Pulp tissue was removed almost to the half-length of the root canal, and after rinsing with saline, good pulpal bleeding control was achieved. The remaining pulp was covered and the root canal was filled with a Ca(OH)$_2$ paste (UltraCal XS, Ultradent). ZOE cement was then placed over this paste, and the cavity was closed with glass ionomer cement (GIC). Temporary restoration was carried out 4 weeks later, using a composite resin. The formation of a dentine bridge with normal root development without any periapical pathology could be observed after 10 months (Figure 3.1.10).

Conclusion

Decision-making in dental trauma is not a simple process, and depends on the knowledge, experience and instincts of the dentist. The intention of this chapter was to highlight the most important facts from evidence-based dentistry and clinical experience in one part of dental traumatology. Every pulp and tooth saved is invaluable – moreso when we consider the age of the patients. Children and adolescents are the most vulnerable age group when affected by dental trauma, especially in young permanent teeth. With good diagnosis and adequate therapy, normal growth and development of the entire oral cavity can be maintained, avoiding difficulties for future dental care and saving greatly on future dental costs.

References

Abd-Elmeguid, A., Yu, D. C. 2009. Dental pulp neurophysiology: Part 1. Clinical and diagnostic implications. *Journal of the Canadian Dental Association*, **75**(1), 55–9.

Andreasen, F. M., Andreasen, J. O. 2007. Crown fractures. In: Andreasen, J.O., Andreasen, F.M., Andersson, L. (eds). *Textbook and Color Atlas of Traumatic*

Injuries to the Teeth, 4th edn. Oxford: Blackwell, pp. 280–305.

Andreasen, F. M., Kahler, B. 2015. Pulpal response after acute dental injury in the permanent dentition: clinical implications – a review. *Journal of Endododontics*, **41**(3), 299–308.

Andrew, D., Matthews, B. 2000. Displacement of the contents of dentinal tubules and sensory transduction in intradental nerves of the cat. *Journal of Physiology*, **529**(3), 791–802.

Aranha, A. M., Zhang, Z., Neiva, K. G., Costa, C. A. S., Hebling, J., Nor, J. E. 2010. Hypoxia enhances the angiogenic potential of human dental pulp cells. *Journal of Endodontics*, **36**(10), 1633–7.

Bakland, L. K. 2009. Revisiting traumatic pulpal exposure: materials, management principles, and techniques. *Dental Clinics of North America*, **53**(4), 661–73.

Belobrov, I., Parashos, P. 2011. Treatment of tooth discoloration after the use of white mineral trioxide aggregate. *Journal of Endodontics*, **37**(7), 1017–20.

Bender, I. B. 2000 Pulpal pain diagnosis – a review. *Journal of Endodontics*, **26**(3), 175–9.

Bimstein, E., Rotstein, I. 2016. Cvek pulpotomy – revisited. *Dental Traumatology*, **32**(6), 438–42.

Byers, M. R. 1984. Dental sensory receptors. *International Review of Neurobiology*, **25**, 39–94.

Byers, M. R., Dong, W. K. 1983. Autoradiographic location of sensory nerve endings in dentin of monkey teeth. *The Anatomical Record*, **205**(4), 441–54.

Byers, M. R., Närhi, M. V. 1999. Dental injury models: experimental tools for understanding neuroinflammatory interactions and polymodal nociceptor functions. *Critical Reviews in Oral Biology and Medicine*, **10**(1), 4–39.

Corbman, A. L. 1947. Pulpotomy, a conservative treatment for exposed vital young permanent teeth. *Journal of Dentistry for Children*, **14**(3), 15–18.

Cvek, M. 1978. A clinical report on partial pulpotomy and capping with calcium hydroxide in permanent incisors with complicated crown fracture. *Journal of Endodontics*, **4**(8), 232–7.

da Rosa, W. L. O., Cocco, A. R., Silva, T. M. D., Mesquita, L. C., Galarça, A. D., Silva, A. F. D., Piva E. 2018. Current trends and future perspectives of dental pulp capping materials: a systematic review. *Journal of Biomedical Materials Research. Part B, Applied Biomaterials*, **106**(3), 1358–68.

Dean, J. A. 2016. Treatment of deep caries, vital pulp exposure, and pulpless teeth. In: Dean, J. E., Jones, J. E., Vinson L. A. W. (eds). *McDonald and Avery's Dentistry for the Child and Adolescent*, 10th edn. St Louis, MO: Elsevier, pp. 221–42.

de Blanco, L. P. 1996. Treatment of crown fractures with pulp exposure. *Oral Surgery, Oral Medicine, Oral Pathology, Oral Radiology and Endododontics*, **82**(5), 564–8.

Diangelis, A. J., Andreasen J. O., Ebeleseder, K. A., Kenny, D. J., Trope, M., Sigurdsson, A., et al. 2012. International Association of Dental Traumatology guidelines for the management of traumatic dental injuries: 1. Fractures and luxations of permanent teeth. *Dental Traumatology*, **28**(1), 2–12.

Eghbal, M. J., Asgary, S., Baglue, R. A., Parirokh M., Ghoddusi, J. 2009 MTA pulpotomy of human permanent molars with irreversible pulpitis. *Australian Endodontic Journal*, **35**(1), 4–8.

Flores, M. T., Andersson, L., Andreasen, J. O., Bakland, L. K., Malmgren, B., Barnett, F., et al. 2007 Guidelines for the management of traumatic dental injuries. *I. Fractures and luxations of permanent teeth. Dental Traumatology*, **23**(2), 66–71.

Fong, C. D., Davis, M. J. 2002 Partial pulpotomy for immature permanent teeth, its present and future. *Pediatric Dentistry*, **24**(1), 29–32.

Garcia-Godoy, F. M. 1984. Prevalence and distribution of traumatic injuries to the permanent teeth of Dominican children from private schools. *Community Dentistry Oral Epidemiology*, **12**(2), 136–9.

Haug, S. R., Heyeraas, K. J. 2006. Modulation of dental inflammation by the sympathetic nervous system. *Journal of Dental Research*, **85**(6), 488–95.

Johnsen, D. C., Harshbarger, J., Rymer, H. D. 1983. Quantitative assessment of neural development in human premolars. *The Anatomical Record*, **205**(4), 421–9.

Josell, S. D. 1995. Evaluation, diagnosis and treatment of the traumatized patient. *Dental Clinics of North America*, **39**(1), 15–24.

Kahler, B., Rossi-Fedele, G., Chugal, N., Lin LM. 2017. An evidence-based review of the efficacy of treatment approaches for immature permanent teeth with pulp necrosis. *Journal of Endodontics*, **43**(7), 1052–7.

Lauridsen, E., Hermann, N. V., Gerds, T. A., Ahrensburg, S. S., Keibor, S., Andreasen, J. O. 2012. Combination injuries 2. The risk of pulp necrosis in permanent teeth with subluxation injuries and concomitant crown fractures. *Dental Traumatology*, **28**(5), 371–8.

Martens, L., Rajasekharan, S., Cauwels, R. 2015. Pulp management after traumatic injuries with a tricalcium silicate-based cement (Biodentine™): a report of two cases, up to 48 months follow-up. *European Archives of Paediatric Dentistry*, **16**(6), 491–6.

Mjör, I. A. 2002. Pulp-dentin biology in restorative dentistry. Part 7: The exposed pulp. *Quintessence International*, **33**(2), 113–35.

Mullaney, T. P., Howell, R. M., Petrich, J. D. 1970. Resistance of nerve fibers to pulpal necrosis. *Oral Surgery, Oral Medicine and Oral Pathology*, **30**(5), 690–3.

Närhi, M., Jyväsjärvi, E., Virtanen, A., Huopaniemi, T., Ngassapa, D., Hirvonen, T. 1992. Role of intradental A- and C-type nerve fibres in dental pain mechanisms. *Proceedings of Finish Dental Society*, **88**(Suppl. 1), 507–16.

Nowicka, A., Lipski, M., Parafiniuk, M., Sporniak-Tutak, K., Lichota, D., Kosierkiewicz, A., et al. 2013. Response of human dental pulp capped with biodentine and mineral trioxide aggregate. *Journal of Endododontics*, **39**(6), 743–7.

Ozçelik, B., Kuraner, T., Kendir, B., Aşan, E. 2000. Histopathological evaluation of the dental pulps in crown-fractured teeth. *Journal of Endodontics*, **26**(5), 271–3.

Pagadala, S., Tadikonda D. C. 2015. An overview of classification of dental trauma. *International Archives of Integrated Medicine*, **2**(9), 157–64.

Škaričić, J., Vuletić, M., Soldo, M., Trampuš, Z., Čuković-Bagić, I., Jurić H. 2014. Causes and prevalence of dental and oral soft tissue injuries in school children in Zagreb, Croatia. *Paediatria Croatica*, **58**(2), 171–5.

Škaričić, J., Vuletić, M., Hrvatin, S., Jeličić, J., Čuković-Bagić, I., Jurić, H. 2016. Prevalence, type and etiology of dental and soft tissue injuries in children in Croatia. *Acta Clinica Croatica*, **55**(2), 209–16.

Spinas, E., Altana, M. 2002. A new classification for crown fractures of teeth. *Journal of Clinical Pediatric Dentistry*, **26**(3), 225–31.

Tran-Hung, L., Laurent, P., Camps, J., About I. 2008. Quantification of angiogenic growth factors released by human dental cells after injury. *Archives of Oral Biology*, **53**(1), 9–13.

Wang, G., Wang, C., Qin M. 2017. Pulp prognosis following conservative pulp treatment in teeth with complicated crown fractures – a retrospective study. *Dental Traumatology*, **33**(4), 255–60.

Zimna, A., Kurpisz, M. 2015. Hypoxia-inducible factor-1 in physiological and pathophysiological angiogenesis: applications and therapies. *BioMed Research International*, **2015**, 549412.

3.2

Pulpectomy with Open Apex

Isabelle Portenier[1,2], Klaus W. Neuhaus[3,4] and Maria Lessani[5,6]

[1] Department of Endodontics, Dental Faculty, University of Oslo, Oslo, Norway
[2] Private dental clinic, Nyon, Switzerland and Oslo, Norway
[3] Clinic of Periodontology, Endodontology and Cariology, University Center for Dental Medicine Basel, University of Basel, Basel, Switzerland
[4] Private dental office, Herzogenbuchsee, Switzerland
[5] School of Dentistry, Birmingham, United Kingdom
[6] Private dental office, London, United Kingdom

Introduction

The practitioner treating teeth with an open apex will have to overcome two major challenges. First, they must clean the thin root canals walls without instrumenting them, in order to avoid weakening them even more. Second, they must fill and obturate the root without overfilling with either gutta-percha or sealer.

Root canal treatment of the nonvital (necrotic or infected) tooth with an open apex has been treated historically with nonsetting calcium hydroxide to induce an apical barrier, often referred to as apexification (Al Ansary et al., 2009). It was thought that the barrier was calcific due to the calcium derived from the calcium hydroxide, but this was investigated using other materials and found to be incorrect (Cooke and Rowbotham, 1960; Ball, 1964; Heithersay, 1970). The tooth had to be repeatedly redressed to gain a hard barrier, which was not always achievable in every case. When it was successful, however, the operator had achieved a barrier that allowed conventional root filling of the tooth with gutta-percha and sealer (Weisenseel et al., 1987).

The advent of mineral trioxide aggregate (MTA) cement represented a great step forward in the filling of open-apex teeth, as it could be placed in the root end as a biocompatible barrier. It was initially used as an apical plug/barrier, allowing obturation of the root canal space with gutta-percha and sealer. This technique was then modified to allow complete canal obturation with MTA.

Recent case reports on regeneration of the root canal contents and root maturation – initially referred to as revascularisation – suggest management with antibiotics and calcium hydroxide (Duggal et al., 2017). This will be covered in the next chapter. Here, we focus on the clinical aspects of the open-apex permanent tooth with MTA cement in cases not suitable for regeneration. This treatment modality can be utilised for anterior and posterior teeth.

Choice of Treatment

The diagnosis of the nonvital tooth is based on information gathered from the patient history, clinical signs and symptoms and

Management of Dental Emergencies in Children and Adolescents, First Edition.
Edited by Klaus W. Neuhaus and Adrian Lussi.
© 2019 John Wiley & Sons Ltd. Published 2019 by John Wiley & Sons Ltd.
Companion website: www.wiley.com/go/neuhaus/dental_emergencies

further investigations, referred to as special tests. These normally include vitality testing, thermal (cold and heat) and electrical testing, imaging with radiographs and, less frequently cone-beam computed tomography (CBCT).

Clinical Procedure

Once it has been established that a tooth is nonvital and the presence of an open apex has been seen on images, the tooth can be treated in the following manner.

Local Anaesthesia and Rubber Dam

A local anaesthesic is ideally administered using a topical agent followed by needle injection of anaesthetic solution. A rubber dam is then applied to isolate the site. Care should be taken to be as atraumatic as possible when applying the dam. Some systems (e.g. wedjets) allow for isolation without the use of clamps, which is especially useful for anterior teeth. When the placement of a clamp directly on the tooth is not possible (e.g. the tooth is still erupting and only the convex part of the clinical crown is exposed), a temporary composite build-up allows for its positioning (Figure 3.2.1).

Access Cavity

As much of the tooth structure as possible should be preserved when considering access cavity design. Immature teeth generally have large pulp chambers, and it is fundamental that the irrigation and debridement of the pulp contents includes the pulp horns. If any necrotic tissue or burnt gutta-percha or cement is left in these areas, it can lead to tooth discolouration postoperatively, which is considered an iatrogenic error.

Some address this problem by creating access cavities that incorporate the whole pulp chamber, including the pulp horns. Others use magnification (e.g. loupes or operating microscopes) to access and debride these areas with ultrasonics and copious irrigation, so as to maintain a minimally

invasive approach for access into the root canal system (Figure 3.2.1).

Working Length Determination

Determination of working length (WL) can be challenging due to the open apex, but the current generation of apex locators is better than ever at addressing this problem.

It is important to follow these main steps:

- Make sure there is no excess fluid in the pulp chamber.
- Use small instruments with a lubrication agent (e.g. ethylenediaminetetraacetic acid (EDTA) gel). It is not necessary to use large instruments (files) to gain contact with the apical walls, which can be fragile, in order to get a predictable reading.
- The predictable reading is the zero reading, which is the reading when the file is just out of the canal space and in contact with the periodontium.
- The WL can be taken as 0.5 mm short of the zero reading in most cases, but with open apices this can be challenging. It is the authors' suggestion that 1 mm short of the zero reading should be used, in order to minimise the risk of extrusion of material (including irrigation, interappointment dressing and obturation).

Disinfection

Disinfection should be carried out mainly via irrigation, although in some cases interappointment dressing can also be applied. The irrigation agent, the delivery system and the activation of the irrigant have been found to be important.

Normally, a needle and syringe is used to deliver the irrigant (mainly sodium hypochlorite, with EDTA as a final rinse), but new delivery systems are being introduced into the dental market. The irrigation needle should be 2 mm short of the WL and should be applied with a small-amplitude vertical movement to allow for agitation of the irrigants.

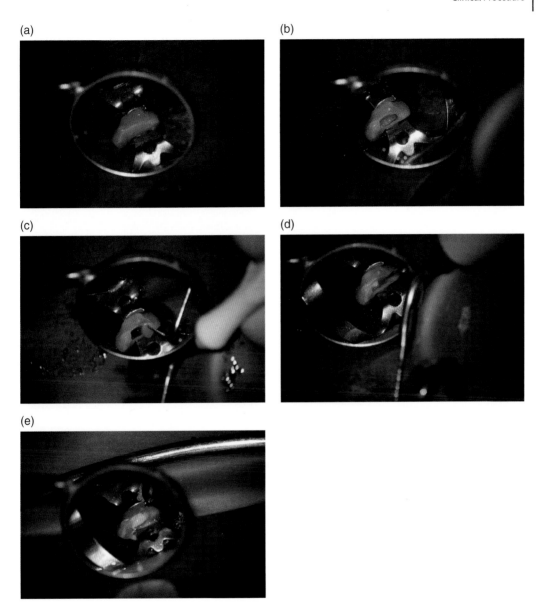

Figure 3.2.1 (a) Preoperative placement of a composite, allowing for use of a rubber dam clamp. (b) Due to the position of the clamp and the early stage of tooth eruption, the access cavity was prepared through the incisal edge. (c) Removal of the necrotic pulp with a microdebrider size 20. (d) Ultrasonic irrigation of the root canal with sodium hypochlorite 3%. (e) Intracanal dressing with calcium hydroxide. (f) Closed access cavity. The presence of a huge cyst can be seen buccally. (g) After cyst removal. The composite build-up is nearly invisible, and was later removed. (h) 6-year recall. The contralateral pulp survived longer, but root canal treatment was indicated as well.

Activation can be carried out using a tapered gutta-percha device (McGill et al., 2008; Bronnec et al., 2010) or with a custom-made instrument such as an XP-endo Finisher (FKG Dentaire, La Chaux-de-Fonds, Switzerland), which is designed not to shape the canal but to aid in cleaning the canal walls, or an Eddy tip (VDW, Munich, Germany) or Irri-Safe tip (Acteon, Merignac, France), which agitate the liquid through sonic or ultrasonic activity.

(f)

(g)

(h)

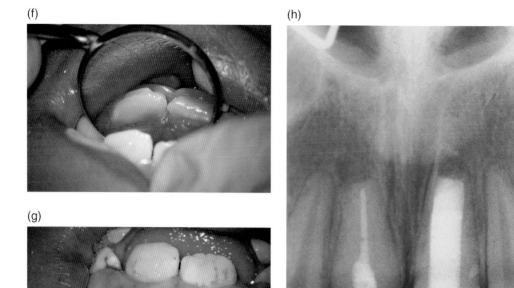

Figure 3.2.1 (Continued)

The use of lasers has been advancing in dentistry, and it seems there is a potential role for lasers in endodontics, although at present the clinical evidence is limited and their use cannot be fully recommended until clinical outcome studies indicate they are of benefit to the disinfection process of the root canal system.

The paper points should be pre-measured so as to avoid leaving parts behind in the apical tissues, causing a foreign-body reaction in the future.

Interappointment Dressing of the Canal

The tooth is either dressed with calcium hydroxide or obturated. The evidence in the literature for single- versus multivisit treatment has been supportive of both modes, although open apices have not been widely studied in this area.

An open apex is commonly found to be associated with root-end exudate, and hence a dressing is recommended. The gold-standard material for a root canal is non-setting calcium hydroxide. The duration of placement is frequently debated. We recommend a minimum of 1 week but ideally 2 and no longer than 1 month, to avoid weakening of the dentine (unless the patient is unable to attend).

Obturation

The tooth is obturated with MTA/bioceramic cement in the apical part.

The various instruments available for this purpose are displayed in Figures 3.2.2–3.2.6. The aim is to facilitate the procedure, but it must be stated that obturating teeth with an open apex is not normally an easy process. The use of delivery guns, ultrasonics (for dense packing) and pluggers (for accurate measurement)

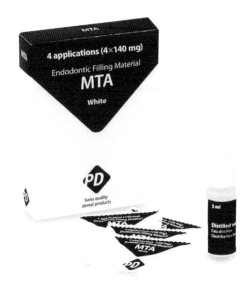

Figure 3.2.2 MTA, the material of choice for direct apexification.

the materials are normally radiopaque and comparable with alveolar bone.

Once the material is in place in the apical 3 mm, there are two main ways the operator can proceed. (i) Obturation of the remainder of the root canal system with gutta-percha and sealer. This normally entails re-dressing of the canal to allow for setting of the MTA unless a fast-set material is used; even then, setting is over 15 minutes in duration. Use of a moist cotton pellet has become increasingly uncommon as it has been found that the humidity from the dentinal tubules and the apical tissues associated with an open apex can be useful in providing moisture for the setting process. (ii) Complete obturation of the canal system with MTA cement. Both methods should terminate the material below the cemento-enamel junction (CEJ) to prevent discolouration of the coronal tooth structure and to provide a good seal for the coronal restoration.

Table 3.2.1 summarises the protocol discussed in this section. The following cases illustrate treatments of open apices with either a direct apexification using a bioceramic cement (Figure 3.2.7) or without additional apexification (Figure 3.2.8).

is fundamental to gaining a dense apical cement barrier without extrusion.

Some operators use a collagen barrier to prevent extrusion of the MTA cement; others feel this can hinder assessment of healing, as

(a)

(b)

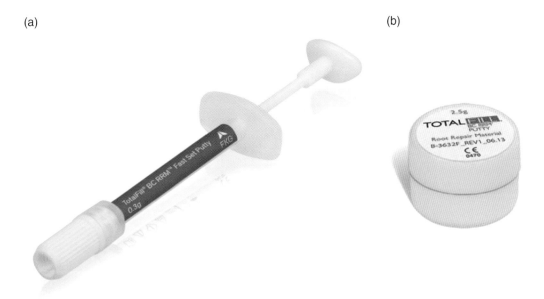

Figure 3.2.3 (a,b) Total Fill RRM premixed: a bioceramic putty material that is easier to apply than hand-mixed MTA, but is also much more expensive.

(a)

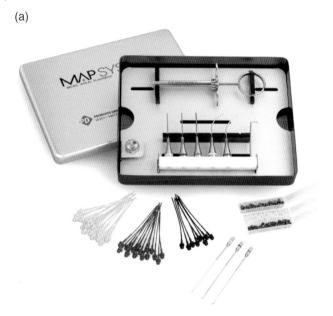

Figure 3.2.4 (a) Delivery system for MTA/bioceramic (MAP System Produits Dentaires Vevey). (b) Kerr amalgam gun for carrying large amounts of cement.

(b)

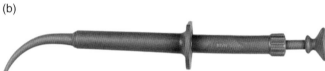

(a)

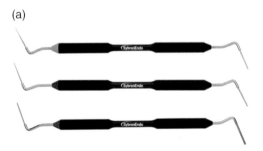

(b)

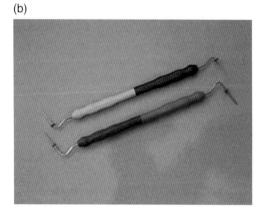

Figure 3.2.5 (a) Buchanan Hand Pluggers for condensation. (b) Machtou Hand Pluggers for condensation of heated gutta-percha.

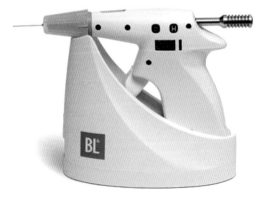

Figure 3.2.6 BL SuperEndo Beta for application of heated gutta-percha during back-fill.

Table 3.2.1 Clinical protocol summary.

Local anaesthesia	• Gel and injection
Rubber dam	• Make application atraumatic as possible
Access cavity	• Straight-line access
	• Incorporating the whole pulp
Working length (WL)	• Apex locator
	• Radiograph
Disinfection	• NaOCl and EDTA
	• Irrigation needle, tapered GP, ultrasound, XP-endo Finisher
Interappointment dressing	• Calcium hydroxide
	• Minimum 2 weeks
Obturation	• 3 mm plug with MTA or bioceramic and GP backfill; or
	• MTA/bioceramic in the whole canal

(a)

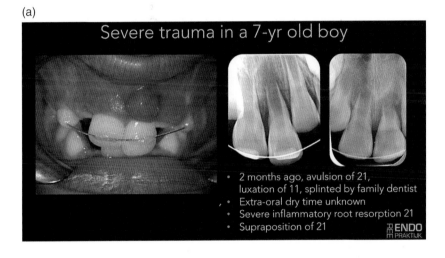

(b)

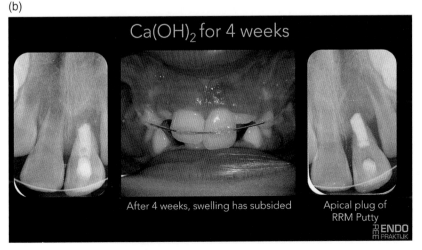

Figure 3.2.7 (a) Preoperative status. (b) 4 weeks' follow-up. (c) Postoperative status. (d) 11 months' follow-up. (e) 2 years' follow-up. *Source: Marga Ree, The Netherlands.*

(c)

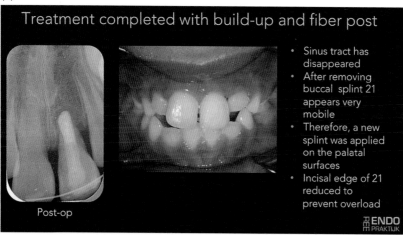

Treatment completed with build-up and fiber post

Post-op

- Sinus tract has disappeared
- After removing buccal splint 21 appears very mobile
- Therefore, a new splint was applied on the palatal surfaces
- Incisal edge of 21 reduced to prevent overload

(d)

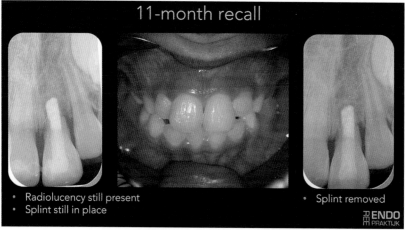

11-month recall

- Radiolucency still present
- Splint still in place

- Splint removed

(e)

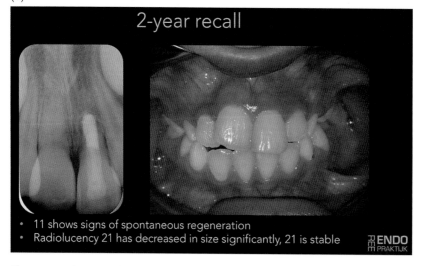

2-year recall

- 11 shows signs of spontaneous regeneration
- Radiolucency 21 has decreased in size significantly, 21 is stable

Figure 3.2.7 (Continued)

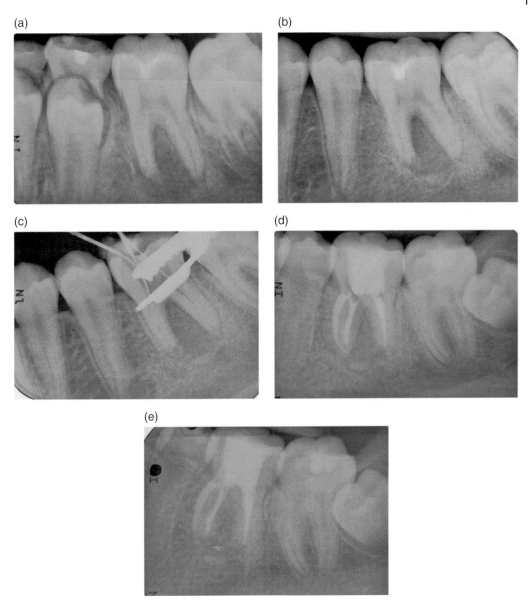

Figure 3.2.8 (a) Periradicular radiolucency on tooth 36 in a 10-year-old boy. The tooth history showed that it was surgically loosened because of ankylosis. The apical part of the mesial root was fractured. No pain, no swelling. (b) Same patient at the age of 13. Indication for root canal treatment was given because of pain. Because the patient was traumatised, the treatment was performed using sedation. (c) The mesial roots had an open apex due to the fracture. Gauging showed an apical diameter of size 35. No indication for MTA placement was given. (d) Immediate postoperative radiograph. (e) 1-year recall. Complete healing, no symptoms.

MTA and Bioceramic

MTA was developed in 1993 by M. Torabinejad and co-workers at the Loma Linda University in California (School of Dentistry, Department of Endodontics), with the patent issued in 1995. After several laboratory tests on cytotoxicity and biocompatibility, MTA was certified by the US Food and Drug Administration (FDA) for application in humans and was introduced on to the market as ProRoot MTA (Tulsa Dental Products, Tulsa/Oklahoma, USA) in 1998. Initially, it was grey, but in 2001 the grey version was replaced by white MTA. The difference between the two is in the composition of aluminium, magnesium and iron (Asgary et al., 2005), and in the fact that white MTA does not contain any aluminium ferrite (Camilleri and Pitt Ford, 2006).

Portland cement (PC) is defined as "hydraulic cement" – a cement that not only hardens by reacting with water but also forms a water-resistant end-product. MTA contains around 75% PC, around 20% bismuth oxide (Bi_2O_3) and around 5% gypsum ($CaSO_4 \times 2\,H_2O$) (Berzins, 2014). PC contains calcium oxide (65%), silicon dioxide (20%), aluminium oxide (5%), ferric oxide (5%) and sulphur oxide (1–4%). The quantity of gypsum (calcium sulphate) determines the setting time. Bismuth oxide is added for its radiopacity.

After mixing with water, tricalcium silicate, dicalcium silicate, tricalcium aluminate and tetracalcium aluminoferrite are formed (Camilleri and Pitt Ford, 2006). When mixing MTA, a sterile glass plate and spatula should be used. The ratio of sterile water to powder is $1:3$ and the powder is added in portions until a creamy consistency is reached. The mixing process should last for at least a minute in order to ensure dissolution of the powder into the liquid.

During the setting process, a gel is formed, which will set within 3 hours (Torabinejad et al., 1995). While setting, calcium silicate and calcium hydroxide are formed; the latter explains the high pH values (around 10–13) of set MTA. Walker et al. (2006) showed that too much liquid increases the porosity and the risk of washing out parts of the cement. If too little is used, the material will be brittle and very difficult to apply; however, the humidity of the dentinal tubules will still allow the cement to set.

Bozeman et al. (2006) showed that hydroxyapatite crystals are formed, which interact with the dentine, allowing a tight bond between the structures (Han and Okij, 2011). Many studies have tested the cytotoxicity of

MTA (Camilleri and Pitt Ford, 2006), and most have found a layer of cells growing over it. A study by Akhavan et al. (2017) showed that, as compared to calcium hydroxide and composite material, MTA had the highest rate of hard tissue formation within 63 days.

Katsamakis et al. (2013) published a review article on the histological reaction of the periodontium to MTA. In general, the studies they analysed showed that MTA had low cytoxicity and regenerative potentials. The latter was negatively influenced by bacterial contamination. Demiriz and Bodrumlu (2017) showed that the extrusion of MTA had no influence on the radiographic prognosis over a 3-year period; in 85% of cases, the amount of material extruded was reduced.

The disadvantages of MTA include its high price and the difficulties in handling it. Its long setting time can also be a disadvantage, as in some situations (e.g. retrograde) the material is washed out when the root surface is cleaned. There is also the presence of bismuth oxide, which is responsible for tooth discolouration. Kohli et al. (2015) showed that products containing bismuth oxide discolour teeth but that products containing zirconium oxide do not.

Bioceramic materials can be either inert (e.g. ceramic oxides) or resorbable. It contains mainly pure tricalcium silicate and not PC. In that way, bioceramic does not contain the aluminate phase. At present, calcium phosphate-based ceramics represent the preferred bone substitute in orthopaedic and maxillofacial surgery (Combes and Rey, 2010). Calcium phosphates usually found in bioceramic include hydroxyapatite (HAP) $Ca_{10}(PO_4)_6(OH)_2$, tricalcium phosphate β (β TCP), $Ca_3 (PO_4)_2$ and mixtures of HAP and β TCP. Calcium phosphates are found in many living organisms, including bone mineral and tooth enamel.

The premixed bioceramic root-repair material and sealer EndoSequence is produced by Brassler (Savannah, GA, USA). In Europe, it is sold as Total Fill RRM (root repair material) by FKG (FKG Dentaire, La Chaux-de-Fonds, Switzerland). It is a hydrophile, insoluble, radiopaque and aluminium-free material based on a calcium phosphate silicate composition. Its setting and hardening reactions require the presence of water from tissue or dentin tubules. As with MTA, the advantages of this new repair material are its high pH (>12.5), high resistance to washout, lack of shrinkage during setting, excellent biocompatibility and superb physical properties. In fact, it has a compressive strength of 50–70 MPa, which approximates that of the currently used root canal repair materials, ProRoot MTA (Dentsply) and BioAggregate (Diadent). In addition, because of the presence of zirconium oxide or tantalum oxide in place of bismuth oxide, it does not discolour teeth.

References

Akhavan, A., Arbabzadeh, F., Bouzari, M., Razavi, S. M., Davoudi, A. 2017. Pulp response following direct pulp capping with dentin adhesives and mineral trioxide aggregate: an animal study. *Iranian Endodontic Journal*, **12**(2), 226–30.

Al Ansary, M. A., Day, P. F., Duggal, M. S., Brunton, P. A. 2009. Interventions for treating traumatized necrotic immature permanent anterior teeth: inducing a calcific barrier & root strengthening. *Dental Traumatology*, **25**(4), 367–79.

Asgary, S., Parirokh, M., Eghbal, M. J., Brink, F. 2005. Chemical differences between white and gray mineral trioxide aggregate. *Journal of Endodontics*, **31**(2), 101–3.

Ball, J. S. 1964 Apical root formation on non-vital immature permanent incisor. *British Dental Journal*, **116**, 166–7.

Berzins, D. W. 2014. Chemical properties of MTA. In: Torabinejad, M. (ed.). *Mineral Trioxide Aggregate Properties and Clinical Applications*. Oxford: Wiley-Blackwell, pp. 17–36.

Bozeman, T. B., Lemon, R. R., Eleazer, P. D. 2006. Elemental analysis of crystal precipitate from gray and white MTA. *Journal of Endodontics*, **32**, 425–8.

Bronnec, F., Bouillaguet, S., Machtou, P. 2010. Ex vivo assessment of irrigant penetration and renewal during the final irrigation regimen. *International Endodontic Journal*, **43**, 663–72.

Camilleri, J., Pitt Ford, T. R. 2006. Mineral trioxide aggregate: a review of the constituents and biological properties of the material. *International Endodontic Journal*, **39**(10), 747–54.

Combes, C., Rey, C. 2010. Bioceramics. In: Boch, P., Niepce, J.-C. (eds). *Ceramic Materials: Processes, Properties and Applications*. London: Wiley.

Cooke, C., Rowbotham, T. C. 1960. Root canal therapy in non-vital teeth with open apices. *British Dental Journal*, **108**, 147–50.

Demiriz, L., Bodrumlu, E. H. 2017. Retrospective evaluation of healing of periapical lesions after unintentional extrusion of mineral trioxide aggregate. *Journal of Applied Biomaterials & Functional Materials*, **15**, 382–6.

Duggal, M., Tong, H. J., Al-Ansary, M., Twati, W., Day, P. F., Nazzal, H. 2017. Interventions for the endodontic management of non-vital traumatised immature permanent anterior teeth in children and adolescents: a systematic review of the evidence and guidelines of the European Academy of Paediatric Dentistry. *European Archives of Paediatric Dentistry*, **18**(3), 139–51.

Han, L., Okiji, T. 2011. Uptake of calcium and silicon released from calcium silicate-based endodontic materials into root canal dentine. *International Endodontic Journal*, **44**, 1081–7.

Heithersay, G. S. 1970. Stimulation of root formation in incompletely developed pulpless teeth. *Oral Surgery Oral Medicine Oral Pathology*, **29**(4), 620–30.

Katsamakis, S., Slot, D. E., van der Sluis, L. W., van der Weijden, F. 2013. Histological responses of the periodontium to MTA: a systematic review. *Journal of Clinical Periodontology*, **40**, 334–44.

Kohli, M. R., Yamaguchi, M., Setzer, F. C., Karabucak, B. 2015. Spectrophotometric analysis of coronal tooth discoloration induced by various bioceramic cements and other endodontic materials. *Journal of Endodontics*, **41**(1), 1862–6.

McGill, S., Gulabivala, K., Mordan, N., Ng, Y. L. 2008. The efficacy of dynamic irrigation using a commercially available system (RinsEndo_R) determined by removal of a collagen "bio-molecular film" from an ex vivo model. *International Endodontic Journal*, **41**, 602–8.

Torabinejad, M., Hong, C. U., McDonald, F., Pitt Ford, T. R. 1995. Physical and chemical properties of a new root-end filling material. *Journal of Endodontics*, **21**(7), 349–53.

Walker, M. P., Diliberto, A., Lee, C. 2006. Effect of setting conditions on mineral trioxide aggregate flexural strength. *Journal of Endodontics*, **32**, 334–6.

Weisenseel, J. A. Jr, Hicks, M. L., Pelleu, G. B. 1987. Calcium hydroxide as an apical barrier. *Journal of Endodontics*, **13**, 1–5.

3.3

Regenerative Endodontic Procedures

Richard Steffen[1,2]

[1] Clinic of Orthodontics and Paediatric Dentistry, University Center for Dental Medicine Basel, University of Basel, Basel, Switzerland
[2] Private dental office, Weinfelden, Switzerland

Introduction

The occurrence of pulpal necrosis in immature permanent teeth, usually front teeth, is a real emergency for young patients. Owing to their thin and underdeveloped roots, classical endodontic treatments such as apexification with calcium hydroxide ($CaOH_2$) and root filling have a bad prognosis. Regenerative endodontic procedures (REPs) (Diogenes et al., 2017) seek a successful continuation of root canal growth by harnessing the stem cells at the apical end of the root, allowing the regrowth of vital tissue. This technique has been used frequently in teeth that have been made nonvital either by caries or by trauma (Duggal et al., 2017).

The theory behind REPs is simple: all you need to do is disinfect the root canal of the nonvital tooth without harming contiguous vital tissue and activate apical stem cells by evoking bleeding into the root canal system (Lovelace et al., 2011), which leads to regrowth of vital tissue and further growth of the root. However, because evidence related to the successful use of REPs is still very weak, this technique should currently only be used in selected cases where the prognosis

of other techniques would be expected to be very poor (Duggal et al., 2017).

In clinics, REDs are in fact challenging and very manipulation-sensitive procedures that require a strict protocol for effective implementation. The careful selection of suitable patients is likewise very important.

Patient Selection

Patients suitable for REPs should be young (6–20 years old), because in older patients mesenchymal stem cells (MSCs) decrease in their capacity for proliferation and differentiation (Yu et al., 2011). Suitable patients should also have immature teeth with wide-open apexes (at least 1.5 mm diameter) (Andreasen et al., 1995) and an aetiology for vitality loss attributable either to caries or, at least, not to serious traumatic injury (Nazzal and Duggal, 2017). The more complicated a traumatic injury of a tooth, the more extensive the damage to the apical tissue and the tooth structures (e.g. to Hertwig's epithelial root sheath) and the poorer the prognosis for REPs (Figure 3.3.1) (Saoud et al., 2014).

Management of Dental Emergencies in Children and Adolescents, First Edition.
Edited by Klaus W. Neuhaus and Adrian Lussi.
© 2019 John Wiley & Sons Ltd. Published 2019 by John Wiley & Sons Ltd.
Companion website: www.wiley.com/go/neuhaus/dental_emergencies

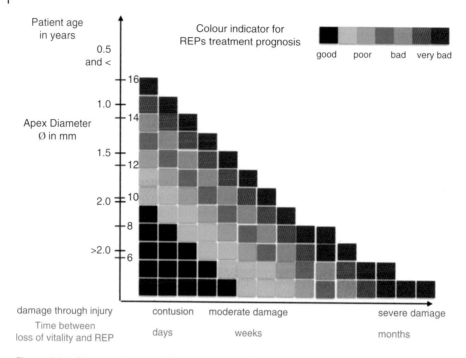

Figure 3.3.1 Diagram showing different aspects of the prognosis of successful REP treatment.

Treatment Protocol

After correct diagnosis of pulpal necrosis (Figure 3.3.2a,b), which is often indicated by a fistula, access to the root canal system of the immature tooth should be established and debridement and disinfection should be carried out (Diogenes et al., 2014). Longer-lasting chemical disinfection with sodium hypochlorite (2.5% NaOCl) with minimal mechanical instrumentation, perhaps with additional ultrasonic activation, will preserve the thin and fragile dentin walls whilst destroying the biofilm and dissolving the remaining organic tissue (Banch and Trope, 2004).

After irrigation followed by careful drying, an intracanal medication for further disinfection should be introduced into the root canal system. Here, $CaOH_2$ has shown more favourable effects than triple or double antibiotic paste (TAP/DAP). Antibiotic pastes in concentrations over 0.1 mg/ml cause heavy stem cell damage (Althumairy et al., 2014), whereas $CaOH_2$ promotes stem cell migration to the root canal (Ruparel et al., 2012).

Intracanal medication should be carefully placed 1 mm above the apex and not overextruded into periapical tissues.

Before access to the root canal system is established for the second visit, normally after 2–4 weeks, successful disinfection should be controlled: there should be no pain, no fistula, no swelling, no gangrenous odour and no sensitivity to palpation and tapping. TAP (with penetration media propylene glycol/macrogol) should be applied as a second medication only if disinfection in the first treatment failed (Diogenes et al., 2017).

At the final (second or third) treatment visit for REPs, the remaining root canal medication should be removed as completely as possible. Irrigation with saline (>20 ml) followed by gentle cleaning with a convenient intracanal brush is recommended (Galler et al. 2015). This is followed by a second rinse with ethylenediaminetetraacetic acid (17% EDTA), which has been shown to release growth factors embedded in dentin (such as TGF-β) and to promote stem cell adhesion to

(a)

(b) (c)

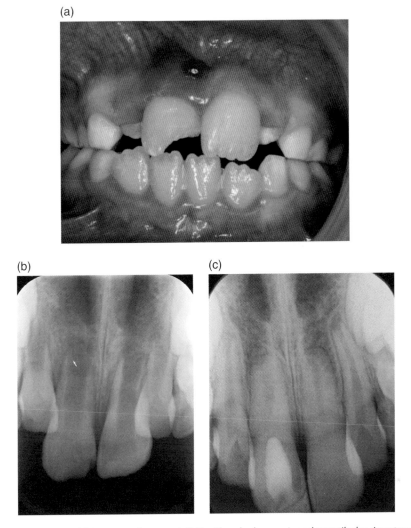

Figure 3.3.2 (a) Immature front tooth (11) with pulpal necrosis and a vestibular sinus tract (fistula). (b) Radiograph of the same tooth at the beginning of REPs. (c) Radiograph of the same tooth 38 months after REPs with a closed apex, growth in the root length and obliteration of the root canal (same signs of healing as tooth 21).

dentin and the differentiation of stem cells into odontoblast-like cell types (Casagrande et al., 2010).

After drying of the root canal system, bleeding is induced by an endodontic instrument (i.e. K-file size 30) 2–3 mm past the apical foramen. If disinfection leads to distinctly suppressed inflammation (most likely with TAP/DAP disinfection), provocation of bleeding is sometimes difficult. Evoked bleeding from the apical papilla brings MSCs into the root canal system. Filling the entire

root canal system with blood as far as the level of the cement–enamel junction forms a clot to serve as an internal matrix for regenerative reorganization (Ulusoy and Cehreli, 2017). Positioning of synthetic or natural scaffolds for stabilisation of this blood clot and other biological agents is still in an academic phase and may promote soft-tissue healing rather than regeneration of pulp tissue (Nazzal and Duggal, 2017).

Instant coronal sealing of the blood clot has to be carried out with a three-component

---

Box 3.3.1 A Recommended Clinical Protocol for REPs

- First visit
- Informed consent, isolation of the working area and pain control
- Access to root canal system, working length determination
- Irrigation of the root canal system with 20 ml 2.5% NaOCl/10 minutes
- 20 ml saline for 5 minutes, with the needle position always approximately 1–2 mm from the apex
- Drying of the canal with paper points
- Root canal system filled with CaOH2 and temporarily sealed with a plug
- Additional visit when signs and symptoms of infection persist
- No hypersensitivity to palpation or contusion, no fistula or signs of inflammation
- Root canal system filled with TAP or DAP (>1 mg/ml) and temporarily sealed with a plug
- Second visit (after 2–3 weeks)
- Success of disinfection (see above)
- Isolation of the working area and pain control (no vasoconstrictor)
- Irrigation with saline and perhaps a brush (intracanal medication: Ca(OH)$_2$, TAP or DAP flushed out)
- Irrigation with 17% EDTA (10 ml/canal, 5 minutes)
- Drying of the canal with paper points
- Induction of bleeding by a sharp sterile instrument with a length 2 mm greater than the root canal
- Continuation of bleeding to fill the root canal
- Stopping of bleeding with a sterile cotton pellet; cleaning of the root canal up to 2 mm apically from the cement–enamel junction
- Sealing with colour-stable HSC as Biodentine® for example or as a stopgap sealing with pure Portland cement (in front teeth: no MTA)
- Covering of HSC/Portland cement with glass ionomer and then with composite resin
- Follow-up
- x-rays: 3 months, 6 months, 1 year and 4 years

---

seal (hydraulic silicate cement/mineral trioxide aggregate (HSC/MTA), glass ionomer cement (GIC) and composite resin). Direct contact of HSC/MTA with the blood clot will stimulate angiogenic growth factor release and related gene expression in stem cells from the apical papilla (Peters et al., 2016). Owing to its tendency to discolour, MTA may be substituted with pure medical Portland cement (PC) or HSC with a colour-stable radiopacifier (Figure 3.3.2c, Box 3.3.1) (Steffen et al., 2011).

Success and Future of REPs

REPs are successful when all signs of pathology are remedied, root development is proceeding lengthwise, walls are thickening and, in the best case, the development of a closed apex can be seen (Nagy et al., 2014). But REPs may be considered successful even with just the resolution of pathological symptoms. It seems possible that a sterile root canal with sterile but vital connective tissue serves as a better biological basis than a root with an HSC/MTA apex plug and root filling; the more so because an apical HSC/MTA plug with root filling may still occur after REP failure with reinfection of the root canal.

Whether stem cell signalling or root canal scaffolds will produce more predictable results is still an open question, but the chance of gaining some deposition of hard tissue through REPs cannot be ignored (Nicoloso et al., 2016).

References

Althumairy, R. I., Teixeira, F. B., Diogenes, A. 2014. Effect of dentin conditioning with intracanal medicaments on survival of stem cells of apical papilla. *Journal of Endodontics*, **40**, 521–5.

Andreasen, J. O., Borum, M. K., Jacobsen, H. L., Andreasen, F. M. 1995. Replantation of 400 avulsed permanent incisors. Factors related to pulpal healing. *Endodontics & Dental Traumatology*, **11**, 59–68.

Banchs, F., Trope, M. 2004. Revascularization of immature permanent teeth with apical periodontitis: new treatment protocol? *Journal of Endodontics*, **30**, 196–200.

Casagrande, L., Demarco, F. F., Zhang, Z., Vacanti, C. A., Nor, J. E. 2010. Dentin-derived BMP-2 and odontoblast differentiation. *Journal of Dental Research*, **89**, 603–8.

Diogenes, A. R., Ruparel, N., Teixeira, F. B., Hargreaves, K. M. 2014. Translational science in disinfection for regenerative endodontics. *Journal of Endodontics*, **40**, 52–7.

Diogenes, A., Chrepa, V., Ruparel, N. B. 2017. Nonvital pulp therapies. In: Waddington, R. J., Sloan, A. (eds). *Tissue Engineering and Regeneration in Dentistry*, 1st edn. Chichester: Wiley Blackwell, pp. 148–55.

Duggal, M., Tong, H. J., Al-Ansary, M., Twati, W., Day, P. F., Nazzal, H. 2017. Interventions for the endodontic management of non-vital traumatised immature permanent anterior teeth in children and adolescents: a systematic review of the evidence and guidelines of European Academy of Paediatric Dentistry. *European Archives of Paediatric Dentistry*, **18**, 139–51.

Galler, K. M., Buchalla, W., Hiller, K., Federlein, M., Eidt, A., Schieferstein, M., Schmalz, G. 2015. Influence of root canal disinfectants on growth factor release from dentin. *Journal of Endodontics*, **41**, 363–8.

Lovelace, T. W., Henry, M. A., Hargreaves, K. M., Diogenes, A. 2011. Evaluation of the delivery of mesenchymal stem cells into the root canal space of necrotic immature teeth after clinical regenerative endodontic procedure. *Journal of Endodontics*, **37**, 133–8.

Nagy, M. M., Tawfik, H. E., Hashem, A. A., Abu-Seida, A. M. 2014. Regenerative potential of immature permanent teeth with necrotic pulp after different regenerative protocols. *Journal of Endodontics*, **40**, 192–8.

Nazzal, H., Duggal, M. S. 2017. Regenerative endodontics: a true paradigm shift or a bandwagon about to be derailed. *European Archives of Paediatric Dentistry*, **18**, 3–15.

Nicoloso, G. F., Potter, I. G., Rocha, R. O., Montagner, F., Casagrande, L. A. 2016. A comparative evaluation of endodontic treatments for immature teeth based on clinical and radiographic outcomes: a systematic review and meta-analysis. *International Journal of Paediatric Dentistry*, **27**, 217–27.

Peters, O. A., Galicia, J., Arias, A., Tolar, M., Ng, E., Shin, J. 2016. Effects of two calcium silicate cements on cell viability, angiogenic growth factor release and related gene expression in stem cells from the apical papilla. *International Endodontic Journal*, **49**, 1132–40.

Ruparel, N. B., Teixeira, F. B., Ferraz, C. C., Diogenes, A. 2012. Direct effect of intracanal medicaments on survival of stem cells of the apical papilla. *Journal of Endodontics*, **38**, 1372–5.

Saoud, T. M., Zaazou, A., Nabil, A., Moussa, S., Lin, L. M., Gibbs, J. L. 2014. Clinical and radiographic outcomes of traumatized immature permanent necrotic teeth after revascularization/revitalization. *Journal of Endodontics*, **40**, 1946–52.

Steffen, R., Fadi, A. A., van Waes, H. J. M. 2011. Pulpotomy – is MTA/Portland cement the future? In: Splieth C (ed.). *Revolutions in Paediatric Dentistry*. London: Quintessenz, pp. 174–83.

Ulusoy, A. T., Cehreli, Z. C. 2017. Regenerative endodontic treatment of necrotic primary molars with missing premolars: a case series. *Pediatric Dentistry*, **39**, E131–4.

Yu, J. M., Wu, X., Gimble, J. M., Guan, X., Freitas, M. A., Bunnell, B. A. 2011. Age-related changes in mesenchymal stem cells derived from rhesus macaque bone marrow. *Aging Cell*, **10**, 66–79.

Unit 4

Management of Open Pulp in Deciduous Teeth

4.1

Pulpotomy

Eirini Stratigaki[1] and Joana Monteiro[2]

[1] Clinic of Orthodontics and Pediatric Oral Health, University Center for Dental Medicine Basel, University of Basel, Basel, Switzerland
[2] Department of Paediatric Dentistry, Eastman Dental Hospital, London, United Kingdom

Introduction

Pulpotomy is the most widely performed vital pulp treatment in deciduous teeth. The aim of this treatment is to remove the coronal pulp tissue, which is thought to be irreversibly inflamed, and apply a medicament to the healthy or reversibly inflamed pulp tissue that is left in situ (Rodd et al., 2006). The benefit of this treatment is that it maintains pulp vitality and preserves arch integrity until eruption of permanent successors (Fuks and Peretz, 2016).

As previously discussed, deciduous tooth pulp consists of a loose connective tissue containing blood vessels, nerves and immune cells. Studies have found deciduous teeth to have a similar histology to young permanent teeth (Sahara et al., 1993; Sari et al., 1999). Furthermore, deciduous teeth seem to maintain structures for tissue repair, and therefore potential for healing, until late stages of root resorption (Monteiro et al., 2009). Comparable histological changes have been observed in carious resorbing teeth, supporting the suggestion that resorbing teeth maintain the potential for healing and repair (Rajan et al., 2014).

High success rates for pulpotomy have consistently been found despite the use of different materials (Fuks et al., 1997; Holan et al., 2005; Huth et al., 2005). Following formaldehyde's classification as carcinogenic to humans by the International Agency for Research on Cancer (IARC, 2004), formocresol's (FC) use has often been considered imprudent (Rodd et al., 2006). High success rates amongst alternative materials, along with concerns over carcinogenicity, have led to reduced clinical use and teaching of this material in Europe (Ni Chaollai et al., 2009; Monteiro et al., 2017). Materials such as ferric sulphate (FS) and mineral trioxide aggregate (MTA) have increasingly been advocated, demonstrating high clinical and radiographic success (Smaïl-Faugeron et al., 2014).

An accurate pulpal diagnosis is determinant prior to all vital pulp treatments, especially in resorbing deciduous teeth. It is crucial to determine the extent of pulp inflammation and to understand the mechanisms of healing, therapies and materials to be used in order to guarantee pulp healing.

Indications and Contraindications

It should be appreciated that clinical decisions for managing carious deciduous teeth should not be focused on the tooth in isolation, but should consider the patient as a whole. Social, medical and dental aspects play equally determinant roles in treatment planning for paediatric patients (Table 4.1.1).

Management of Dental Emergencies in Children and Adolescents, First Edition.
Edited by Klaus W. Neuhaus and Adrian Lussi.
© 2019 John Wiley & Sons Ltd. Published 2019 by John Wiley & Sons Ltd.
Companion website: www.wiley.com/go/neuhaus/dental_emergencies

Table 4.1.1 Indications and contraindications for pulpotomy in primary molars.

Indications for pulpotomies	Contraindications for pulpotomies
Medical indications • Children with coagulation disorders that may be at increased risk of bleeding following extraction	*Medical contraindications* • Children at increased risk of infective endocarditis • Immunocompromised children
Dental indications • Hypodontia. These children may benefit from maintenance of the primary tooth at least until a definitive, multidisciplinary treatment plan can be made • Orthodontic reasons. In order to maintain arch integrity and prevent mesialisation of the first permanent molar • Iatrogenic exposure • Pulp exposure on a vital tooth with a healthy or reversibly inflamed pulp	*Dental contraindications* • Unrestorable tooth • Irreversible pulpitis • Periapical periodontitis or necrosis (including radiographic signs of infection or pathological resorption) • Teeth close to exfoliation[a]

[a] A risk/benefit assessment should be made in this scenario. Although the tooth pulp retains potential for healing, it may be unwarranted to perform a pulpotomy and restoration on an exfoliating tooth. Furthermore, care should be taken to prevent iatrogenic damage to the permanent successor.

Table 4.1.2 Different pulpotomy materials and their action on the pulp.

	Devitalising	Preserving	Regenerating
Formocresol	×		
Electrosurgery	×		
Laser	×		
Sodium hypochlorite		×	
Glutaraldehyde		×	
Ferric sulphate (FS)		×	
Calcium hydroxide			×
Mineral trioxide aggregate (MTA)			×
Portland cement			×
Biodentine			×

Pulpotomy Techniques

Buckley's FC has been considered the gold standard for decades, since it was first introduced in the 1930s as the medicament of choice for nonvital deciduous teeth. Concerns regarding carcinogenicity and further studies on pulp therapies led to the increased use of alternative materials (Kuo et al., 2018). The search for an optimal material dictated the need to classify the vital pulp therapy according to its effect on the remaining radicular pulp (Table 4.1.2, Figure 4.1.1a,b). An updated Cochrane Review on pulp therapy for deciduous teeth found no superior pulpotomy medicament or technique, but the authors consider that MTA and FS may be preferable to others (Smaïl-Faugeron et al., 2014).

Ferric Sulphate

FS is a well-known and widely used agglutinating agent for gingival retraction and endodontic haemorrhage control. The main

(a)

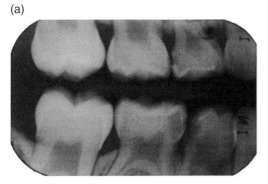

(b)

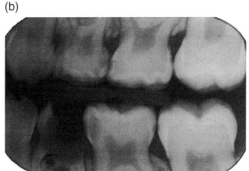

Figure 4.1.1 (a,b) Preoperative bitewing radiographs.

advantage of its use is the reduced likelihood of clot breakdown, as once in contact with blood, it forms a ferric ion–protein complex, sealing the amputated blood vessels mechanically. As a result of this mechanical seal, the risk of an undesired inflammatory response is limited. On that basis, Landau and Johnson (1988) and Fei et al. (1991) conducted the first studies on FS as a pulpotomy agent, showing histologically a favourable response of the pulp to the FS, as well as clinically and radiographically higher success rates (96.6%) than FC (77.8%). Following these preliminary studies, a great number of authors attempted to compare FS to the gold-standard but already condemned FC, presenting similar success rates and thus rendering FS an economically viable alternative. Despite radiographic findings of internal resorption, good success rates and ease of application rendered FS a treatment of choice, especially in countries where the use FC was discouraged (Fuks et al., 1997; Ibricevic and Al-Jame, 2003). The technique for using FC in pulpotomy is as follows:

1) Access the pulp chamber with a high-speed diamond bur.
2) Remove the coronal pulp with a slow-speed round bur or an excavator (Figure 4.1.2).
3) Rinse with saline and dry with a sterile cotton wool pellet (Figure 4.1.3). Should the bleeding persist, it is an indication of hyperaemia and thus pulpectomy or extraction should be performed.

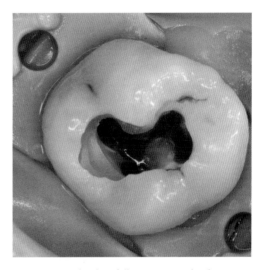

Figure 4.1.2 Bleeding following coronal pulp removal.

4) Apply a 15.5% FS solution (commercially known as Astringident, Ultradent, USA) to the pulp stumps with a cotton pellet for 15 seconds (Figure 4.1.4a,b).
5) Place a thick paste of zinc oxide eugenol (ZOE), MTA or Portland cement (PC) in the pulp chamber. Immediately restore the tooth with composite or a preformed crown (Figures 4.1.5 and 4.1.6).

Mineral Trioxide Aggregate

MTA was first introduced by Lee et al. (1993) as a repair material for lateral root perforations. It contains fine hydrophilic particles of tricalcium silicate, tricalcium aluminate, tricalcium

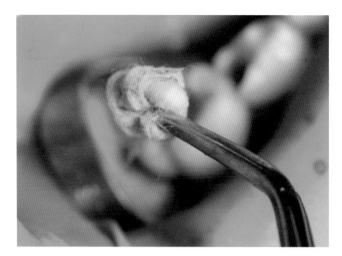

Figure 4.1.3 Use of a wet cotton pellet to induce haemostasis by application of pressure.

(a)

(b)

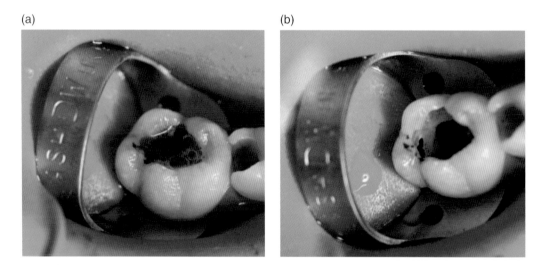

Figure 4.1.4 (a) Application of FS. (b) Pulp stumps following application of FS.

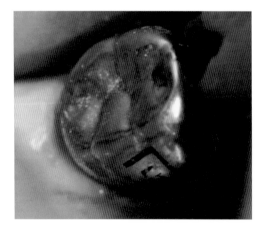

Figure 4.1.5 Final restoration using a preformed metal crown.

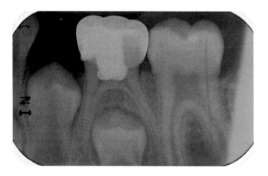

Figure 4.1.6 Post-operative periapical radiograph showing a pulpotomy on a primary molar restored with a preformed metal crown.

oxide, silicate oxide, tetracalcium alumino-ferrite, gypsum and bismuth oxide. It is bio-compatible, radiopaque, has a pH of 12.5 (and therefore is bactericidal), provides an enhanced seal over the amputated pulp and is nonre-sorbable (Torabinejad et al., 1995 Torabinejad and Chivian, 1999; Ford et al., 1996). The high demand for a biocompatible pulpotomy medicament led to a great number of research-ers focusing on this very promising material. Its higher clinical and radiographic success rates (95–100% at 24 months' follow-up) when compared to all other pulpotomy agents have been confirmed by a considerable number of studies (Eidelman et al., 2001; Agamy et al., 2004; Moretti et al., 2008; Doyle et al., 2010; Erdem et al., 2011) and a recent Cochrane Review, where MTA showed an overall superi-ority in most of the aspects considered (Smaïl-Faugeron et al., 2014). In the most recent American Academy of Pediatric Dentistry (Dhar et al., 2017) guidelines on pulp therapy in deciduous teeth, MTA is recommended as the medicament of choice. The main draw-backs of the material are its high cost, extended setting times (3–4 hours) and discolouration due to bismuth oxide. The technique for using MTA in pulpotomy is as follows:

1) Access the pulp chamber with a high-speed diamond bur.
2) Remove the coronal pulp with a slow-speed round bur or an excavator.
3) Rinse with saline and dry with a sterile cotton wool pellet. Should the bleeding persist, it is an indication of hyperaemia and thus pulpectomy or extraction should be performed.
4) Mix 3 : 1 MTA to sterile saline into a paste and place in the pulp chamber.
5) Place a second layer of glass ionomer cement (GIC) over the MTA. Immediately restore the tooth with composite or a preformed crown.

Portland Cement

PC is a fine powder produced by grinding cement clinker, comprising 65% lime, 20% silica, 10% alumina and ferric oxide and 5% other compounds (Steffen and van Waes, 2009). It is the primary component of MTA and has been the focus of great interest as a more cost-efficient alternative to that mate-rial. It also doesn't contain bismuth oxide, so it causes less discolouration. The lack of bis-muth oxide, however, renders PC radiolucent. The levels of arsenic contained in limestone have been proven to be comparable to those present in MTA, so there is no contraindica-tion to its use in clinical practice (Duarte et al., 2005). Recently, an increasing number of studies have given a solid basis to its suitabil-ity (94–100% clinical success rate at 24 months' follow-up) as an alternative to MTA (Holland et al., 2001; Min et al., 2007; Conti et al., 2009; Yildirim et al., 2016). The technique for using PC in pulpotomy is as follows:

1) Access the pulp chamber with a high-speed diamond bur.
2) Remove the coronal pulp with a slow-speed round bur or an excavator.
3) Rinse with saline and dry with a sterile cotton wool pellet. Should the bleeding persist, it is an indication of hyperaemia and thus pulpectomy or extraction should be performed.
4) Mix PC and water into a paste and place in the pulp chamber (Figure 4.1.7).
5) Add a second layer of GIC. Immediately restore the tooth with composite or a preformed crown (Figure 4.1.8).

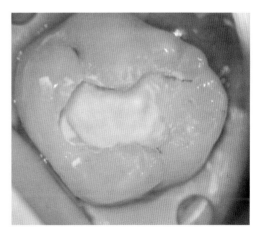

Figure 4.1.7 Application of Portland cement paste in the pulp chamber.

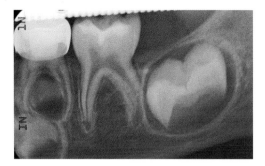

Figure 4.1.8 Postoperative radiograph after final restoration with a preformed metal crown. *Source:* Photographs by Dr.med dent. Richard Steffen.

Other Techniques and Materials

Formocresol

The ability of FC to mummify the radicular pulp tissue within a 5 minute application made it the most used medicament in the treatment of inflamed deciduous pulp for many years. Its success rate ranged from 55 to 95% (Fuks and Peretz, 2016). However, Rolling and Lambjerg-Hansen (1978) showed that teeth clinically successfully treated with FC presented histologically with severe radicular inflammation adjacent to the inflammation site, with signs of necrosis within the remaining pulp tissue and no evidence of pulp fixation. Despite these findings, FC carried on being the treatment of choice, as well as the gold standard against which any new medicaments were compared. Nadin et al. (2003) published a Cochrane Review on pulp materials for deciduous teeth, which found there was lack of evidence for a superior pulp medicament. A year later, the IARC (2004) declared formaldehyde carcinogenic to humans, leading to a clear shift towards researching new medicaments. For this reason, the authors do not recommend FC as a pulpotomy medicament.

Laser

Erbium lasers were introduced as an alternative to FC. Their decontaminating and superficial coagulating actions, with no effect on the underlying pulp, made them seem a promising lead. A number of animal studies, however, showed conflicting results in terms of pulpal healing. Although Shoji et al. (1985) found no detectable change in the remaining radicular pulpal tissue, Jukic et al. (1997) reported carbonisation, necrosis, inflammatory infiltration, oedema and haemorrhage in the remaining pulpal tissue. Saltzman et al. (2005) compared diode laser-MTA to FC-ZOE pulpotomy, raising concerns over the low success rates in the laser-MTA group due to the potential masking of hyperaemia through ablation of the pulp tissue. Because of its precise technique, laser pulpotomy involves a learning curve, is time-consuming and is highly costly. These factors, along with concerns regarding the status of the remaining pulp tissues, must be taken into account when considering laser as a pulpotomy technique.

Calcium Hydroxide

A number of studies on calcium hydroxide as a pulpotomy medicament confirmed the formation of a dentine bridge in an amputated pulp, which morphologically was very close to osteodentine. Thus, it was presumed that calcium hydroxide could promote either preservation or mineralisation of the remaining pulp tissue. Unfortunately, internal resorption was also described in most studies (Huth et al., 2012; Oliveira et al., 2013). Through an "embolisation" process (Heilig et al., 1984), particles of calcium hydroxide induce focal points of inflammation in the pulp tissue (Zurn and Seale, 2008). Success rates for pulpotomies using calcium hydroxide range from 36 (Doyle et al., 1962) to 77% (Waterhouse et al., 2000). Tooth selection criteria have to be very strict in order for calcium hydroxide to be considered an acceptable alternative to FC (Waterhouse et al., 2000).

Glutaraldehyde

Glutaraldehyde, a dialdehyde with superior fixative properties to FC, a self-limiting penetration ability and low antigenicity, was first introduced by Kopel et al. (1980). Garcia-Godoy (1986) used a 2% glutaraldehyde formulation over the amputated pulp with a success rate of 98% after 19–42 months. This was significantly reduced when ZOE was incorporated (Garcia-Godoy and Ranly, 1987). However, Fuks et al. (1986) found that success rates reduced from 94.3% at 6 months to 82% at 25 months, thus rendering glutaraldehyde a weak alternative to conventional FC pulpotomy.

Electrosurgery

One of the first attempts to introduce electrosurgery into the treatment of deciduous molars was made by Anderman (1982). This method aimed to create a barrier of coagulative necrosis between the healthy radicular tissue and the lining material after the carbonisation and denaturation of the inflamed carious coronal pulp. It was described as time-efficient and lacking in toxic effects. However, the limited number of studies and small sample size (and the fact the studies were mainly conducted on primates) meant that electrosurgery failed to show any clear benefits compared to FC (Ruemping et al., 1983; Shaw et al., 1987; Shulman et al., 1987).

Sodium Hypochlorite

Sodium hypochlorite (NaOCl) is a well-established antibacterial irrigation agent used in various concentrations (1–5% solution) in nonvital root canals of permanent teeth with closed or open apex. Vargas et al. (2006) showed comparable outcomes to FS in a preliminary evaluation of the use of sodium hypochlorite in pulpotomies over a 12-month period. Other studies have followed, with success rates ranging between 82 and 95% (Vostatek et al., 2011). However, longer-term studies are needed before NaOCl can be considered a valid alternative to the existing pulpotomy techniques.

Conclusion

There is a constant call for more biocompatible patient- and clinician-friendly materials. In the light of this, new bioceramic materials like Biodentine and EndoSequence are being launched on to the market in an attempt to overcome the known drawbacks of MTA and PC. However, the few clinical cases (Grewal et al., 2016) and even fewer trials (El Meligy et al., 2016) are not yet strong enough to substantiate the use of these agents in deciduous molar pulpotomies.

References

Agamy, H. A., Bakry, N. S., Mounir, N. M., Avery, D. R. 2004. Comparison of mineral trioxide aggregate and formocresol as pulp-capping agents in pulpotomized primary teeth. *Pediatric Dentistry*, **26**(4), 302–9.

Anderman, I. I. 1982. Indications for use of electrosurgery in pedodontics. *Dental Clinics of North America*, **26**, 711–28.

Conti, T. R., Sakai, V. T., Fornetti, A. P., Moretti, A. B. S., Oliveira, T. M., Lourenco Neto, N., et al. 2009. Pulpotomies with Portland cement in human primary molars. *Journal of Applied Oral Sciences*, **17**, 66–9.

Dhar V, Marghalani AA, Crystal YO, et al. 2017. Use of vital pulp therapies in primary teeth with deep caries lesions. *Pediatr Dent*, **39**(5), E146–E159.

Doyle, T. L., Casas, M. J., Kenny, D. J., Judd, P. L. 2010. Mineral trioxide aggregate produces superior outcomes in vital primary molar pulpotomy. *Pediatric Dentistry*, **32**(1), 41–7.

Doyle, W. A., McDonald, R. E., Mitchell, D. F. 1962. Formocresol versus calcium hydroxide in pulpotomy. *Pediatric Dentistry*, **29**, 86–97.

Duarte, M. A. H., Demarchi, A. C. C. O., Jamashita, J. C., Kuga, M. C., Fraga, S. C. 2005.

Arsenic release provided by MTA and Portland Cement. *Oral Surgery Oral Medicine Oral Pathology Oral Radiology and Endodontics*, **99**, 648–50.

Eidelmann, E., Holan, G., Fuks, A. B. 2001. Mineral trioxide aggregate versus formocresol in pulpotomized primary molars: a preliminary report. *Pediatric Dentistry*, **23**(1), 15–18.

El Meligy, O. A., Allazzam, S., Alamoudi, N. M. 2016. Comparison between biodentine and formocresol for pulpoomy of primary teeth: a randomized clinical trial. *Quintessence International*, **47**(7), 571–80.

Erdem, A. P., Guven, Y., Balli, B., Ilhan, B., Sepet, E., Ulukapi, I., Aktoren, O. 2011. Success rates of mineral trioxide aggregate, ferric sulphate and formocresol pulpotomies: a 24-month study. *Pediatric Dentistry*, **33**(2), 165–70.

Fei, A. L., Udin, R. B., Johnson, R. 1991. A clinical study of ferric sulphate as a pulpotomy agent in primary teeth. *Pediatric Dentistry*, **13**(6), 327–30.

Ford, T. R., Torabinejad, M., Abedi, H. R., Bakland, L. K., Kariyawasam, S. P. 1996. Using mineral trioxide aggregate as a pulp capping material. *Journal of the American Dental Association*, **127**, 1491–4.

Fuks, A. B., Peretz, B. 2016. *Pediatric Endodontics, Current Concepts in Pulp Therapy for Primary and Young Permanent Teeth*. Heidelberg: Springer.

Fuks, A. B., Bimstein, E., Kelin, H. 1986. Assessment of a 2 percent buffered glutaraldehyde solution in pulpotomized primary teeth of school children: a preliminary report. *Journal of Pedodontics*, **10**, 323–30.

Fuks, A. B., Holan, G., Davis, J. M., Eidelman, E. 1997. Ferric sulphate versus dilute formocresol in pulpotomized primary molars: long-term follow-up. *Pediatric Dentistry*, **19**, 327–30.

Garcia-Godoy, F. 1986. A 42-month evaluation of glutaraldehyde pulpotomies in primary teeth. *Journal of Pedodontics*, **10**, 148–55.

Garcia-Godoy, F., Ranly, D. M. 1987. Clinical evaluation of pulpotomies with ZOE as the

vehicle for glutaraldehyde. *Pediatric Dentistry*, **9**(2), 144–6.

Grewal, N., Salhan, R., Kaur, N., Patel, H. B. 2016. Comparative evaluation of calcium silicate-based dentine substitute (Biodentine) and calcium hydroxide (Pulpdent) in the formation of reactive dentine bridge in regenerative pulpotomy of vital primary teeth: triple-blind randomized clinical trial. *Contemporary Clinical Dentistry*, **7**(4), 457–63.

Heilig, J., Yates, J., Siskin, M., McKnight, J., Turner, J. 1984. Calcium hydroxide pulpotomy for primary teeth: a clinical study. *Journal of the American Dental Association*, **108**, 775–8.

Holan, G., Eidelman, E., Fuks, A. B. 2005. Long-term evaluation of pulpotomy in primary molars using mineral trioxide aggregate or formocresol. *Pediatric Dentistry*, **27**(2), 129–36.

Holland, R., de Souza, V., Murata, S. S., Nery, M. J., Bernabé, P. F., Otoboni Filho, J. A., Déjan, E. Jr. 2001. Reaction of rat connective tissue to implanted dentin tube filled with mineral trioxide aggregate, Portland cement or calcium hydroxide. *Brazilian Dental Journal*, **12**(2), 109–13.

Huth, K. C., Paschos, E., Hajek-Al-Khatar, N., Hollweck, R., Crispin, A., Hickel, R., Folwaczny, M. 2005. Effectiveness of 4 pulpotomy techniques – randomized controlled trial. *Journal of Dental Research*, **84**(12), 1144–8.

Huth, K. C., Hajek-Al-Khatar, N. H., Wolf, P., Ilie, N., Hicker, R., Paschos, R. 2012. Long-term effectiveness of four pulpotomy techniques: 3-year randomised controlled trial. *Clinical Oral Investigation*, **16**(4), 1243–50.

Ibricevic, H., Al-Jame, Q. 2003. Ferric sulphate and formocresol in pulpotomy of primary molars: long-term follow-up study. *European Journal of Paediatric Dentistry*, **4**(1), 28–32.

International Agency for Research on Cancer (IARC). 2004. IARC classifies formaldehyde as carcinogenic to humans. World Health Organization Press Release No. 153, June 15. Available from: https://web.archive.org/

web/20180419023944/https://www.iarc.fr/
en/media-centre/pr/2004/pr153.html
(last accessed January 30, 2019).

Jukic, S., Anic, I., Koba, K., Najzar-Fleger, D.,
Matsumoto, K. 1997. The effect of
pulpotomy using CO2 and Nd: YAG lasers
on dental pulp tissue. *International
Endodontic Journal*, **30**, 175–80.

Kopel, H. M., Bernick, S., Zachrisson, E.,
De Romero, S. A. 1980. The effects of
glutaraldehyde on primary pulp tissue
following coronal amputation: an in vivo
histological study. *Journal of Dentistry for
Children*, **47**, 425–30.

Kuo, H. Y., Lin, J. R., Huang, W. H., Chiang, M. L.
2018. Clinical outcomes for primary molars
treated by different types of pulpotomy: a
retrospective cohort study. *Journal of the
Formosan Medical Association*, **117**(1), 24–33.

Landau, M. J., Johnson, D. C. 1988. Pulpal
response to ferric sulphate in monkeys.
Journal of Dental Research, **67**, 215.

Lee, S. J., Monsef, M., Torabinejad, M. 1993.
Sealing ability of a mineral trioxide aggregate
for repair of lateral root perforation. *Journal
of Endodontics*, **19**, 541–4.

Min, K. S., Kim, H. I., Park, H. J., Pi, S. H.,
Hong, C. U., Kim, E. C. 2007. Human pulp
cells response to Portland cement in vitro.
Journal of Endodontics, **33**, 163–6.

Monteiro, J., Day, P., Duggal, M., Morgan, C.,
Rodd, H. 2009. Pulpal status of human
primary teeth with physiological root
resorption. *International Journal of
Paediatric Dentistry*, **19**(1), 16–25.

Monteiro, J., Ní Chaollaí, A., Duggal, M. 2017.
The teaching of management of the pulp in
primary molars across Europe. *European
Archives of Paediatric Dentistry*, **18**(3),
203–8.

Moretti, A. B., Sakai, V. T., Oliveira, T. M.,
Fornetti, A. P., Santos, C. F., Machado, M.
A., Abdo, R. C. 2008. The effectiveness of
mineral trioxide aggregate, calcium
hydroxide and formocresol for pulpotmies
in primary teeth. *International Endodontic
Journal*, **41**, 547–55.

Nadin, G., Goel, B. R., Yeung, C. A., Glenny, A.
M. 2003. Pulp treatment for extensive decay

in primary teeth. *Cochrane Database of
Systematic Reviews*, **1**, CD003220.

Ni Chaollai, A., Monteiro, J., Duggal, M. S.
2009. The teaching of management of the
pulp in primary molars in Europe: a
preliminary investigation in Ireland and the
UK. *European Archives of Paediatric
Dentistry*, **10**(2), 98–103.

Oliveira, T. M., Moretti, A. B. S., Sakai, V. T.,
Lourenco Neto, N., Santos, C. F., Machado,
M. A. A. M. 2013. Clinical, radiographic and
histologic analysis of the effects of pulp
capping materials used in pulpotomies of
human primary teeth. *European Archives of
Paediatric Dentistry*, **14**, 65–71.

Rajan, S., Day, P. F., Christmas, C.,
Munyombwe, T., Duggal, M., Rodd, H. D.
2014. Pulpal status of human primary molars
with coexisting caries and physiological root
resorption. *International Journal of
Paediatric Dentistry*, **24**(4), 268–76.

Rodd, H. D., Waterhouse, P. J., Fuks, A. B.,
Fayle, S. A., Moffat, M. A. 2006. Pulp therapy
for primary molars. *International Journal of
Paediatric Dentistry*, **116**(Suppl. 1), 15–23.

Rolling, I., Lambjerg-Hansen, H. 1978. Pulp
condition of successfully formocresol-
treated primary molars. *Scandinavian
Journal of Dental Research*, **86**(4), 267–72.

Ruemping, D. R., Morton, T. H., Anderson,
M. W. 1983. Electrosurgical pulpotomy in
primates – a comparison with formocresol
pulpotomy. *Pediatric Dentistry*, **5**, 14–18.

Sahara, N., Okafuji, N., Toyoki, A., Ashizawa, Y.,
Yagasaki, H., Deguchi, T., Suzuki, K. 1993.
A histological study of the exfoliation of
human deciduous teeth. *Journal of Dental
Research*, **72**, 634–40.

Saltzmann, B., Sigal, M., Clokie, C., Rukavina,
J., Titley, K., Kulkarni, G. V. 2005.
Assessment of a novel alternative to
conventional formocresol-zinc oxide
eugenol pulpotomy for the treatment of
pulpally involved human primary teeth:
diode laser-mineral trioxide aggregate
pulpotomy. *International Journal of
Paediatric Dentistry*, **15**, 437–47.

Sari, S., Aras, S., Gunham, O. 1999. The effect
of physiological root resorption on the

histological structure of primary tooth pulp. *Journal of Clinical Pediatric Dentistry*, **23**, 221–5.

Shaw, D. W., Sheller, B., Barrus, B. D., Morton Jr., T. H. 1987. Electrosurgical pulpotomy – a 6-month study in primates. *Journal of Endodontics*, **13**, 500–5.

Shoji, S., Nakamura, M., Horiuchi, H. 1985. Histopathological changes in dental pulps irradiated by CO2 laser: a preliminary report on laser pulpotomy. *Journal of Endodontics*, **11**, 379–84.

Shulman, E. R., McIver, F. T. I., Burkes, E. J. 1987. Comparison of electrosurgery and formocresol as pulpotomy techniques in monkey primary teeth. *Pediatric Dentistry*, **9**, 189–94.

Smaïl-Faugeron, V., Courson, F., Durieux, P., Muller-Bolla, M., Glenny, A. M., Fron Chabouis, H. 2014. Pulp treatment for extensive decay in primary teeth. *Cochrane Database of Systematic Reviews*, **8**, CD003220.

Steffen, R., van Waes, H. 2009. Understanding mineral trioxide aggregate/Portland cement: a review of literature and background factors. *European Archives of Paediatric Dentistry*, **10**, 93–7.

Torabinejad, M., Chivian, N. 1999. Clinical applications of mineral trioxide aggregate. *Journal of Endodontics*, **25**, 197–205.

Torabinejad, M., McDonald, F., Pitt Ford, T. R. 1995. Physical and chemical properties of a new root-end filling material. *Journal of Endodontics*, **21**, 349–53.

Vargas, K., Packham, B., Lowman, D. 2006. Preliminary evaluation of sodium hypochlorite for pulpotomies in primary molars. *Pediatric Dentistry*, **28**, 511–17.

Vostatek, S., Kanellis, M., Weber-Gasparoni, K., Gregorsok, R. 2011. Sodium hypochlorite pulpotomies in primary teeth: a retrospective study. *Pediatric Dentistry*, **33**, 327–32.

Waterhouse, P. J., Nunn, J. H., Whitworth, J. M. 2000. An investigation of the relative efficacy of Buckley's formocresol and calcium hydroxide in primary molar vital pulp therapy. *British Dental Journal*, **188**, 32–6.

Yildirim, C., Basak, F., Akgun, O. M., Polat, G. G., Altun, C. 2016. Clinical and radiographic evaluation of the effectiveness of formocresol, mineral trioxide aggregate, Portland cement, and enamel matrix derivative in primary teeth pulpotomies: a two-year follow-up. *Journal of Clinical Pediatric Dentistry*, **40**(1), 14–20.

Zurn, D., Seale, N. S. 2008. Light-cured calcium hydroxide versus formocresol in human primary molar pulpotomies: a randomized controlled trial. *Pediatric Dentistry*, **30**(1), 34–41.

4.2

Pulpectomy of Deciduous Teeth

Klaus W. Neuhaus[1,2] and Jan Kühnisch[3]

[1] Clinic of Periodontology, Endodontology and Cariology, University Center for Dental Medicine Basel, University of Basel, Basel, Switzerland
[2] Private dental office, Herzogenbuchsee, Switzerland
[3] Department of Conservative Dentistry and Periodontology, Ludwig-Maximilians-University, Munich, Germany

Introduction

The majority of dental emergencies in paediatric clinics relate to dental caries, which have been reported to account for about three-quarters of all dental paediatric patients (Lygidakis et al., 1998; Wong et al., 2012). As outlined in Chapter 1.4, there may be a long history of pain in the patient, and care should be taken to support the diagnosis by listening carefully to what they or their parents/guardians have to say. Because at some point in the development of the dental arch the deciduous teeth fulfil the function of dental arch space maintenance for the succeeding permanent teeth (see Chapter 5.4), preservation of deciduous teeth with pulpectomy should be in the armamentarium of any dentist treating children. If no permanent successor is present at all, pulpectomy of deciduous molars is mandatory upon indication.

Indication of Pulpectomy

The main clinical indication of pulpectomy in deciduous teeth is caries sequelae: irreversible pulpitis, pulp necrosis or (a)symptomatic apical periodontitis. Further possible indications refer to dental trauma: crown fractures with pulp involvement or pulp necrosis after traumatic incidences. The goal of pulpectomy is to get rid of inflamed pulp and any bacteria that have already entered the root canal system. Sometimes, the decision to perform a pulpectomy is taken after the primary intention of performing a pulpotomy when bleeding from the root canal orifices cannot be controlled (see Chapter 4.1). Figure 4.2.1 shows such a case, where a pulpotomy was sufficient for the mesial root due to suspended bleeding, but pulpectomy was necessary in the distal root canal due to pulp necrosis.

A prerequisite before we can perform a pulpectomy in deciduous teeth is an intraoral radiograph of the complete tooth, including the apical area. Such a radiograph will show the presence or absence of the permanent successor, the degree of physiological or pathological root resorption and the developmental stage of the Foramen apicale, and it will allow for an initial working length (WL) estimation. It further shows a possible periapical osteolysis and the caries extension in relation to the pulp. If no radiograph can be taken in the young patient for whatever reason, a pulpectomy is contraindicated. Further contraindications are an incomplete root development with an open apex,

Management of Dental Emergencies in Children and Adolescents, First Edition.
Edited by Klaus W. Neuhaus and Adrian Lussi.
© 2019 John Wiley & Sons Ltd. Published 2019 by John Wiley & Sons Ltd.
Companion website: www.wiley.com/go/neuhaus/dental_emergencies

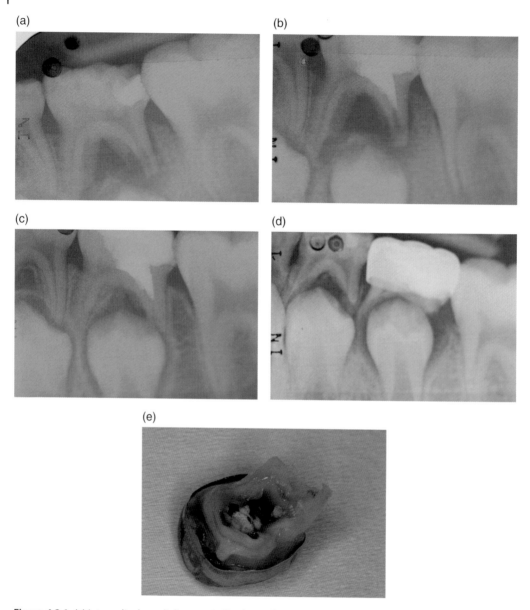

Figure 4.2.1 (a) Interradicular radiolucency indicating pulp necrosis after treatment of a deep caries lesion. (b) Because only the distal canal was necrotic, whilst the bleeding in the mesial canals stopped, the distal root received a pulpectomy (intracanal dressing: calcium hydroxide/iodoform paste), whilst the mesial portion of the pulp was treated with pulpotomy. (c) Healing of the interradicular lesion, control after 3 months. (d) Further healing after application of a stainless-steel crown. (e) Tooth after natural exfoliation. The "imperfect" crown margins are no problem for the gums. However, it is important to prevent reinfection of the root canal system, and in deciduous teeth a resorpbable root canal dressing must be applied.

physiological root resorption involving the apical endodont, internal and external pathological root resorptions, an apical unrestorable crown, increased tooth mobility and an expected natural exfoliation within the next year. Noncompliance of the patient is not per se a contraindication, because with sedative measures a pulpectomy might be performed nevertheless. In some countries, the prospective costs of treatment might also be a contraindication for pulpectomy in deciduous teeth. It should then be considered whether extraction in combination with a space maintainer should be preferred, perhaps with a stainless-steel crown as permanent restoration.

The placement of rubber dam is also mandatory for pulpectomy procedures in deciduous teeth, just as it is in permanent teeth, because it protects the patient against ingestion or inhalation of endodontic instruments or irrigation solutions, and the pulp space against (re)infection with oral bacteria. If no rubber dam or an equal isolation can be applied, pulpectomy should not be carried out. A buccal swelling per se is not a contraindication for pulpectomy, but it does require a critical consideration. Due to the anatomy of deciduous molars, a swelling occurs relatively early in the process of pulp nectrotisation (Figure 4.2.2) (Schaffner et al., 2012). In cases with short-term symptoms and a minimal periapical inflammation, joint decision-making between the dentist and the parents/guardians should be the foundation for treatment. In situations of an extensive osteolysis – especially with an involvement of the permanent tooth germ – extraction should be the treatment of choice.

One- versus Two-Visit Treatment

There has been a considerable debate over whether pulpectomy in permanent teeth should be completed in one or two visits. In children, the situation is simpler: their limited attention span results in limited compliance, so a one-visit treatment is preferable. If teeth receive pulpectomy due to irreversible pulpitis, the root canals will presumably be sterile, especially if the treatment itself is done under sterile conditions. It is then unproblematic to finalise the treatment in one session. If there is pulp necrosis and buccal or apical abscess and swelling, an effective disinfection of the root canal system is necessary. Fortunately, the obturation material is the same as the interappointment medicament. It is therefore also advisable to attempt a one-visit treatment in infected cases, and decide whether or not to reenter the root canals upon reevaluation after a few weeks (Moskovitz et al., 2005; Farokh-Gisour et al., 2018). Most often, the symptoms will be gone, and it will be safe simply to observe the tooth regularly.

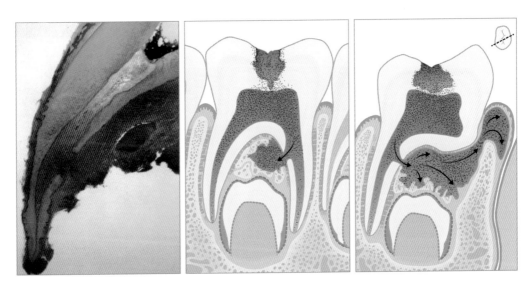

Figure 4.2.2 Deciduous teeth often have accessory lateral canals, which facilitate the spreading of infection in the interradicular area, as well as a buccal swelling at a relatively early stage.

Clinical Procedure

Local Anaesthesia

Local anaesthetics should be provided carefully (see Chapter 1.4). Even in cases where a complete pulp necrosis can be expected, a local anaesthesia helps calm the patient (and the dentist), and it anaesthetises the gums where the rubber dam clamp exerts pressure. It might also be practical to place an injection in the oral mucosa, preferably entering through the buccal papilla when buccal anaesthesia has been accomplished.

Isolation and Caries Removal

After rubber dam isolation, complete caries removal must be performed. If necessary, an adhesive preendodontic build-up is placed on clean dentine using a one-step adhesive system and a bulk-fill composite. This is tighter and more stable than conventional cements, and more durable than resin-modified glass ionomer cements (GICs). A preendodontic build-up is indicated where tooth substance loss through caries or trauma would result in considerable leakage during root canal irrigation (Figure 4.2.3). In highly inflamed pulps, local anaesthesia might be insufficient, and the young patient might suffer from persisting strong pain. In such cases, one should refrain from completing treatment in a single session, and a second visit is advocated, once the pulp is less acutely inflamed. In order to relieve the pain, placement of a cotton or foam pellet soaked with an antibiotic/

(a)　　　　　　　　(b)　　　　　　　　(c)

(d)　　　　　　　　(e)

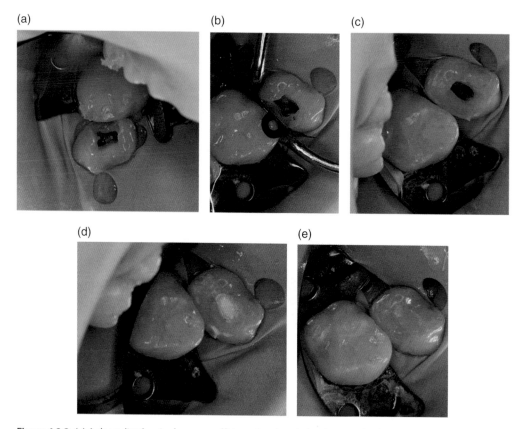

Figure 4.2.3 (a) A deep distal caries hampers efficient cleaning during intenend pulpectomy: there is no reservoir, and the rubber dam is not as tight as it should be. (b) Preparation of a preendodontic build-up: finalising caries excavation (leave no infected dentine behind!) and application of a sectional matrix. (c) Restoration of the distal wall with self-etch adhesive and bulk-fill composite. Especially in paediatric dentistry, time matters. Safe irrigation is now possible. (d) After application of Vitapex and Coltosol. (e) Temporary filling with GIC. If, after clinical and radiographic reevaluation, the tooth remains stable, a permanent restoration is required.

corticosteroid paste (e.g. Ledermix, Odontopaste) inside the pulp chamber might subdue the symptoms. The second appointment should be 1 week later, and the parents/guardians should be reminded that the treatment is not yet complete.

Shaping

Because the roots of deciduous molars can be resorbed by the succeeding permanent teeth at a much higher level than the radiographic apex (Figure 4.2.4), an arbitrary WL of around

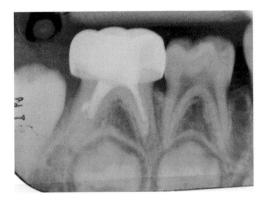

Figure 4.2.4 Only the upper two-thirds of the root canals of deciduous roots need instrumentation, in order to avoid complications with the permanent teeth.

two-thirds of the radiographic length should be aimed for. If it is radiographically safe, instrumentation up to 2 mm short of WL might be considered, although this increases the risk of strip perforation, especially in the roots of deciduous molars. Root canal instrumentation with simultaneous electronic length control further prevents unwanted preparation and is therefore strongly recommended in clinical practice. Pulpectomy of deciduous front teeth often does not require further enlargement of the root canal (Figure 4.2.5). Nevertheless, sometimes there is a need to enlarge the orifices in order to improve accessibility and instrumentation (Figure 4.2.6). Irrigation after pulp extraction should be sufficient. In deciduous molars, the root canal anatomy can be complex, including extremely curved roots (see Chapter 1.1), confluent root canals and accessory canals (Figure 4.2.7). Because the orifices of the root canals can be tiny, good magnification and good coaxial illumination are a tremendous support for the operating dentist. When using rotary instruments, the insertion of an orifice-shaping device as a single instrument is often appropriate (Figure 4.2.8). If no rotary instruments are used, 21 mm hand instruments should be applied in decreasing ISO

(a)

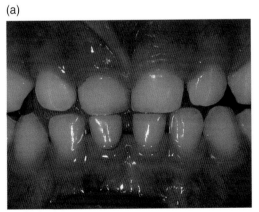

(b)

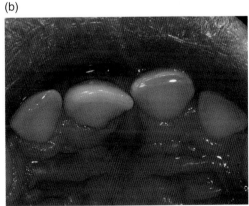

Figure 4.2.5 (a,b) Traumatic luxation of tooth 51 in a 5-year-old boy with loss of vitality due to disruption of the pulp at the apical endodont. (c) Preoperative apical radiograph showing no signs of physiological or pathological tooth resorption. (d,e) Aiming at maintaining the deciduous incisor reposition, splinting and pulpectomy was indicated and performed. (f,g) 0.5-year-follow-up revealed a symptom-free incisor, although the calcium hydroxide dissolved in the root canal. (h) An apical inflammation was diagnosed just before exfoliation around 3 years after initial treatment, which resulted in extraction of tooth 51.

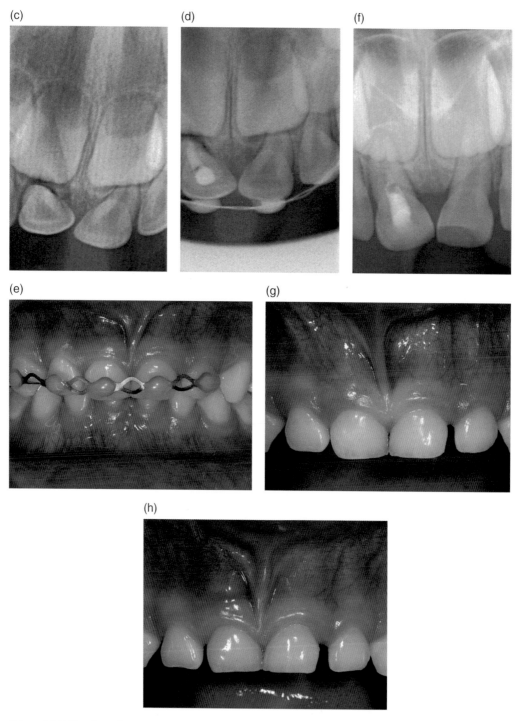

Figure 4.2.5 (Continued)

(a)

(b)

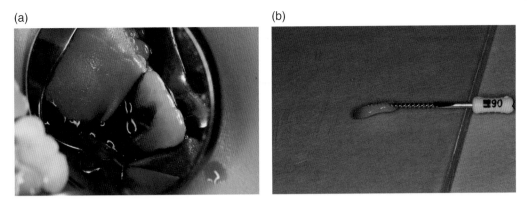

Figure 4.2.6 (a) Hyperaemia of a trauma tooth after trephination. Especially in young patients, the pulp space is wide, requiring a not-too-small trephination cavity that allows for (b) quick (manual) pulpectomy and prevents blocking of the needle during irrigation.

(a)

(b)

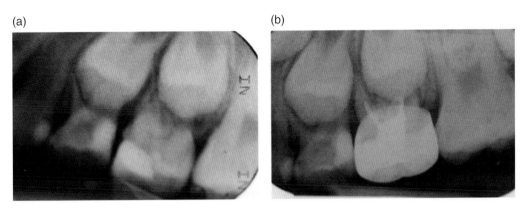

Figure 4.2.7 (a) Pain and swelling around tooth 65. Because tooth preservation was deemed critical at this stage, a pulpectomy was planned. (b) Irrigation with sodium hypochlorite was necessary to remove infected soft tissue. A C-shaped canal was cleaned and filled with Vitapex.

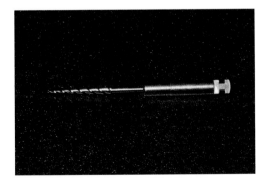

Figure 4.2.8 In deciduous endodontics, a crown-down technique is often advised. Short rotary instruments with a large taper save time because they can often be used as single instruments during root canal preparation.

sizes (40.02, 35.02, 30.02, 25.02) for the crown-down instrumentation, which often will be sufficient to reach the middle of the root. It should be remembered that it is not the shaping procedure that cleans the root canal system, but the irrigation procedure (Zehnder et al., 2003).

Disinfection

If a rubber dam is applied, irrigation is performed using sodium hypochlorite. Some dentists are afraid of using sodium hypochlorite in deciduous teeth because of complications occurring after unwanted extrusion of the irrigation solution. This cannot happen when the indication is warranted – closed apex – and the irrigation needle is thinner than the root canal. A 30G side-vented needle should be used, and blocking of the root canal with the needle must be avoided. The pressure of the tissue is greater than the pressure of the irrigation solution when the solution has a way to escape at the orifice. Even irrigation solutions with sonic (Neuhaus et al., 2016), ultrasonic (Basrani, 2011) or laser (Koch et al., 2016) systems can be activated without risking extrusion of the irrigation solution (see Chapter 3.2). Chlorhexidine solution is also an effective antibacterial agent, but it has no tissue-dissolving capacities (Zehnder et al., 2003). If chlorhexidine solution is used in the root canal, it must not mix with sodium hypochlorite because the two will immediately react, precipitating toxic chloric aniline.

Oburation/Intracanal Dressing

After drying the root canals with isometric sterile paper points, dressing is performed, preferably using a syringe system with a backfill technique. The material of choice in obturating deciduous root canals is calcium-hydroxide/iodoform paste. A clinical success rate of 100% at 6 months and 96% at 12 months has been described (Trairatvorakul and Chunlasikaiwan, 2008). Zinc oxide eugenol (ZOE)-based pastes can also be applied, but have somewhat lower success rates after 6 and 12 months (Trairatvorakul and Chunlasikaiwan, 2008). Both pastes are resorbable and radiopaque, and both fulfil their purpose as long-term root canal dressings up to exfoliation of the tooth. Calcium hydroxide products might also be used in clinical practice, but as aqueous solutions, these can dissolve more rapidly over time. Thus, silicone oil-based root canal filling materials are preferred. To date, there is no clear evidence from well-designed clinical trials to favour one root canal dressing over another, so the choice is a matter of clinician discretion (Smaïl-Faugeron et al.,

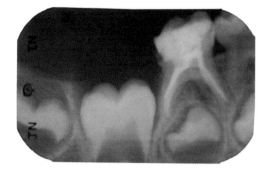

Figure 4.2.9 Apical protrusion of the root canal dressing due to condensation of cement at the pulp floor, despite the roots being instrumented only to the middle part.

2018). In order to separate the obturated root canals from the pulp chamber, a cement is condensed at the pulp chamber floor. This may contribute to some apical protrusion of the root canal paste, which is not unwanted (Figure 4.2.9).

Final Restoration

Reinfection through coronal leakage can best be prevented using adhesive fillings, or in the case of greater tooth substance loss, by cementation of stainless-steel crowns on top of a preferably adhesive build-up. The placement of costlier restorations should not be postponed; it should be done as soon as the clinical signs of inflammation have vanished (Moskovitz et al., 2005). A postoperative radiograph is mandatory.

Conclusion

Pulpectomy in the deciduous dentition is a complex and expensive means of treating teeth with extensive decay. If the cost–compliance–benefit estimation is in favour of maintaining the deciduous tooth, all precautions should be taken to safely disinfect the root canal system and prevent reentry of oral microorganisms. Tooth survival until exfoliation can then be expected.

References

Basrani, B. 2011. Irrigation in endodontic treatment. *Alpha Omegan*, **104**, 18–25.

Farokh-Gisour, E., Parirokh, M., Kheirmand Parizi, M., Nakhaee, N., Aminizadeh, M. 2018. Comparison of postoperative pain following one-visit and two-visit vital pulpectomy in primary teeth: a single-blind randomized clinical trial. *Iranian Endodontic Journal*, **13**, 13–19.

Koch, J. D., Jaramillo, D. E., Divito, E., Peters, O. A. 2016. Irrigant flow during photon-induced photoacoustic streaming (PIPS) using particle image velocimetry (PIV). *Clinical Oral Investigatons*, **20**, 381–6.

Lygidakis, N. A., Marinou, D., Katsaris, N. 1998. Analysis of dental emergencies presenting to a community paediatric dentistry centre. *International Journal of Paediatric Dentistry*, **8**, 181–90.

Moskovitz, M., Sammara, E., Holan, G. 2005. Success rate of root canal treatment in primary molars. *Journal of Dentistry*, **33**, 41–7.

Neuhaus, K. W., Liebi, M., Stauffacher, S., Eick, S., Lussi, A. 2016. Antibacterial efficacy of a new sonic irrigation device for root canal disinfection. *Journal of Endodontics*, **42**, 1799–803.

Schaffner, M., Neuhaus, K. W., Lussi, A. 2012. Endodontology in the primary dentition. In: Lussi, A., Schaffner, M. (eds.) *Advances in Restorative Dentistry*. Berlin: Quintessence.

Smaïl-Faugeron, V., Glenny, A. M., Courson, F., Durieux, P., Muller-Bolla, M., Fron Chabouis, H. 2018. Pulp treatment for extensive decay in primary teeth. *Cochrane Database of Systematic Reviews*, **5**, CD003220.

Trairatvorakul, C., Chunlasikaiwan, S. 2008. Success of pulpectomy with zinc oxide-eugenol vs calcium hydroxide/iodoform paste in primary molars: a clinical study. *Pediatric Dentistry*, **30**, 303–8.

Wong, N. H., Tran, C., Pukallus, M., Holcombe, T., Seow, W. K. 2012. A three-year retrospective study of emergency visits at an oral health clinic in south-east Queensland. *Australian Dental Journal*, **57**, 132–7.

Zehnder, M., Lehnert, B., Schönenberger, K., Waltimo, T. 2003. Irrigants and intracanal medicaments in endodontics. *Schweizerische Monatsschrift für Zahnmedizin*, **113**, 756–63.

4.3

Tooth Extraction

Hubertus van Waes

Clinic of Orthodontics and Pediatric Dentistry, Center of Dental Medicine, University of Zurich, Zurich, Switzerland

Introduction

Due to the limited value of deciduous teeth, the decision to extract them can be easier than in the permanent dentition. One should always keep in mind, however, that a deciduous tooth is important for food consumption, aesthetics and speech, and that it acts as a space maintainer for the permanent dentition. Loss of a deciduous tooth can therefore cause a variety of problems and create the need for further treatment to enable a normal development of the dentition. On the other hand, leaving an infected deciduous tooth in situ can harm the permanent successor. Accidental damage of the permanent tooth bud is always a factor when performing an extraction of a deciduous tooth. For that reason, it is generally not indicated to remove any granulation tissue after the extraction of a deciduous tooth. Once the origin of infection is eliminated, granulation tissue will disappear, so there is no need to put a tooth germ in danger by scraping in that area. The same is true for fistulas.

In the case of multiple extractions, such as in situations with early childhood caries, it can be useful to apply sutures or haemostatic sponges to eliminate the danger of postoperative bleeding, which can be dramatic and traumatising for the child. Extractions of molars with very divergent roots may result

in a widening of the alveolar bone and sometimes in the disruption of the soft tissues. In these cases, careful compression of the alveolae and sutures may be indicated (Figure 4.3.1).

Prior to each intervention, an x-ray of the tooth is necessary in order to evaluate the state and shape of root resorption and the topographic relation to the permanent successor. Depending on these findings, different approaches can be chosen, such as splitting a molar in a mesial and distal part.

Anchylosed molars pose a special challenge. Their roots are subject to replacement resorption with loss of the periodontal space and failure of vertical growth of the alveolar process in this area. These teeth can be far from the occlusal plane and can even be submerged under the gingiva, which makes it very difficult to grab them with extraction forceps and mobilise them. Due to the replacement resorption, it is very likely that root remnants will stay in place after an extraction. It has then to be decided whether they can be left behind or if their complete removal is necessary to allow orthodontic movement of neighbouring teeth. Usually, such remnants will be resorbed if a permanent tooth erupts in this area, but will resist resorption and remodelling in the case of orthodontic movements. In such a case, orthodontic movement of a tooth into the extraction site may be severely hampered.

Management of Dental Emergencies in Children and Adolescents, First Edition.
Edited by Klaus W. Neuhaus and Adrian Lussi.
© 2019 John Wiley & Sons Ltd. Published 2019 by John Wiley & Sons Ltd.
Companion website: www.wiley.com/go/neuhaus/dental_emergencies

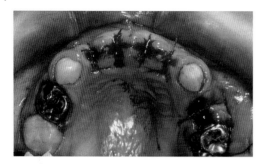

Figure 4.3.1 Resorbable sutures after multiple extractions in a small child treated under general anaesthesia.

Extraction of Incisors

Because of their anatomic shape, extraction of deciduous incisors is usually quite simple, involving a rotary movement with a forceps after cutting the superficial periodontal fibres. Because of the close proximity to their permanent successors, however, it is important not to move the crown too far labially, because this will result in a movement of the root tip to the palatal side, where the permanent tooth is located (Figure 4.3.2).

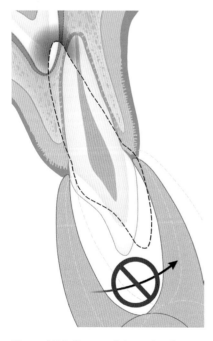

Figure 4.3.2 Danger of damaging the permanent tooth by excessive labial movement of the crown.

Extraction of Molars

Whilst the extraction of incisors is usually a quick and easy task, deciduous molars can be very difficult to extract (Van Waes, 2001). Especially in young patients with minor physiologic resorptions, the very long and often divergent roots can be difficult to luxate. Due to their relatively small diameter and curved shape, fractures of roots are very common.

Because molars with long or even anchylosed roots are so difficult to luxate, extreme care should be taken when using elevators placed between the deciduous molar and a freshly erupted and not yet fully grown permanent tooth. With the interdental force generated by the elevator, it is easy to unintentionally luxate the permanent neighbour instead of the deciduous molar (Figure 4.3.3).

Therefore, extractions of deciduous molars are usually performed by using a forceps and applying forces to move the tooth to buccal and lingual. The force should be applied for some time, in order to widen the alveolar socket and create room for the large and divergent roots to come out.

During the extraction of a deciduous molar, the germ of the permanent successor, which is often located between its curved roots, can be accidentally damaged or even extracted. This underlines the importance of

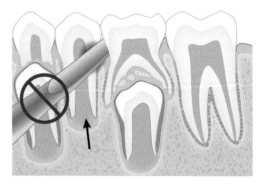

Figure 4.3.3 Elevators should not be used against a freshly erupted tooth, because it might be luxated instead of the target deciduous molar. Elevators should always be supported by bone.

a preoperative radiograph and a careful approach. Particularly in the lower jaw, it may be necessary to split a deciduous molar with a bur and then take out the mesial and distal parts separately (Figure 4.3.4). The cutting has to be done with care in cases where the permanent tooth is very close to the bifurcation of the deciduous molar. If the cut is not deep and large enough, luxation of the fragments may be difficult; if it is extended into the furcation area, the permanent tooth may be damaged (Figure 4.3.5).

This can also happen in cases with severely destroyed crowns, where special forceps which grab into the furcation of a molar are used because there is no bone above the permanent successor.

Extractions in Emergency Situations

Deciduous teeth with infected pulps (e.g. due to profound carious lesions) can be the origin of local abscesses or oedemas. Unlike in adults, incision is rarely necessary in the deciduous dentition and is unlikely to produce pus, because the visible and sometimes impressive swelling is primarily an oedema. In the case of an abscess, extraction of the deciduous tooth will solve the problem, because the source of infection is more superficial than in adults. In general, the extraction is technically easy, because the bone of children rapidly disappears due to inflammation and the teeth can become very mobile. The main concerns for the dentist are pain control and patient cooperation. In order to gain time, improve cooperation and improve conditions for local anaesthesia, prescription of antibiotics and pain killers may be indicated (American Academy of Pediatric Dentistry, 2017).

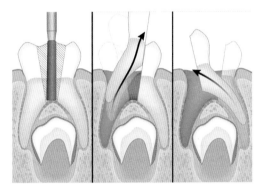

Figure 4.3.4 Schematic procedure of splitting a lower deciduous molar prior to extraction. The cut has to go all the way down to the furcation, without damaging the permanent tooth.

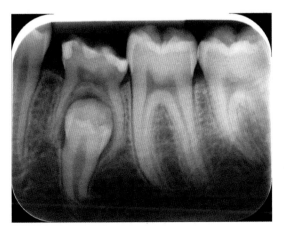
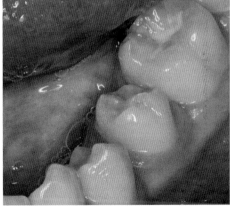

Figure 4.3.5 Radiograph of an ankylosed lower second deciduous molar. It was decided by the dentist to split the tooth by slicing it with a bur. After eruption of the successor, damage to the buccal cusp caused by the bur became evident.

References

American Academy of Pediatric Dentistry. 2017. Guideline on management considerations for pediatric oral surgery and oral pathology. *Pediatric Dentistry*, **39**(6), 279–88.

Van Waes, H. 2001. Chirurgie bei Kindern und Jugendlichen. In: Van Waes, H., Stöckli, P. (eds). *Kinderzahnmedizin, Farbatlanten der Zahnmedizin Bd 17*. Stuttgart: Thieme, pp. 227–52.

Unit 5

Management of Missing Teeth

5.1

Reconstructive Considerations: Temporary and Long-Term Treatment Options

Nicola U. Zitzmann and Nadja Rohr

Department of Reconstructive Dentistry, University Center for Dental Medicine Basel, University of Basel, Basel, Switzerland

Introduction

Tooth loss in the anterior region requires immediate replacement by a temporary or definitive restoration for aesthetic and functional reasons (Zitzmann et al., 2015b). Particularly in children and adolescents, anterior tooth loss usually occurs through accidents or from complications arising from previous trauma (e.g. external root resorption, ankylosis). The maxillary central incisors are the teeth most frequently affected by trauma (Andreasen, 1992; Borum and Andreasen, 2001). The second most common teeth to lose are the lateral incisors, which additionally show aplasia in 1–3% of the population (Kavadia et al., 2011; Andrade et al., 2013). Space closure with the patient's own tooth material is the treatment of choice, in order to avoid lifelong restorative needs.

Thorough diagnostics and treatment planning are required when autotransplantation or orthodontic space closure is considered. Due to the potential for complications with implant infraposition, particularly in the maxillary anterior region in young women and in patients with a hyperdivergent growth pattern, single-tooth implants should be postponed to mature adulthood (Zitzmann et al., 2015a). During this time, which is particularly critical when puberty is affected,

a noninvasive long-term temporary restoration should be planned, until an implant is indicated.

When orthodontic space closure is not indicated but orthodontic treatment is still required, denture teeth provided with a bracket can be easily included in the multi-band fixed appliance during this period. For anterior tooth replacement in young patients, resin-bonded fixed dental prostheses (FDPs) are preferable, which offer the possibility to rehabilitate the growing patient with a minimally invasive temporary, semipermanent or even definitive restoration. Further, a single crown with a cantilever or even an FDP ("three-unit bridge") can be considered, depending on the conditions of the adjacent teeth. With any reconstructive treatment applied in adolescence, the least invasive treatment option should be selected, since repeated treatment needs are likely during the patient's lifetime.

Treatment Plan for Managing Anterior Tooth Loss during Growth

When a permanent tooth is lost in the mixed dentition during adolescence, a thorough clinical examination must be performed,

Management of Dental Emergencies in Children and Adolescents, First Edition.
Edited by Klaus W. Neuhaus and Adrian Lussi.
© 2019 John Wiley & Sons Ltd. Published 2019 by John Wiley & Sons Ltd.
Companion website: www.wiley.com/go/neuhaus/dental_emergencies

Table 5.1.1 Factors evaluated during clinical examination and via panoramic radiograph.

Factor	Criteria	Clinical implication
Dentition and tooth development	Normal Aplasia in the affected jaw Premolars already extracted	Orthodontic space closure in normal mixed or permanent dentition; Space closure is not indicated if teeth are already missing in the affected jaw
Facial morphology and the skeletal situation	Orthognathic Prognatic Retrognatic	Orthodontic space closure restricted with retrogantic maxilla, but anterior space closure while opening a space in premolar region is considerable
Skeletal growth	Normal/mesocephal Hyperdivergent Hypodivergent	Postpone implant treatment with hyperdivergent growth pattern (Zitzmann et al. 2015a)
Dental morphology of maxillary incisors and canines	Matching form, contour and colour Great differences in colour and shape	Consider potential of transformation of lateral incisors into centrals or of canines into lateral incisors with composite fillings as required after orthodontic space closure (Stenvik and Zachrisson, 1993; Czochrowska et al., 2003; Zachrisson, 2007)

supplemented by a panoramic radiograph to evaluate potential aplasia (Table 5.1.1).

When mesialisation of the entire dentition is not feasible or not indicated (e.g. with retrognathic maxilla or aplasia of premolars), space closure can be achieved in the anterior whilst space is opened for a single-tooth implant in the area of the first or second premolar, where the potential for implant infrapositioning is less critical (Zachrisson, 2006). When neither autotransplantation nor orthodontic space closure is indicated, the single-tooth gap has to be maintained with some sort of restoration, so that migration of the adjacent teeth into the space can be avoided (Zitzmann et al., 2015b).

Reconstructive Treatment Options

Resin-bonded restorations facilitate a minimally invasive treatment option that allows re-treatment during adulthood or delay of implant placement to an older age (Zitzmann et al., 2010, 2015a; Kern and Sasse, 2011; Kern, 2017). One must be aware that any reconstructive treatment in the aesthetic zone in adolescents is likely to require re-treatment, particularly due to changes from gingival maturation with 1–2 mm recession in young adults (Hujoel et al. 2005).

1) Short-term provisionals can be fabricated chairside using the coronal tooth portion of the extracted tooth (Figure 5.1.1a–d), a denture tooth or a composite build-up in combination with a glass-fibre reinforcement adhesively fixed at the mesial and/or distal (Figure 5.1.2a–f) adjacent teeth (van Heumen et al., 2009). Fibre-reinforced composite resin-bonded restorations show limited indication as long-term provisionals, due to reduced survival rates of 73% after 4.5 years (van Heumen et al., 2009), or 90% after 4 years in patients with a history of periodontal disease (Li et al., 2016). The simplest design for an indirect resin-bonded provisional is the Rochette type, with a coarse perforated metal reinforcement cemented to the adjacent teeth without any preparation (Figure 5.1.3a,b) (Rochette, 1973).

2) Due to achievements in adhesive cementation techniques, metal-reinforced or full-ceramic resin-bonded restorations are used as long-term provisionals or

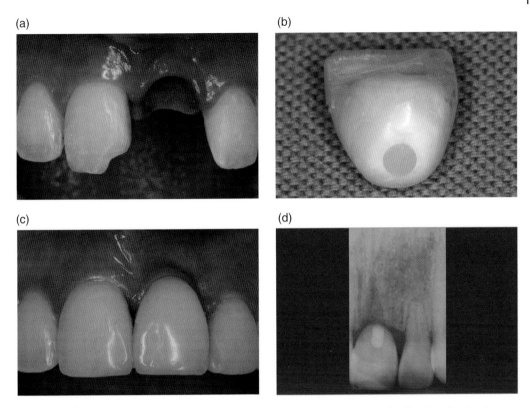

Figure 5.1.1 (a–d) Short-term provisional adhesive restoration with patient's tooth adhesively fixed at the adjacent tooth. *Source:* Courtesy of Prof. Dr. Gabriel Krastl.

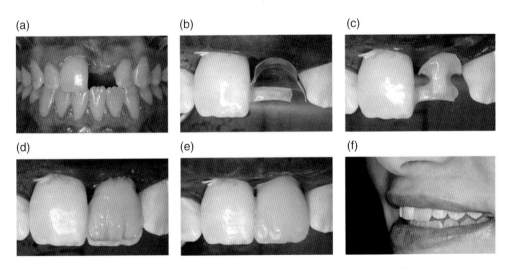

Figure 5.1.2 (a–f) Short-term provisional adhesive restoration with a glass-fibre reinforcement and composite build-up. *Source:* Courtesy of Prof. Dr. Gabriel Krastl.

(a) (b)

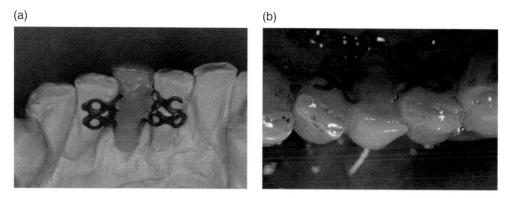

Figure 5.1.3 (a,b) Rochette-type adhesive restoration.

(a) (b) (c) (d)

(e) (f) (g) (h)

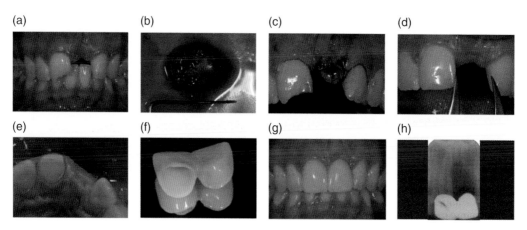

Figure 5.1.4 (a–h) Situation with reduced space width (area 21) and coronal fracture of tooth 11, ridge augmentation with connective tissue graft, minimal crown preparation and veneered zirconia cantilevered restoration.

even as permanent solutions. For these indirect restorations fabricated by the dental technician, a minimally invasive preparation is indicated, comprising removal of undercuts, a defined finishing line and a palatal rest that facilitates clear final positioning during the cementation procedure. In addition to cement adhesion, metal frameworks allow a retentive preparation with thin grooves and pins, which cannot be reproduced in ceramics.

3) When the adjacent tooth is discoloured or requires changes in form and contour, or the space width has decreased whilst orthodontic realignment is refused, a cantilevered single crown may be considered (Figure 5.1.4a–h).

4) Root canal-treated adjacent teeth may indicate a conventional three-unit FDP (e.g. with full-ceramic and adhesive cementation), allowing for minimal preparation and preservation of the coronal tooth structure (Figure 5.1.5a–f).

Design and Material Selection of Resin-Bonded Restorations

For resin-bonded FDPs, metal or ceramic frameworks can be used, veneered with feldspar ceramic. Metal resin-bonded FDPs can be designed with one or two wings (single or

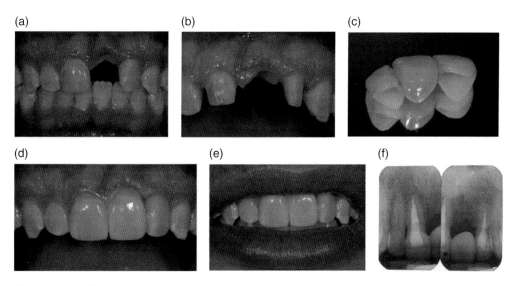

Figure 5.1.5 (a–f) 18-year-old patient (trauma experienced at age 8) with missing tooth 21 and extended root canal treatment at adjacent teeth, lithium disilicate FDP.

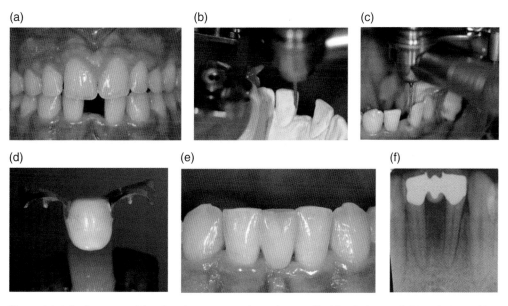

Figure 5.1.6 (a–f) 15-year-old patient (trauma experienced at age 8) with missing teeth 31 and 41, requiring retention after orthodontic treatment, diagnostic and intraoral preparation of guiding grooves with Parallel-A-Prep and metal-reinforced resin-bonded FDP.

double retainers), with retention at a mesial or distal abutment tooth (Figure 5.1.6a–f). They can replace one or more missing teeth with up to four pontics (i.e. when the lower incisors have to be replaced and the canines serve as abutments, Table 5.1.2) (Zitzmann

et al., 2015b). A retentive preparation facilitates retention of the metal resin-bonded FDP in addition to the adhesive cementation and can be particularly indicated when the enamel structure on the lingual surface of the abutment tooth is compromised (e.g. in

Table 5.1.2 Options and indications for one- and two-wing metal or full ceramic resin-bonded FDPs.

Location	Number of pontics/teeth to be replaced	Number of abutments (one or two wings)	Material	Indications
Anterior	1	1	Full ceramics[a]	Short- or long-term, clearance of 0.7-1.0mm required
		1 or 2	Metal	Long-term, clearance of 0.3-0.5mm required, retentive preparation feasible while enamel layer may be compromised. Fullfills splinting requirement (e.g. after orthodontic tooth movements)
	2	2	Metal	Long-term, stable splinting
		2 × 1-wing	Full ceramics[a]	Short- or long-term, sufficient clearance
	3–4	2	Metal	Lower central incisors
Posterior	1	2	Metal	
			Zirconia	Not routinely

[a] Lithium disilicate or zirconia.
Source: Modified from Zitzmann et al. (2015b).

elderly patients). The preparation should ideally be performed with an intraoral parallelometer (Parallel-A-Prep, Dentatus, USA). This involves the establishment of parallel walls to house the parallel guiding grooves, the elimination of undercuts to make use of the entire enamel surface, the preparation of grooves to facilitate a retention and resistance form against bucco-oral forces, an occlusal/palatal rest and sufficient palatal clearance (Marinello et al., 1991).

For the application of an intraoral parallelometer, a diagnostic preparation on a situation cast is recommended, in order to select a similar path of insertion for the preparation of the parallel guiding grooves. These grooves have to be positioned and aligned so that they are surrounded by the metal framework and are not visible from the labial aspect, their incisal end is aligned to the palatal, in order not to end too closely at the incisal edge and the incisal third of the abutment tooth can be kept free from any metal coverage. During the provisional period, up until the final restoration is fabricated, the grooves can be covered with white gutta-percha (DeTrey Dentsply, Konstanz,

Germany). For metal resin-bonded FDPs, precious and nonprecious alloys (chrome-moly) can be used. These require waxing on investment models to facilitate casting of the thin pins and grooves. Whilst precious alloys allow the use of conventional ceramic materials, nonprecious alloys facilitate thin attachments and small connectors due to their high elastic modulus, but necessitate the use of a gold layer to cover the discoloured oxide surface before ceramic veneering.

Early studies documented reduced survival rates for resin-bonded FDPs, with 88% survival after 5 years and loss of retention in 19% of restorations (Pjetursson et al., 2008). Applying a retentive preparation, however, provided better results than the nonretentive design, so that a survival rate of 95% was achieved after 10 years (Rammelsberg et al., 1993; Behr et al., 1998). According to a recent review, no difference was found in the debonding rate of two versus three-unit adhesive metal restorations (Wei et al., 2016), but two-unit metal restoration was preferable to three-unit FDP in restoring maxillary incisors (Botelho et al., 2016).

Full-ceramic restorations are pressed or milled and made from lithium disilicate ceramics (IPS e.max Press/IPS e.max CAD; Ivoclar Vivadent, Schaan, Liechtenstein), glass-infiltrated aluminiumoxide (In-Ceram Alumina; Vita, Bad Säckingen, Germany) or zirconia (e.g. LAVA; 3M ESPE, St Paul, MN, USA). Since these materials do not allow the replication of thin grooves or pins, fixation relies solely on the adhesion of the resin composite cement material to sound enamel (Figure 5.1.7a–f). The preparation comprises removal of undercuts with a slight approximal wrap-around, delineation of a clear marginal demarcation line and a cingulum rest to enable exact positioning during the cementation procedure. To ensure accurate positioning during cementation, a splint resting on the adjacent teeth can be prepared using flowable light-curing composite resin (Stimmelmayr et al., 2016). A palatal clearance of 0.7 mm is required for zirconia, and at least 1 mm is needed for lithium disilicate. These requirements may interfere with the need for a sound enamel structure along the entire lingual surface, since only 0.5 mm enamel thickness is present in this area (Atsu et al., 2005), and adhesion to dentin is reduced (Özcan and Mese, 2012).

Given this discrepancy, a deep bite situation may be an indicator against full-ceramic attachments, whilst metal – particularly nonprecious alloys – can be designed with thinner layers of 0.3–0.5 mm thickness. The indication for lithium disilicate is restricted to anterior tooth replacement, due to its limited fracture resistance and the dimensions required for the connector, which should measure at least 8 mm^2. For zirconia resin-bonded FDP, a connector surface of 6–8 mm^2 has been recommended.

Whilst two-wing full-ceramic resin-bonded FDPs (In-Ceram) had a survival rate of 74% at 10 years, 94% survival was achieved with one-wing restorations (Kern and Sasse, 2011). Failures with two-wing restorations were related to fractures in the connector region at one side, and restorations were kept as one-wing resin-bonded FDPs (Kern and Sasse, 2011; Wei et al., 2016; Kern, 2017). To avoid excessive load from the lever arm in one-wing restorations, occlusal and functional contacts at the cantilever should be minimised. Ceramic chippings, but no fractures or debonding, were reported with lithium disilicate one-wing resin-bonded FDPs, which were mainly inserted in the anterior region with large connector sizes of 16 mm^2

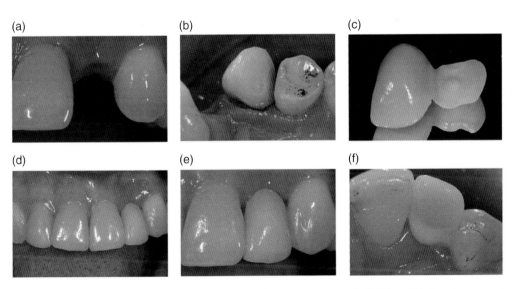

(a) (b) (c)

(d) (e) (f)

Figure 5.1.7 (a–f) 22-year-old patient showing minimal preparation at tooth 23 (11 and 21 already crowned). Lithium disilicate one-wing restoration was used, with no occlusal or functional contact on cantilever.

(Sailer et al., 2013). With zirconia one-wing resin-bonded FDP, early debonding occurred in 2 out of 15 restorations, which were successfully recemented, providing 100% survival after 4 years (mean 53 months) (Sailer and Hämmerle, 2014). Knowing that the position of the dentition is not completely stable even in adults and even with healthy periodontal conditions, the approximal contact area between the cantilever and the adjacent tooth should be enlarged.

Adhesive Cementation of Resin-Bonded FDPs

The improvements in the long-term results of resin-bonded FDPs are mainly related to new technologies in the cementation process (Zitzmann et al., 2015b). The adhesion obtained relies both on micromechanical retention and on chemical interaction of specific monomers with the bonding substrate. Resin composite cement systems containing 10-methacryloyloxydecyl dihydrogen phosphate (MDP) are thereby preferable (i.e. Panavia F2.0 or V5 (Kuraray, Kurashiki, Japan) or RelyX Ultimate (3M ESPE)). Certainly, opaque cement materials have to be selected for any metal restoration to avoid any grey shine-through and discolouration, whilst tooth-coloured cements are used for full-ceramic restorations. On the tooth surface, the best mechanical retention can be achieved following etching of the enamel surface with phosphoric acid (35–37% for 30–60 seconds), and any subsequent contact with saliva has to be avoided. Irrespective of the restoration material used, cleaning and degreasing of the surfaces should be performed after the final try-in using chloroform or isopropanol with cotton pellets (Table 5.1.3) (Zitzmann et al., 2015b; Rohr and Fischer, 2017).

Zirconia is a polycrystalline ceramic material that is free of silica and hence presents inferior adhesion to resin-based cements as compared to its glass-ceramic or metallic framework counterparts (Özcan and Vallittu,

2003). Both zirconia and metal alloy frameworks require previous surface conditioning for adequate adhesion (Rohr et al., 2017). Air abrasion is commonly recommended to produce a microretentive surface. Amongst the different abrasives used for airborne particle abrasion, the so-called tribochemical silica coating provides the most durable results. This involves sandblasting with 30 μm silica-coated aluminiumoxide particles and then applying a silane coupling agent (Kern and Thompson, 1993; Özcan et al., 2008a, 2008b). The airborne particle abrasion is applied either chairside (e.g. CoJet; 3M ESPE) or with relevant laboratory facilities (Rocatec soft; 3M ESPE). This silicatisation process not only roughens the surface, but also leaves a silica layer on the restoration surface, which may facilitate a chemical bond to the resin composite cement through the corresponding silane containing primer. The primers used for zirconia are commonly based on γ-methacryloxypropyltrimethoxysilane (MPS), MDP or a combination of the two, and create covalent bonds between the crystalline ceramics and the resin composite cement. In addition, some primers also contain methacrylate monomers, fillers and solvents, which affect their wettability properties (Inokoshi et al., 2014).

For high precious alloys lacking a superficial layer of metal oxides, the adhesion mechanism relies mainly on the chemical interaction between the resin composite cement and the silane coupling agent after tribochemical silica coating of the restoration surface. As an alternative means of bonding to noble metals, dedicated metal primers containing thiophosphoric methacrylates are available. The mechanisms of adhesion then depend on a chemical interaction of the organic sulphur compounds and noble metal elements (Ikemura et al., 2012).

Adhesion to glass matrix ceramics such as lithium disilicate is well established. Hydrofluoric acid (HF) removes the glass matrix selectively and exposes the crystalline ceramic structure, producing a microretentive surface. Unlike with conventional glass

Table 5.1.3 Cementation of metal and full-ceramic resin-bonded FDPs. *Source:* Modified from Zitzmann et al. (2015b).

Restoration material	Resin composite cement	Cleaning/microretention at restoration (after try-in)	Conditioning of restoration	Pretreatment of enamel
General procedure		Cleaning and degreasing (chloroform, isopropanol) Surface roughening and modification Water spray or ultrasonic bath and air dry		Enamel etching (phosphoric acid 35–37%, 30–60 sec.)
Zirconia	MDP containing resin composite cement system (e.g. Panavia V5, RelyX Ultimate)	Airborne particle abrasion with alumina particles, optionally coated with silica (e.g. Cojet 30 μm or Siljet 30 μm)	Ceramic primer containing MDP and silane coupling agent (e.g. Clearfil Ceramic Primer plus, Scotchbond Universal Adhesive)	Bonding agent (e.g. Panavia V5 tooth primer, Scotchbond Universal Adhesive)
Lithium disilicate glass ceramics (etchable)	MDP containing resin composite cement system (e.g. Panavia V5, RelyX Ultimate) or Conventional BIS-GMA-based resin composite cement (e.g. Variolink II Esthetic)	Hydrofluoric acid etching (e.g. 5%, 20 sec.)	Silane coupling agent (e.g. Clearfil Ceramic primer plus, Scotchbond Universal Adhesive, Monobond Plus)	Bonding agent (e.g. Panavia V5 tooth primer, Scotchbond Universal Adhesive, Syntac Classic)
High-precious or nonprecious (chrom-moly) alloys	MDP containing resin composite cement system (e.g. Panavia V5, RelyX Ultimate)	Airborne particle abrasion with alumina particles, optionally coated with silica (e.g. Cojet 30 μm or Siljet 30 μm)	Coupling agent (e.g. alloy primer, Scotchbond Universal Adhesive)	Bonding agent (e.g. Panavia V5 tooth primer, Scotchbond Universal Adhesive)
Fibre-reinforced composites	MDP containing resin composite cement system (e.g. Panavia V5, RelyX Ultimate) or Conventional BIS-GMA-based resin composite cement (e.g. Variolink II Esthetic)	Airborne particle abrasion with alumina particles, optionally coated with silica (e.g. Cojet 30 μm or Siljet 30 μm)	Silane coupling agent (e.g. Clearfil Ceramic Primer Plus, Scotchbond Universal Adhesive, Monobond Plus)	Bonding agent (e.g. Panavia V5 tooth primer, Scotchbond Universal Adhesive, Syntac Classic)

MDP, 10-methacryloyloxydecyl dihydrogen phosphate.

ceramics, it is recommended to reduce the etching time to 20 seconds (4.9% HF gel) for lithium disilicate ceramic. Again, a ceramic primer containing silane is used to increase wettability and to promote chemical bonding to the silica surface.

To simplify the cementation procedure and, simultaneously, create a reliable adhesion to different restorative materials, universal primers have been introduced which combine silane methacrylates and phosphoric methacrylates (e.g. Clearfil Ceramic Primer Plus, Kuraray), and possibly also thiophosphoric methacrylates (e.g. Monobond Plus, Ivoclar Vivadent) (Attia and Kern, 2011). As an additional step towards simplification, a universal adhesive (Scotchbond Universal, 3M ESPE) has been introduced, in which the same monomer is applied on the restoration and the hard-tissue surfaces. However, data on the effectiveness of this approach are scarce.

After accomplishing the microretentive surface on the inner aspects of the attachments, the resin-bonded FDP is cleaned using water spray or an ultrasonic bath and dried with pressurised air. For the final conditioning, the corresponding primer is applied to the restoration and the etched enamel surface, and the resin composite cement is applied (Table 5.1.3). The polymerisation of dual-cured resin composite cement is catalysed by a chemical (peroxide)- and a light (e.g. Camphorquinone)-activated initiator. The polymerisation reaction starts with the mixing of base and catalyst paste, activating the chemical initiator. Hence, the processing time is limited. Light initiation allows the polymerisation reaction to be advanced at the time the restoration is correctly placed and any cement excess is removed. When metal frameworks are used and the interface on the labial aspect is slightly visible after cementation, this area can be covered by a thin layer of composite resin, applied after the cement excess has been removed and the surface has been etched and bonded as for a conventional filling (Figure 5.1.6d).

Conclusion

New technologies in adhesive cementation have facilitated improved long-term data for resin-bonded FDPs, which can be applied as an interim or final treatment option. Whilst one-wing full-ceramic resin-bonded FDPs are preferably used to replace a single missing anterior tooth, metal-ceramic resin-bonded FDPs with one or two wings can be used to replace one or more teeth, particularly when retention is required in addition to the adhesive cementation.

Acknowledgements

The authors would like to thank the master dental technicians Alwin Schönenberger, Zürich and Clemens Gessner, Basel for the restorative work.

References

Andrade, D. C., Loureiro, C. A., Araujo, V. E., Riera, R., Atallah, A. N. 2013. Treatment for agenesis of maxillary lateral incisors: a systematic review. *Orthodontics & Craniofacial Research*, **16**, 129–36.

Andreasen, J. O. 1992. *Atlas of Replantation and Transplantation of Teeth*. Philadelphia, PA: Saunders.

Atsu, S. S., Aka, P. S., Kucukesmen, H. C., Kilicarslan, M. A., Atakan, C. 2005. Age-related changes in tooth enamel as measured by electron microscopy: implications for porcelain laminate veneers. *Journal of Prosthetic Dentistry*, **94**, 336–41.

Attia, A., Kern, M. 2011. Long-term resin bonding to zirconia ceramic with a new universal primer. *Journal of Prosthetic Dentistry*, **106**, 319–27.

Behr, M., Leibrock, A., Stich, W., Rammelsberg, P., Rosentritt, M., Handel, G. 1998. Adhesive-fixed partial dentures in anterior and posterior areas. Results of an on-going prospective study begun in 1985. *Clinical Oral Investigations*, **2**, 31–5.

Borum, M. K., Andreasen, J. O. 2001. Therapeutic and economic implications of traumatic dental injuries in Denmark: an estimate based on 7549 patients treated at a major trauma centre. *International Journal of Paediatric Dentistry*, **11**, 249–58.

Botelho, M. G., Chan, A. W., Leung, N. C., Lam, W. Y. 2016. Long-term evaluation of cantilevered versus fixed-fixed resin-bonded fixed partial dentures for missing maxillary incisors. *Journal of Dentistry*, **45**, 59–66.

Czochrowska E. M., Skaare A. B., Stenvik A., Zachrisson B. U. 2003 Outcome of orthodontic space closure with a missing maxillary central incisor. *American Journal of Orthodontics and Dentofacial Orthopedics*, **123**, 597–603.

Hujoel PP, Cunha-Cruz J, Selipsky H, Saver BG. Abnormal pocket depth and gingival recession as distinct phenotypes. Periodontology 2000, Vol. 39, 2005, 22–29.

Ikemura, K., Endo, T., Kadoma, Y. 2012. A review of the developments of multi-purpose primers and adhesives comprising novel dithiooctanoate monomers and phosphonic acid monomers. *Dental Materials Journal*, **31**, 1–25.

Inokoshi, M., Poitevin, A., De Munck, J., Minakuchi, S., Van Meerbeek, B. 2014. Bonding effectiveness to different chemically pre-treated dental zirconia. *Clinical Oral Investigations*, **18**, 1803–12.

Kavadia, S., Papadiochou, S., Papadiochos, I., Zafiriadis, L. 2011. Agenesis of maxillary lateral incisors: a global overview of the clinical problem. *Orthodontics: The Art and Practice of Dentofacial Enhancement*, **12**, 296–317.

Kern, M. 2017. Fifteen-year survival of anterior all-ceramic cantilever resin-bonded fixed dental prostheses. *Journal of Dentistry*, **56**, 133–5.

Kern, M., Sasse, M. 2011. Ten-year survival of anterior all-ceramic resin-bonded fixed dental prostheses. *Journal of Adhesive Dentistry*, **13**, 407–10.

Kern, M., Thompson, V. P. 1993. Sandblasting and silica-coating of dental alloys: volume loss, morphology and changes in the surface composition. *Dental Materials*, **9**, 151–61.

Li, J., Jiang, T., Lv, P., Fang, X., Xiao, Z., Jia, L. 2016. Four-year clinical evaluation of GFRC-RBFPDs as periodontal splints to replace lost anterior teeth. *International Journal of Prosthodontics*, **29**, 522–7.

Marinello, C. P., Soom, U., Schärer, P. 1991. Tooth preparation in adhesive dentistry. *Dentistry Today*, **10**(8), 46, 48–51.

Özcan, M., Mese, A. 2012. Adhesion of conventional and simplified resin-based luting cements to superficial and deep dentin. *Clinical Oral Investigations*, **16**, 1081–8.

Özcan, M., Vallittu, P. K. 2003. Effect of surface conditioning methods on the bond strength of luting cement to ceramics. *Dental Materials*, **19**, 725–31.

Özcan, M., Kerkdijk, S., Valandro, L. F. 2008a. Comparison of resin cement adhesion to Y-TZP ceramic following manufacturers' instructions of the cements only. *Clinical Oral Investigations*, **12**, 279–82.

Özcan, M., Nijhuis, H., Valandro, L. F. 2008b. Effect of various surface conditioning methods on the adhesion of dual-cure resin cement with MDP functional monomer to zirconia after thermal aging. *Dental Materials Journal*, **27**, 99–104.

Pjetursson, B. E., Tan, W. C., Tan, K., Brägger, U., Zwahlen, M., Lang, N. P. 2008. A systematic review of the survival and complication rates of resin-bonded bridges after an observation period of at least 5 years. *Clinical Oral Implants Research*, **19**, 131–41.

Rammelsberg, P., Pospiech, P., Gernet, W. 1993. Clinical factors affecting adhesive fixed partial dentures: a 6-year study. *Journal of Prosthetic Dentistry*, **70**, 300–7.

Rochette, A. L. 1973. Attachment of a splint to enamel of lower anterior teeth. *Journal of Prosthetic Dentistry*, **30**, 418–23.

Rohr, N., Fischer, J. 2017. Tooth surface treatment strategies for adhesive cementation. *Journal of Advanced Prosthodontics*, **9**, 85–92.

Rohr, N., Brunner, S., Martin, S., Fischer, J. 2017. Influence of cement type and ceramic primer on retention of polymer-infiltrated ceramic crowns to a one-piece zirconia implant. *Journal of Prosthetic Dentistry*, **119**(1), 138–45.

Sailer, I., Hämmerle, C. H. 2014. Zirconia ceramic single-retainer resin-bonded fixed dental prostheses (RBFDPs) after 4 years of clinical service: a retrospective clinical and volumetric study. *International Journal of Periodontics & Restorative Dentistry*, **34**, 333–43.

Sailer, I., Bonani, T., Brodbeck, U., Hämmerle, C. H. 2013. Retrospective clinical study of single-retainer cantilever anterior and posterior glass-ceramic resin-bonded fixed dental prostheses at a mean follow-up of 6 years. *International Journal of Prosthodontics*, **26**, 443–50.

Stenvik, A., Zachrisson, B. U. 1993. Orthodontic closure and transplantation in the treatment of missing anterior teeth. *An overview. Endodontics & Dental Traumatology*, **9**, 45–52.

Stimmelmayr, M., Stangl, M., Kremzow-Stangl, J., Krennmair, G., Beuer, F., Edelhoff, D., Guth, J. F. 2016. Precise placement of single-retainer resin-bonded fixed dental prostheses with an innovative splint design. *Journal of Prosthodontics*, **26**(5), 359–63.

van Heumen, C. C., Kreulen, C. M., Creugers, N. H. 2009. Clinical studies of fiber-reinforced resin-bonded fixed partial dentures: a systematic review. *European Journal of Oral Sciences*, **117**, 1–6.

Wei, Y. R., Wang, X. D., Zhang, Q., Li, X. X., Blatz, M. B., Jian, Y. T., Zhao, K. 2016. Clinical performance of anterior resin-bonded fixed dental prostheses with different framework designs: a systematic review and meta-analysis. *Journal of Dentistry*, **47**, 1–7.

Zachrisson, B. U. 2006. Single implant-supported crowns in the anterior maxilla – potential esthetic long-term (>5 years) problems. *World Journal of Orthodontics*, **7**, 306–12.

Zachrisson, B. U. 2007. Improving the esthetic outcome of canine substitution for missing maxillary lateral incisors. *World Journal of Orthodontics*, **8**, 72–9.

Zitzmann, N. U., Krastl, G., Hecker, H., Walter, C., Waltimo, T., Weiger, R. 2010. Strategic considerations in treatment planning: deciding when to treat, extract or replace a questionable tooth. *Journal of Prosthetic Dentistry*, **104**, 80–91.

Zitzmann, N. U., Arnold, D., Ball, J., Brusco, D., Triaca, A., Verna, C. 2015a. Treatment strategies for infraoccluded dental implants. *Journal of Prosthetic Dentistry*, **113**, 169–74.

Zitzmann, N. U., Özcan, M., Scherrer, S. S., Bühler, J. M., Weiger, R., Krastl, G. 2015b. Resin-bonded restorations: a strategy for managing anterior tooth loss in adolescence. *Journal of Prosthetic Dentistry*, **113**, 270–6.

5.2

Management of Avulsed Teeth

Andrea Zürcher and Andreas Filippi

Department of Oral Surgery and Center of Dental Traumatology, University Center for Dental Medicine Basel, University of Basel, Basel, Switzerland

Introduction

While avulsed teeth in the primary dentition are usually not replanted (Filippi and Krastl, 2007; Andersson et al., 2012), children and adolescents in the permanent dentition often lack alternatives to tooth preservation. Therefore, avulsed permanent teeth should be replanted, even if the prognosis is not always ideal (Andersson et al., 2012).

In a dental trauma, the anterior teeth of the maxilla are predominantly affected (von Arx et al., 2000). The crown fracture is the most common injury in the permanent dentition (Filippi and Krastl, 2007), an avulsion is observed in 0.5-3% of the cases (Glendor et al., 1996; Andreasen and Andreasen, 2007). In the case of an avulsion, the tooth completely leaves the alveolus disrupting its periodontal ligament together with the pulp. Possible concomitant injuries may affect the bone and soft tissue as well as tooth fractures (Andreasen and Andreasen, 2007).

While trauma associated tooth loosening, lateral dislocation and extrusion do not always occur in combination with the pulp being torn off and larger periodontal defects, the need for periodontal and pulpal treatment is highest in cases of avulsion and intrusion (Andreasen and Andreasen, 2007). In contrast to an intrusion, the periodontal prognosis of an avulsed tooth is decided by the rescue chain of the tooth where the accident took place (von Arx et al., 2000; Filippi, 2009b; Andersson et al., 2012). Unphysiological storage, dehydration, disinfection or cleaning of the root surface all irreversibly destroy the periodontal cells on the root surface (cementoblasts, periodontal fibroblasts) (Pongsiri et al., 1990). The tooth is subsequently lost through a replacement root resorption (Andreasen et al., 1995b; Andersson and Malmgren, 1999; Kawanami et al., 1999; Filippi et al., 2000b). In addition to the rescue chain of the tooth, survival of the pulp also correlates with the diameter of the apical foramen (Andreasen et al., 1995a). If this is clearly smaller than 2 mm, revascularization is not possible and an early endodontic intervention is required.

In contrast to some other dental accidents, the avulsion of permanent teeth should be considered a dental emergency that needs immediate attention and treatment (Andersson et al., 2012).

Terminology

The avulsion is classified as one of the accidental dislocation injuries of the teeth and describes the complete loss of the periodontal anchorage.

Management of Dental Emergencies in Children and Adolescents, First Edition.
Edited by Klaus W. Neuhaus and Adrian Lussi.
© 2019 John Wiley & Sons Ltd. Published 2019 by John Wiley & Sons Ltd.
Companion website: www.wiley.com/go/neuhaus/dental_emergencies

Terms used in the orthopedic field such as "luxation", "total luxation", "eluxation" and "exarticulation" should therefore not be used in modern dental traumatology (Filippi, 2009a).

Behavior at the Scene of the Accident

Immediately after avulsion of a permanent tooth, it should be searched for as quickly as possible and placed in a cell-physiological medium. About 80% of all dental accidents, up to the age of 16, happen within a 100 m radius of the school and home (Onetto et al., 1994). Therefore, it is important that the respective supervisors (parents and teachers) are informed about immediate measures of how to act after a tooth is avulsed (Lieger et al., 2009). The Center of Dental Traumatology in Basel has repeatedly published information posters for public institutions, which today should hang wherever frequent dental accidents may occur, such as: primary schools, swimming pools and gyms (Figure 5.2.1) (Filippi, 2009b). The best cell-physiological environment for avulsed teeth is a tooth-rescue box (Dentosafe, Medice, Iserlohn, Germany or miradent SOS Zahnbox, Hager & Werken, Duisburg, Germany), which contains an organ transplantation fluid. This allows the periodontal cells on the root surface to survive extraorally for at least 24 hours at room temperature (Pohl et al., 1999). If a tooth-rescue box is not immediately available, cold milk or cling film may be a short-term alternative (Blomlöf, 1981; Andersson et al., 2012, Zeissler-Lajtman et al., 2017). Here, the cells mentioned can survive for up to two hours. Unphysiological storage in saliva or water are generally not recommended (Pongsiri et al., 1990).

Procedure in the Dental Practice

Medical History and Diagnosis

If a patient with an avulsed permanent tooth enters the dental practice, the storage media should be checked. If the tooth is not in the media of a tooth-rescue box, it should be relocated immediately to one.

The special medical history includes the details of the accident and possible signs of craniocerebral trauma. This can be suspected when certain symptoms may be reflected during the checkup, such as: amnesia, nausea or vomiting as well as severe headache. If suspicion arises, further medical investigations should be arranged. The status of tetanus immunization should also be clarified (von Arx et al., 2000; Andreasen and Andreasen, 2007; Trope, 2011; Andersson et al., 2012).

The clinical-dental diagnosis includes all extra- and intra-oral findings in order to get an overview of the injury. The procedure according to the HEPAG classification is important: The five tissues potentially affected by a dental accident should be independently evaluated: hard dental tissue, endodontic system, periodontal ligament (PDL), alveolar bone, gingiva/oral mucosa (HEPAG) (Figure 5.2.2) (Ebeleseder et al., 1998; Filippi et al., 2000a; von Arx et al., 2000). In addition a radiological examination of the empty alveolus and surrounding adjacent teeth (intraoral dental film) is performed (Figure 5.2.3). Panoramic Radiograph or Digital Volume Tomography are only indicated in specific clinical situations (von Arx et al., 2000).

The following clinical treatment is determined by the condition of the PDL and the diameter of the apical foramen (Andersson et al., 2012).

General Therapy

After local anesthesia, the coagulum in the alveolus must be completely removed before the tooth is replanted. This should be done primarily by rinsing with sterile isotonic saline solution (Figure 5.2.4). If the accident happened further in the past, this can be supported by curettage. The complete removal of the coagulum is important, otherwise the tooth can only be replanted with pressure, which results in additional PDL cell death. A soft tissue wound around the socket should

Zahnunfall

Zahnunfälle passieren zu Hause, in der Freizeit oder beim Sport – junge Menschen sind besonders betroffen. Richtig erkannt und behandelt, können auch schwer verletzte Zähne häufig erhalten werden. Deshalb:

1. **Ruhe bewahren – Zahnerhalt ist meistens möglich, wenn Sie richtig handeln!**

2. **Sofort Zahnarztpraxis oder Zahnklinik aufsuchen – bei jedem Zahnunfall!**

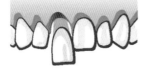

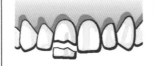

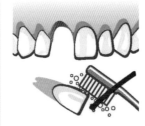

Zahn locker oder verschoben

Den Zahn in seiner Position belassen und umgehend einen Zahnarzt aufsuchen.

Zahn abgebrochen

Das abgebrochene Zahnstück suchen, in Wasser legen und damit zum Zahnarzt gehen.

Zahn ausgeschlagen

Den ausgeschlagenen Zahn in eine Zahnrettungsbox legen (erhältlich in Apotheken oder Zahnarztpraxen). Falls nicht verfügbar, Zahn in kalte Milch legen oder in Frischhaltefolie einwickeln. Sofort den Zahnarzt oder eine Zahnklinik aufsuchen!

Niemals den Zahn reinigen oder trocken lagern!

www.uzb.ch
www.zahnunfallzentrum.ch

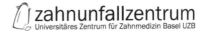

zahnunfallzentrum
Universitäres Zentrum für Zahnmedizin Basel UZB

Figure 5.2.1 Dental trauma poster published by the Center of Dental Traumatology, Basel (poster in German language).

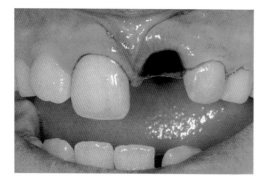

Figure 5.2.2 Clinical situation after avulsion and fracture in the enamel on the upper left central incisor of a 9-year-old patient (additional loosening of the upper right central incisor).

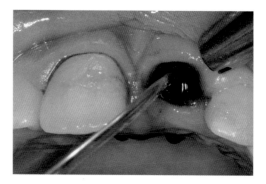

Figure 5.2.4 Removal of the coagulum by rinsing with sterile isotonic saline solution.

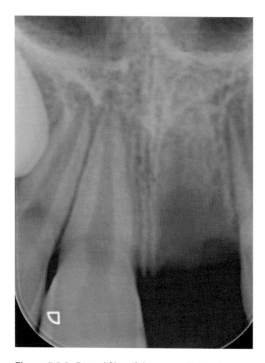

Figure 5.2.3 Dental film of the upper first incisor region (taken outside of the clinic).

be closed with thin, monofilament sutures prior to replantation of the tooth. If the buccal bone wall is fractured and the fragment has detached itself from the periosteum, it must be removed. Bone fragments fixed on the periosteum can be repositioned back into its original place (von Arx et al., 2000; Trope, 2011; Andersson et al., 2012).

Antiresorptive and Regenerative Therapies

If the root's surface is visibly contaminated it should be rinsed with sterile isotonic saline solution until it is macroscopically clean (Andersson et al., 2012). Before replanting the tooth, root surface and torn pulp stump are pretreated with medication. This treatment concept is based on four pillars: By storing the tooth in the organ transplantation medium of the tooth-rescue box, the surviving cells should be preserved, damaged cells regenerate and tissue decay products of destroyed tissue or their toxins should be washed away from the root surface (Cvek et al., 1974). To do this, the tooth must have been in the tooth-rescue box for a minimum of 30 minutes and occasionally swiveled so that these toxins can break away from the root surface and prevent diffusion bridges to build. In addition, an antibiotic-steroid mixture is inserted into the medium of the tooth rescue box (NoResorb, Medcem, Weinfelden, Switzerland) (Figures 5.2.5 and 5.2.6) (Pohl et al., 2005a, 2005b; Filippi and Krastl, 2007; Werder et al., 2011). This has a positive effect on the periodontal healing and revascularization probability of the pulp (Cvek et al., 1990; Sae-Lim et al., 1998; Pohl et al.,

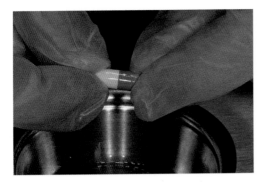

Figure 5.2.5 Opening of a NoResorb capsule.

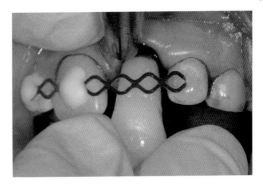

Figure 5.2.7 Replantation of an upper left central incisor (in this case, the titanium trauma splint (TTS) was fixed to adjacent teeth not injured by the accident and to the loosened first upper right central incisor prior to replantation of the avulsed tooth).

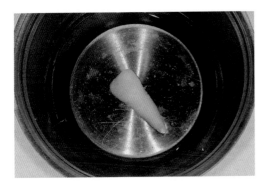

Figure 5.2.6 Storage of an avulsed upper left central incisor in the medium of a tooth rescue box after addition of antibiotics and steroids (NoResorb capsule).

2005a, 2005b), as long as the diameter of the foramen apicale is not smaller than 2 mm. The medication should be applied to the root's surface for at least 10 minutes. In the case of an unfavorable but not entirely hopeless rescue chain, an enamel matrix protein (Emdogain, Straumann, Basel, Switzerland) can additionally be applied to the root surface before replanting the tooth. This is able to repair small-scale cement defects (Hammarström, 1997). If all cells on the root surface have died through an unphysiological tooth rescue, the use of Emdogain is not indicated.

Replantation

After medical pretreatment and complete removal of the coagulum, the avulsed tooth is replanted with the fingers and returned to its original position (Figure 5.2.7). Uninjured adjacent teeth serve as a reference, and if incisors are not fully erupted, recent photographs of the patient (e.g. on a smartphone) can serve as a guide. Mispositions, forced positions or even early contacts must be prevented.

Splinting

The tooth must be protected from recurrent avulsion, significant mobility or dislocation. For this purpose, a fixation on each one not increased mobile adjacent tooth right and left is sufficient. The splint should not be rigid. It is fixed on the buccal surface of the teeth and the adhesive surfaces should be kept as small as possible. It should be attached away from the gingiva. Rigid wires, plastic nets or approximal fixations are no longer recommended today. The titanium trauma splint (TTS), an only 0.2 mm thin splint with attachment holes, has proven to be the material of choice worldwide (von Arx et al., 2001a, 2001b; Filippi et al., 2002). This very soft splint does not have to be pre-bent with forceps but can simply be pressed against the teeth. Their plasticity prevents forced positions due to compressive or tensile forces (Mazzoleni

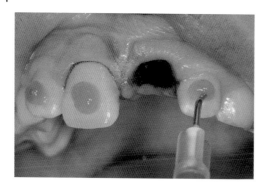

Figure 5.2.8 Etching of the enamel.

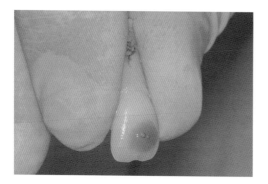

Figure 5.2.9 Etching of the enamel of the upper left central incisor conducted extraorally prior to replantation.

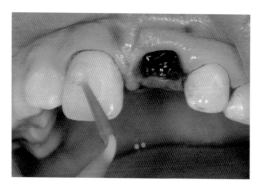

Figure 5.2.10 Conditioning of the enamel.

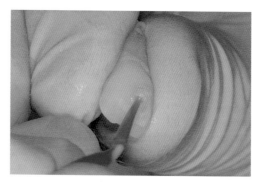

Figure 5.2.11 Conditioning of the enamel of the upper left central incisor conducted extraorally prior to replantation.

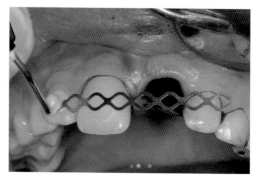

Figure 5.2.12 Fixation of the TTS with a composite of low viscosity (in this case, prior to replantation of the avulsed tooth).

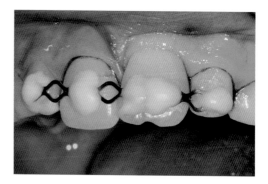

Figure 5.2.13 Upper left central incisor following replantation and fixation of the TTS.

et al., 2010). The fixation is carried out by means of an acid-etching technique and flowable composite (Figures 5.2.8–5.2.12) so the upper lip is not traumatized from the inside during the period when it is worn. For the same reason, the sharp-edged ends of the splint are covered with the same composite (Figure 5.2.13).

Medication and Postoperative Behaviour

In addition to an age-appropriate, body weight and possible allergies-dependent analgesic treatment, a systemic antibiotic treatment is required after avulsion of permanent teeth. As in all severe dislocation injuries such as avulsion, intrusion and a lateral dislocation (> 5mm), a systemic doxycycline intake is recommended. The dosage is based on body weight. The maximum duration of the therapy is 1 week (Andersson et al., 2012). An additional chemical plaque control by means of a mouthwash solution may be useful over a few days, depending on the extent of possible accompanying injuries. More important, however, is the best possible oral hygiene with a soft toothbrush, especially during the first few days after replantation, to achieve a fast and secure dento-gingival junction. The dietary recommendations should not provoke unnecessary plaque accumulation. This means that the patient should not eat anything soft and sticky, and instead continue with normal diet. A lege artis fixed splint tolerates this without any problems.

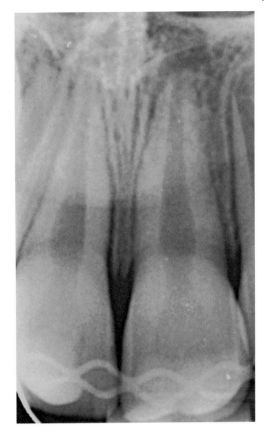

Figure 5.2.14 Dental film of the upper left central incisor as control after 2 days.

First Control after Replantation

The first wound control should be done within 48 hours. If no control dental film could be made on the day of the accident after replantation and splinting, this should be done now (Figure 5.2.14). This radiograph will serve as a reference for the rest of the recall, especially in detecting possible root resorptions. If the diameter of the apical foramen of the replanted tooth is less than 2 mm and/or the tooth had been unphysiologically rescued, the trepanation of the tooth and pulpal exstirpation should occur as soon as possible (Andreasen and Andreasen, 2007; Trope, 2011; Andersson et al., 2012). The definite root canal filling can already be done during this treatment, but sometimes it has to be postponed due to soft tissue swelling or local pain. In this case, a corticoid paste (Odontopaste, Australian Dental Manufacturing, Brisbane, Queensland, Australia) is recommended, which can be left for several weeks. The aim of this paste is not to disinfect the root canal (because on the second day it is not contaminated yet), but to diffuse the corticosteroid into the PDL to support the healing (Abbott et al., 1989; Kirakozova et al., 2009). Calcium hydroxide as medicament is contraindicated at this time because the high pH value provokes additional periodontal damage (Vanderas, 1993).

During the first control appointment the patient's oral hygiene should be checked and if necessary instructions are repeated.

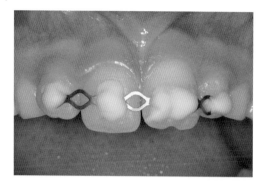

Figure 5.2.15 Clinical situation after 1 week. In the meantime, trepanation of the upper left central incisor was conducted and a medicament (Odontopaste) was placed in the root canal.

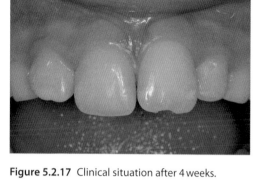

Figure 5.2.17 Clinical situation after 4 weeks.

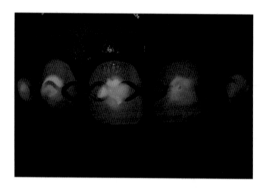

Figure 5.2.16 Composite with fluorescence, which can be made visible with the aid of a polymerisation light.

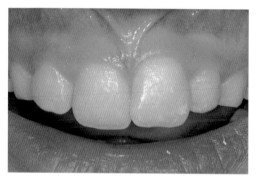

Figure 5.2.18 Clinical situation after 3 months, when root canal treatment was completed and the upper right central incisor was reconstructed with composite.

Control after 1 Week

If soft tissue injuries needed stitches on the day of the accident, they are removed after about a week (Figure 5.2.15). In individual cases, the splint can already be removed at this time. However, it is usually left for 2–4 weeks (Hinckfuss and Messer, 2009; Andersson et al., 2012).

Splint Removal

The removal of the splint should be done as carefully as possible. The fixation composite is removed above the splint with a diamond bur. Once it has been done at all fixation points, the splint can be removed like a sticker or simply lifted off. The remaining composite residues are to be selectively removed with maximum enamel preservation. Today, modern dental traumatology uses composites with fluorescence, which can be visualized with a polymerization lamp (Figure 5.2.16). After everything is removed and polished, a fluoridation is indicated.

Further Controls

Generally, the recall interval for dental accidents is selected depending on the type of injury, the clinical and radiological progress, as well as the age of the patient. Since an avulsion is always associated with pulpal and periodontal tissue damage, it is not uncommon that a long-term consequence may occur. To detect these early, regular clinical

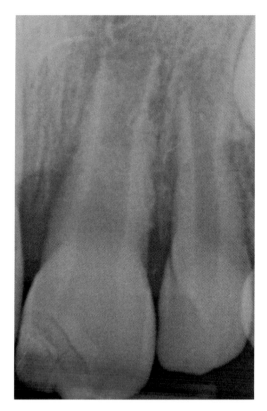

Figure 5.2.19 Infection-related root resorption on the upper left central incisor. Radiographic situation 4 weeks after avulsion (taken outside of the clinic).

and radiological controls are necessary. Controls have proven to be effective after 1 (Figure 5.2.17), 3 (Figure 5.2.18), 6 and 12 months (Andersson et al., 2012).

Prognosis

After a severe dislocation injury pulp necrosis can be treated successfully by early endodontic intervention or revascularization of the pulp. Usually pulp necrosis following dental trauma does not lead to the loss of the tooth. If endodontic intervention is delayed after an avulsion or intrusion, in almost every case an infection-related root resorption occurs (Figure 5.2.19), which rapidly leads to a loss of the tooth within the growing jaw (Filippi et al., 2000b; Andreasen and Andreasen, 2007; Andersson et al., 2012;

Filippi, 2014). About 1 week after the accident, the microorganisms or their toxins, which resides in the necrotic pulp, diffuse through the dentinal tubules to the periodontium and lead to root and bone resorptions. Delayed endodontic intervention must therefore be avoided after severe dislocation injuries, as the teeth can no longer be rescued after a certain progression of root and bone loss.

The survival of the PDL, and thus the possibility of periodontal healing, is primarily determined by the rescue chain of the tooth (von Arx et al., 2000; Filippi, 2009b; Andersson et al., 2012). In the case of a physiologic tooth rescue (insertion of the tooth within a few minutes after the accident into a

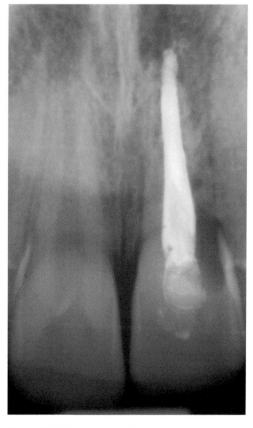

Figure 5.2.20 Osseous replacement in the upper left central incisor. Radiographic situation 18 months after avulsion.

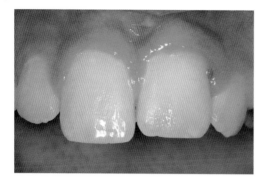

Figure 5.2.21 Infraposition of the upper left central incisor by ankylosis. Clinical situation 18 months after avulsion.

tooth-rescue box) the possibility for a normal periodontal healing, which does not affect the growth development of the anterior jaw, increases.

Many avulsed teeth are not physiologically stored and the periodontal healing results in ankylosis (Figure 5.2.20). The affected tooth is involved in the remodeling of the alveolar bone and is lost by osseous replacement. In the growing anterior jaw this process inhibits the local development of the jaw (Ebeleseder et al., 1998; Andreasen et al., 1995b; Andersson and Malmgren, 1999; Kawanami et al., 1999; Filippi et al., 2000b). In compari-son to the uninjured adjacent teeth, the affected teeth come into infraposition and lose their proximal placeholder function (Figure 5.2.21) (Kawanami et al., 1999; Filippi et al., 2000b). Such teeth should be strictly removed in the growing jaw once an infraposition of 1 mm has been reached, to prevent any aesthetically compromising gingival recession with a corresponding vertical bone loss in the aesthetically visible area. The individual therapy following the tooth removal depends on factors such as age, progression of the mixed dentition, presence of anodontia, need for orthodontic treatment or shape and color of the adjacent teeth. Implants should preferably not be inserted in patients with a high smile line and/or thin gingivabiotype before the age of 30, since the infraposition of implants and thus vertical bone and gingiva loss often occur in people older than the age of 25 (Jemt et al., 2007).

It is important that the affected children and adolescents are offered a different therapy. The decision should be determined and outweighed interdisciplinary, between orthodontic gap closure and tooth transplantation (Lang et al., 2003; Andersson et al., 2012). The lifelong prognosis of both mentioned treatment options are excellent.

References

Abbott, P. V., Hume W. R., Heithersay, G. S. 1989. Effects of combining Ledermix and calcium hydroxide pastes on the diffusion of corticosteroid and tetracycline through human tooth roots in vitro. *Endodontics and Dental Traumatology*, **5**, 188–92.

Andersson, L., Malmgren, B. 1999. The problem of dentoalveolar ankylosis and subsequent replacement resorption in the growing patient. *Australian Endodontic Journal*, **25**, 57–61.

Andersson, L., Andreasen, J. O., Day, P. Heithersay, G., Trope, M., DiAngelis, A. J., et al. 2012. International Association of Dental Traumatology guidelines for the management of traumatic dental injuries: 2. Avulsion of permanent teeth. *Dental Traumatology*, **28**, 88–96.

Andreasen, J. O., Andreasen, F. M. 2007. Avulsions. In: Andreasen, J. O., Andreasen, F. M., Andersson, L. (eds). *Textbook and Color Atlas of Traumatic Injuries to the Teeth*. Oxford: Wiley-Blackwell, pp. 444–88.

Andreasen, J. O., Borum, M. K., Jacobsen, H. L., Andreasen, F. M. 1995a. Replantation of 400 avulsed permanent incisors. 2. Factors related to pulpal healing. *Endodontics & Dental Traumatology*, **11**, 59–68.

Andreasen, J. O., Borum, M. K., Jacobsen, H. L., Andreasen F. M. 1995b. Replantation of 400 avulsed permanent incisors. 4. Factors related to periodontal ligament healing. *Endodontics & Dental Traumatology*, **11**, 76–89.

Blomlöf, L. 1981. Storage of human periodontal ligament cells in a combination of different media. *Journal of Dental Research*, **60**, 1904–6.

Cvek, M., Granath, L. E., Hollender, L. 1974. Treatment of non-vital permanent incisors with calcium hydroxide. 3. Variation of occurrence of ankylosis of reimplanted teeth with duration of extra-alveolar period and storage environment. *Odontologisk Revy*, **25**, 43–56.

Cvek, M., Cleaton-Jones, P., Austin, J., Lownie, J., Kling, M., Fatti, P. 1990. Effect of topical application of doxycycline on pulp revascularization and periodontal healing in reimplanted monkey incisors. *Endodontics & Dental Traumatology*, **6**, 170–6.

Ebeleseder, K. A., Friehs, S., Ruda, C., Pertl, C., Glockner, K., Hulla, H. 1998. A study of replanted permanent teeth in different age groups. *Endodontics & Dental Traumatology*, **14**, 274–8.

Filippi, A. 2009a. Unfallbedingte Zahnverletzungen – Klassifikation, Terminologie und Risikofaktoren. *Quintessenz*, **60**, 525–9.

Filippi, A. 2009b. Verhalten am Unfallort nach Zahntrauma. *Quintessenz*, **60**, 541–5.

Filippi, A. 2014. Infection-related root resorption. *Swiss Dental Journal*, **124**, 144–5.

Filippi, A., Krastl, G. 2007. Traumatologie im Milch- und Wechselgebiss. *Quintessenz*, **58**, 739–52.

Filippi, A., Tschan, J., Pohl, Y., Berthold, H., Ebeleseder, K. 2000a. A retrospective classification of tooth injuries using a new scoring system. *Clinical Oral Investigations*, **4**, 173–5.

Filippi, A., von Arx, T., Buser, D. 2000b. External root resorption following tooth trauma: its diagnosis, sequelae and therapy. *Schweizerische Monatsschrift für Zahnmedizin*, **110**, 712–29.

Filippi, A., von Arx, T., Lussi, A. 2002. Comfort and discomfort of dental trauma splints – a comparison of a new device (TTS) with three commonly used splinting techniques. *Dental Traumatology*, **18**, 275–80.

Glendor, U., Halling, A., Andersson, L., Eilert-Petersson, E. 1996. Incidence of traumatic tooth injuries in children and adolescents in the county of Västmanland, Sweden. *Swedish Dental Journal*, **20**, 15–28.

Hammarström, L. 1997. Enamel matrix, cementum development and regeneration. *Journal of Clinical Periodontology*, **24**, 658–68.

Hinckfuss, S. E., Messer, L.B. 2009. Splinting duration and periodontal outcomes for replanted avulsed teeth: a systematic review. *Dental Traumatology*, **25**, 150–7.

Jemt, T., Ahlberg, G., Henriksson, K., Bondevik, O. 2007. Tooth movements adjacent to single-implant restorations after more than 15 years of follow-up. *International Journal of Prosthodontics*, **20**, 626–32.

Kawanami, M., Andreasen, J. O., Borum, M. K., Schou, S., Hjørting-Hansen, E., Kato, H. 1999. Infraposition of ankylosed permanent maxillary incisors after replantation related to age and sex. *Endodontics & Dental Traumatology*, **15**, 50–6.

Kirakozova, A., Teixeira, F. B., Curran, A. E., Gu, F., Tawil, P.Z., Trope, M. 2009. Effect of intracanal corticosteroids on healing of replanted dog teeth after extended dry times. *Journal of Endodontics*, **35**, 663–7.

Lang, B., Pohl, Y., Filippi, A. 2003. Tooth transplantation. *Schweizerische Monatsschrift für Zahnmedizin*, **113**, 1178–99.

Lieger, O., Graf, C., El-Maaytah, M., von Arx, T. 2009. Impact of educational posters on the lay knowledge of school teachers regarding emergency management of dental injuries. *Dental Traumatology*, **25**, 406–12.

Mazzoleni, S., Meschia, G., Cortesi, R., Bressan, E., Tomasi, C., Ferro, R., Stellini, E. 2010. In vitro comparison of the flexibility of different splint systems used in dental traumatology. *Dental Traumatology*, **6**, 30–6.

Onetto, J. E., Flores, M. T., Garbarino, M. L. 1994. Dental trauma in children and adolescents in Valparaiso, Chile. *Endodontics & Dental Traumatology*, **10**, 223–7.

Pohl, Y., Tekin, U., Boll, M., Filippi, A., Kirschner, H. 1999. Investigations on a cell culture medium for storage and transportation of avulsed teeth. *Australian Endodontic Journal*, **25**, 70–5.

Pohl, Y., Filippi, A., Kirschner, H. 2005a. Results after replantation of avulsed permanent teeth. II. Periodontal healing and the role of physiologic storage and antiresorptive-regenerative therapy (ART). *Dental Traumatology*, **21**, 93–101.

Pohl, Y., Filippi, A., Kirschner, H. 2005b. Is antiresorptive regenerative therapy working in case of replantation of avulsed teeth? *Dental Traumatology*, **21**, 347–52.

Pongsiri, S., Schlegel, D., Zimmermann, M. 1990. Survival rate of periodontal ligament cells after extraoral storage in different media. *Deutsche Zeitschrift für Mund-, Kiefer- und Gesichtschirurgie*, **14**, 364–8.

Sae-Lim, V., Metzger, Z., Trope, M. 1998. Local dexamethasone improves periodontal healing of replanted dogs' teeth. *Endodontics & Dental Traumatology*, **14**, 232–6.

Trope, M. 2011. Avulsion of permanent teeth: theory to practice. *Dental Traumatology*, **27**, 281–94.

Vanderas, A. P. 1993. Effects of intracanal medicaments on inflammatory resorption or occurrence of ankylosis in mature traumatized teeth: a review. *Endodontics & Dental Traumatology*, **9**, 175–84.

von Arx, T., Filippi, A., Buser, D. 2000. The avulsion of the permanent teeth: the diagnostic, clinical and therapeutic aspects. *Schweizerische Monatsschrift für Zahnmedizin*, **110**, 731–44.

von Arx, T., Filippi, A., Buser, D. 2001a. Splinting of traumatized teeth with a new device: TTS (titanium trauma splint). *Dental Traumatology*, **17**, 180–4.

von Arx, T., Filippi, A., Lussi, A. 2001b. Comparison of a new dental trauma splint device (TTS) with three commonly used splinting techniques. *Dental Traumatology*, **17**, 266–74.

Werder, P., von Arx, T., Chappuis, V. 2011. Treatment outcome of 42 replanted permanent incisors with a median follow-up of 2.8 years. *Schweizerische Monatsschrift für Zahnmedizin*, **121**, 312–20.

Zeissler-Lajtman, A., Connert, T., Kühl, S., Filippi, A. 2017. Cling film as storage medium for avulsed teeth. An in vitro pilot study. *Swiss Dental Journal*, **127**, 954–9.

5.3

Autotransplantation: Ankylosis and External Root Resorption after Trauma

Manfred Leunisse[1], Dick S. Barendregt[2,3], Marcel L. E. Linssen[3] and Edwin Eggink[3]

[1] *Clinic for Orthodontics, Rotterdam, Netherlands*
[2] *Department of Periodontology, ACTA, Amsterdam, Netherlands*
[3] *Private dental office Proclin Rotterdam, Netherlands*

Introduction

When an ankylotic tooth is tapped with a dental instrument, a "high-pitched" sound can be heard, which differs from the sound on tapping the neighbouring teeth and is caused by a lack of resilience. Eruption occurs and resilience exists because of a functional periodontal ligament (PDL). A healthy PDL has a turnover rate of 7–14 days, on average (Beertsen et al., 1997). When the PDL is partially or completely destroyed, the root surface comes into direct contact with the alveolar bone, and its dentin is replaced by alveolar bone.

Extensive studies on traumatology by Andreasen in Denmark (Andreasen et al., 1990a, 1990b) and experimental studies by Sture Nyman's group on the healing process around teeth (Nyman et al., 1980) provide clear answers on the subject of periodontal repair. If a tooth has a vital PDL, it will reattach regularly to the alveolar bone after replantation, and the gingiva will redevelop. However, if no PDL is present, initial contact with the dentin will be made by osteoclasts. Nyman's experimental studies showed that direct contact with gingival tissues resulted in root resorption with invagination of soft

tissues, whilst contact with osteoclasts led to a bony connection.

Trauma and the PDL

After trauma, changes often occur in the activity of the PDL. Replacement resorption is one of the most frequently diagnosed reactions. The tooth becomes ankylosed, and the dentin is replaced by alveolar bone. In the long term, the majority of the dentin is transformed, and the traumatised teeth are lost. In young patients (between 6 and 12 years of age), the role of the dentist is crucial here. Together with an orthodontist, they must assess the complete dentoskeletal status in order to determine what treatment options are available.

We analysed the case of a 10-year-old girl who fell on a sidewalk whilst riding her bicycle. Teeth 11 and 21 were avulsed and replanted by her dentist within 20 minutes. Because both teeth responded to cold-sensitivity tests during subsequent control appointments and did not show any pathology periapically, no endodontic treatment was planned. After intervals of 3 and 6 weeks, no indications were visible intraorally (pain or swelling) or

Management of Dental Emergencies in Children and Adolescents, First Edition.
Edited by Klaus W. Neuhaus and Adrian Lussi.
© 2019 John Wiley & Sons Ltd. Published 2019 by John Wiley & Sons Ltd.
Companion website: www.wiley.com/go/neuhaus/dental_emergencies

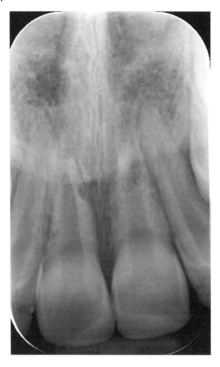

Figure 5.3.1 12 weeks after replantation, external root resorption becomes visible in a periapical radiograph.

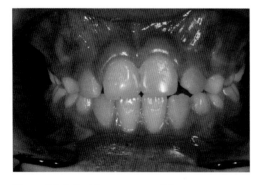

Figure 5.3.2 Positive response of the two upper front teeth to sensitivity testing.

on intraoral radiographs (signs of external inflammatory resorption) to suggest that interventions of any type should be performed. After 12 weeks, the dentist noted that resorption lacunas had formed on both teeth, but the pulps still responded positively to sensitivity testing (Figures 5.3.1 and 5.3.2).

Subsequently, the patient was referred to an endodontist in our clinic. On clinical evaluation, a positive response to sensitivity testing was observed, in addition to a different sound upon percussion of teeth 11 and 21 compared to the neighbouring teeth. Both teeth appeared to be ankylosed.

Since it was too early to start orthodontic treatment because mixed dentition was still present, we decided to monitor the situation. During this time, the external replacement resorption clearly progressed, as shown on the intraoral radiographs obtained by the endodontist at 6 months (Figure 5.3.3a–c). The future loss of the affected teeth was predictable.

Several options existed for replacing the central incisors. The patient was too young for implants, and temporary fixed prosthodontics would lead to bone loss over several years. Another option would be to wait until she had become fully grown and orthodontic space closure could be possible. The disadvantage of this option is that in many cases, it leads to a compromised aesthetic result, with a high incidence of apical root resorption of the lateral incisors. Additionally, the canines will end at the lateral incisor position, which is not optimal. The ideal result of orthodontic treatment would be a stable front contact with canine guidance on the cuspids in a class I occlusion. In our opinion, a sustainable result could be obtained only by transplanting the premolars to the central incisor location. With transplanted premolars, the normal development of the gums and alveolar bone would be promoted in this young patient.

Autotransplantation

One treatment option that is not well known amongst dental practitioners is autotransplantation. In the 1980s and '90s, much research on this subject was conducted, especially in Denmark (Andreasen et al., 1990a) and Norway (Slagsvold and Bjercke, 1978). In the Netherlands, the oral- and maxillofacial surgeons Ralf Voorsmit of Nijmegen and Jacques Baart of Amsterdam frequently employed this method and became outspoken advocates of its use.

(a)   (b)   (c)

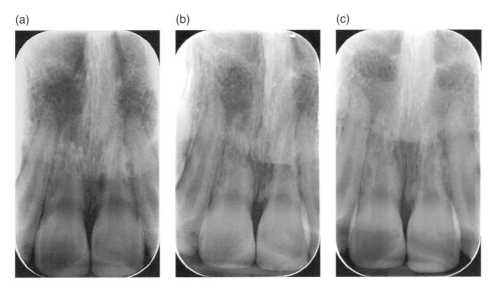

Figure 5.3.3 (a–c) Progression of external root resorptions over 6 months.

In our patient, a tooth size discrepancy (TSD) was also present, which was an important aspect in treatment planning. By choosing to replace the two central incisors through transplantation with two premolars, the space created in the premolar region allowed better interdigitation and the desired class I occlusion of the canines.

Because the apices of the premolars where not yet fully developed, we could perform autotransplantation aiming for the revascularisation of the vital teeth (Czochrowska et al., 2000) (Figures 5.3.4–5.3.7). The timing of transplantation with an open apex is important in this respect. Although roots

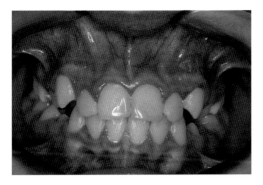

Figure 5.3.4 Tooth size discrepancy of the upper front teeth.

with a length of up to half the expected length can be successfully transplanted, the development of root length is often impaired (Myrlund et al., 2004). Therefore, the Danish option with two-thirds to three-quarter root development, as proposed by Paulsen and Andreasen, creates a more predictable outcome of a favourable root length at the recipient site (Andreasen et al., 1990b). A recent study showed that even with an apical diameter of 0.34 mm, revascularisation is possible (Laureys et al., 2013). After the extraction of teeth 11 and 21, both incisors were preserved, and acted as a template for the transformation of the premolars into central incisors (Figure 5.3.8a,b).

The sutures were removed 1 week following transplantation. A control appointment was scheduled for 3 weeks to monitor the clinical healing by periodontal probing and check the development of the PDL via a radiograph. A lack of deepened pockets indicated that optimal healing was occurring.

If such a situation remains consistent at the 6-week appointment, the orthodontist can start to engage the transplanted teeth in orthodontic treatment and place the new incisors under orthodontic loading (Figure 5.3.9). The early literature shows

(a)　　　　　　　　　(b)

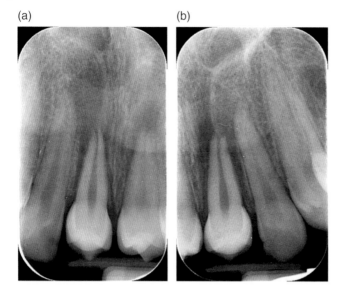

Figure 5.3.5 (a,b) Autotransplantation of two premolars with open apex.

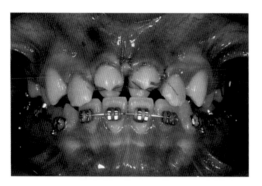

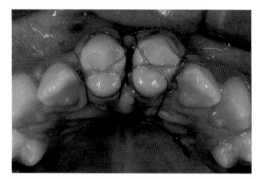

Figure 5.3.6 Clinical situation directly after surgery. The position of the transplanted premolars is secured with cross-sutures.

Figure 5.3.7 Same patient as in Figure 5.3.6, occlusal view.

(a)　　　　　　　　　(b)

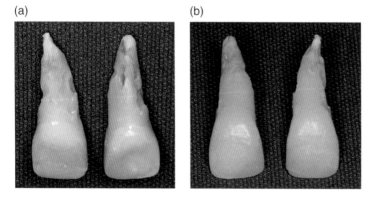

Figure 5.3.8 (a,b) The extracted front teeth give important information for the future composite build-up. Their form can be copied using silicon.

that previous colleagues were much more prudent and advised waiting at least 3 months before starting orthodontic loading. However, based on recent literature and our experience over the last 10 years, it is evident that after 6 weeks, sufficient stability exists to enable a good finishing point (Yang et al., 2012; Lu et al., 2013).

After a little repositioning, we remodelled the transplanted teeth into central incisors using composites, rebounded the brackets in the correct position and continued the orthodontic phase (Figure 5.3.10a–c). The additional advantage of this sequence is that during the orthodontic phase, no delay will occur due to the uncertainty of the shape of the new teeth 11 and 21. The brackets can be bonded directly in the correct position, which results in adequate forces on each tooth. On average, 4 mm of composite must be added on top of the buccal cusp of the transplanted premolar to reach the same length as the extracted incisor. Properly placing a bracket is impossible if the transplant is not transformed into the incisor it replaces prior to bracket placement.

The intraoral radiographs taken at the 6-month appointment showed that the

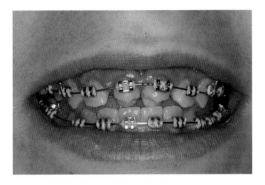

Figure 5.3.9 6 weeks after autotransplantation, the teeth can be moved aorthodontically.

(a)

(b)

(c)

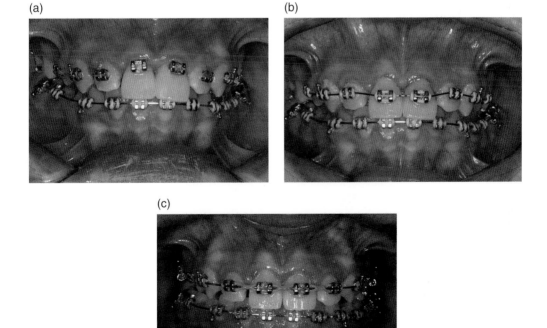

Figure 5.3.10 (a–c) Remodelling the premolars into upper incisors, and continuation of the orthodontic therapy.

(a)　　　　　　　　　(b)

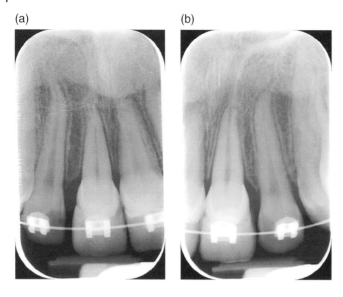

Figure 5.3.11 (a,b) 6 months after autotransplantation, the periapical radiographs show an increasing obliteration of the pulp (which is a sign of pulp vitality) and continuing apical root formation.

obliteration of the pulp chamber was in progress, which is a sign of pulp vitality. They also showed that the apices continued to develop (Figure 5.3.11a,b).

Traumatic Injuries in Later Life

Unfortunately, traumatic injuries are not exclusively reserved for children aged 6–12 years, when autotransplantation of a tooth with an open apex can usually be performed. In the next case, a 15-year-old patient visited our clinic seeking a prosthetic solution to improve the aesthetics of a traumatised tooth 11 (Figure 5.3.12a,b).

The trauma occurred when she was 7 years of age. The orthodontic treatment plan of her former orthodontist involved keeping the traumatised tooth 11 in situ and postponing prosthetic replacement until completion of facial growth had occurred. At the time of

(a)　　　　　　　　　　　　　　　　　(b)

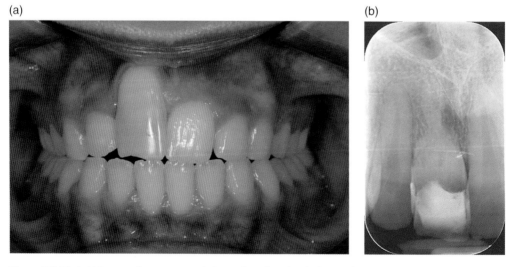

Figure 5.3.12 (a,b) 8 years after trauma, ankylosis of tooth 11 has led to undesired dental aesthetics, mainly due to missing vertical bone growth in the region of the ankylosed tooth.

her first visit to our clinic, and due to the vertical growth and development of her face since tooth 11 had become ankylosed, a large vertical defect of soft and bony tissues had developed. This vertical defect implied that an implant-driven prosthetic and restorative treatment would be very complex and aesthetically compromising. The vertical augmentation of such a loss of bony tissue in an attempt to place either a dental implant or an adhesive bridge is unpredictable, even without considering soft-tissue management. Additionally, the expected further (vertical) development of the facial structures would result in an unsatisfactory aesthetic solution over time.

It was decided to use the PDL of a transplanted tooth to restore both the soft and the bony tissue defect. Although the patient had previously been treated orthodontically, optimal interdigitation and canine guidance were not present, and a considerable amount of tooth wear was already visible. By choosing autotransplantation, it was possible to reach class I canine occlusion and a class II occlusion of one premolar width on the molars, giving a functional and stable finished result. Two premolars could act as spare parts, one of which was chosen as the donor to replace the traumatised tooth 11.

Before transplantation, the donor tooth underwent endodontic treatment. Because root formation was complete, it was highly unlikely that revascularisation would occur. When a vital tooth is treated endodontically, a 98% success rate can be expected (Friedman, 2004). The transplantation of teeth with fully developed roots is as successful as the transplantation of teeth with an open apex (Yoshino et al., 2012).

Using a composite veneer, the premolar was transformed into a central incisor similar to tooth 21, 6 weeks after transplantation and loaded orthodontically to extrude the tooth (Figures 5.3.13–5.3.16). After completion of the orthodontic treatment, tooth 11 was monitored every 3 years by clinical examination and intraoral radiographs.

Conclusion

The PDL can act as a "bioengineer" when treated with care and exposed to favourable conditions. Soft-tissue closure after transplantation and healing in an uninfected environment will induce cell growth, resulting in a new PDL, alveolar bone and gingiva; therefore, a completely new dento-alveolar complex can be generated.

(a)   (b)

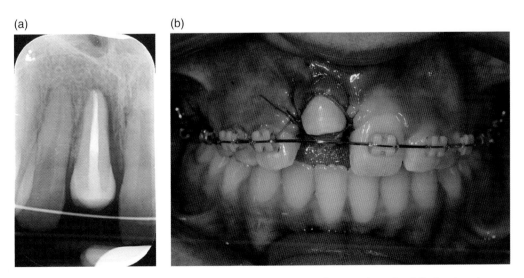

Figure 5.3.13 (a,b) Root canal treatment and autotransplantation of a premolar with a fully developed apex.

(a)　　　　　(b)

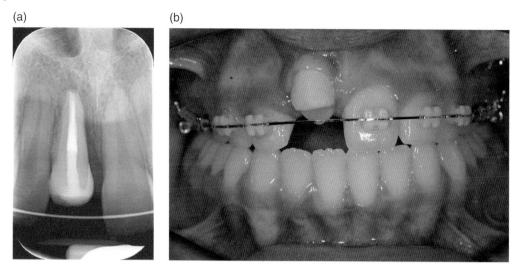

Figure 5.3.14 (a,b) 6 weeks after autrotransplantation, there are no pockets at the transplanted premolar, and orthodontic treatment can commence.

(a)　　　　　(b)

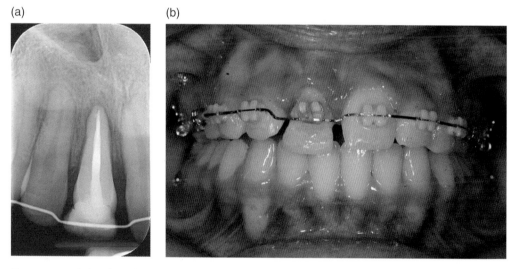

Figure 5.3.15 (a,b) After adding a provisional composite veneer, the tooth can be orthodontically extruded and loaded.

The long-term success rates of donor teeth with open apices and completely closed roots are comparable (95 and 98% survival after 10 years, respectively; the success rate after an average of 25 years has been reported to be 80%, Czochrowska et al., 2002). When the PDL is injured as a result of trauma in such a manner that external (replacement) resorption or ankylosis occurs, autotransplantation can offer an alternative first choice in aesthetic areas (Andersson et al., 2016). Due to the biological reactions that occur, a tooth with an intact PDL has a better long-term prognosis than do implants. This approach fits extremely well with the contemporary idea of finding biomimetic solutions for dental problems.

(a)   (b)

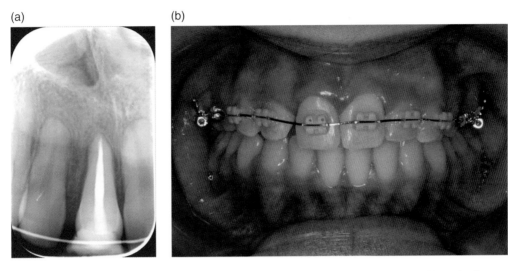

Figure 5.3.16 (a,b) Final composite veneer. The vertical bone defect has been resubstituted by orthodontic extrusion of the transplanted premolar. Clinical and radiographic recall every 3 years is advised.

References

Andersson, L., Andreasen, J. O., Day, P., Heithersay, G., Trope, M., DiAngelis, A. J., et al. 2016. Guidelines for the management of traumatic dental injuries: 2. Avulsion of permanent teeth. *Pediatric Dentistry*, **38**, 369–76.

Andreasen, J. O., Paulsen, H. U., Yu, Z., Ahlquist, R., Bayer, T., Schwartz, O. 1990a. A long-term study of 370 autotransplanted premolars. Part I. Surgical procedures and standardized techniques for monitoring healing. *European Journal of Orthodontics*, **12**, 3–13.

Andreasen, J. O., Paulsen, H. U., Yu, Z., Bayer, T. 1990b. A long-term study of 370 autotransplanted premolars. Part IV. Root development subsequent to transplantation. *European Journal of Orthodontics*, **12**, 38–50.

Beertsen, W., McCulloch, C. A., Sodek, J. 1997. The periodontal ligament: a unique, multifunctional connective tissue. *Periodontology 2000*, **13**, 20–40.

Czochrowska, E. M., Stenvik, A., Album, B., Zachrisson, B. U. 2000. Autotransplantation of premolars to replace maxillary incisors: a comparison with natural incisors. *American Journal of Orthodontics and Dentofacial Orthopedics*, **118**, 592–600.

Czochrowska, E. M., Stenvik, A., Bjercke, B., Zachrisson, B. U. 2002. Outcome of tooth transplantation: survival and success rates 17-41 years posttreatment. *American Journal of Orthodontics and Dentofacial Orthopedics*, **121**, 110–19, quiz 193.

Friedman, S. M., C. 2004. The success of endodontic therapy – healing and functionality. *Journal of the Californian Dental Association*, **32**, 493–503.

Laureys, W. G., Cuvelier, C. A., Dermaut, L. R., De Pauw, G. A. 2013. The critical apical diameter to obtain regeneration of the pulp tissue after tooth transplantation, replantation, or regenerative endodontic treatment. *Journal of Endodontics*, **39**, 759–63.

Lu, L., Sun, H. F., Xue, H., Guo, J., Chen, Y. X. 2013. Effects of orthodontic load on the periodontium of autogenously transplanted teeth in beagle dogs. *Journal of Zhejiang University Science B*, **14**, 1025–32.

Myrlund, S., Stermer, E. M., Album, B., Stenvik, A. 2004. Root length in transplanted premolars. *Acta Odontologica Scandinavica*, **62**, 132–6.

Nyman, S., Karring, T., Lindhe, J., Planten, S. 1980. Healing following implantation of periodontitis-affected roots into gingival connective tissue. *Journal of Clinical Periodontology*, **7**, 394–401.

Slagsvold, O., Bjercke, B. 1978. Applicability of autotransplantation in cases of missing upper anterior teeth. *American Journal of Orthodontics*, **74**, 410–21.

Yang, Y., Bai, Y., Li, S., Li, J., Gao, W., Ru, N. 2012. Effect of early orthodontic force on periodontal healing after autotransplantation of permanent incisors in beagle dogs. *Journal of Periodontology*, **83**, 235–41.

Yoshino, K., Kariya, N., Namura, D., Noji, I., Mitsuhashi, K., Kimura, H., et al. 2012. A retrospective survey of autotransplantation of teeth in dental clinics. *Journal of Oral Rehabilitation*, **39**, 37–43.

5.4

Orthodontic Aspects of Missing Teeth at Various Ages

Carlalberta Verna[1] and Birte Melsen[2]

[1] Department of Orthodontics and Paediatric Dentistry, University Center for Dental Medicine Basel, University of Basel, Basel, Switzerland
[2] Department of Orthodontics, University of Western Australia, Perth, Australia

Introduction

The orthodontic management of missing teeth differs according to their aetiology. The absence of teeth may be a result of either acquired or congenital factors. In the former case, the situation is referred to as "early tooth loss", since the teeth were previously present in the oral cavity, whilst in the latter it is referred to as "congenitally missing teeth", as the teeth were never formed.

Early Tooth Loss

Deciduous Dentition

Early tooth loss in the deciduous dentition can be observed as a consequence of dental trauma in the anterior region. The early loss of one or two incisors does not usually have consequences per se on the masticatory function, and the aesthetic impairment rarely affects the self-esteem of the child. During this phase of dental and facial development, the role of the orthodontist is mostly limited to monitoring the development of major dental arch asymmetry and controlling other factors that might increase the risk of dental crowding, such as thumb-sucking and low tongue posture, which are associated with a narrow palate. Once the permanent teeth start erupting, the orthodontist must make a thorough clinical and radiographic analysis to evaluate whether the eruption has been impaired by the trauma and to establish a customised treatment plan for the individual patient.

Early loss of deciduous teeth may also occur as a consequence of premature exfoliation of the teeth associated with severe systemic disorders, such as metabolic issues, connective tissue disorders and neoplastic diseases (Duggal et al., 2013).

Mixed Dentition

During the mixed dentition phase, other causes of tooth loss can occur in addition to dental trauma, such as pathological conditions and crowding.

Tooth Loss Due to Trauma

As in the deciduous dentition, the most commonly affected teeth are the upper incisors. In cases where teeth are congenitally missing, the anterior region is a major concern because, apart from the aesthetics, the height and width of the alveolar process must be preserved until a permanent solution can

Management of Dental Emergencies in Children and Adolescents, First Edition.
Edited by Klaus W. Neuhaus and Adrian Lussi.
© 2019 John Wiley & Sons Ltd. Published 2019 by John Wiley & Sons Ltd.
Companion website: www.wiley.com/go/neuhaus/dental_emergencies

be reached at the end of growth. A thorough treatment planning based on comprehensive orthodontic records (dental casts, intra- and extraoral pictures, panoramic and lateral head films) and the input from other colleagues who are going to finalise the treatment at the end of growth is essential. In the presence of an overjet of maxillary origin, the closure of the avulsion space through orthodontic treatment will address both the overjet and the lack of front teeth (Figures 5.4.1 and 5.4.2). In cases where no overjet is present, the orthodontic treatment will shift the space created by the avulsed teeth from the front region to a more posterior one, where the risk of alveolar bone collapse is less, and the tension of the supracrestal fibres maintains a better vertical and buccolingual width (Southard et al., 1992; Ostler and Kokich, 1994). If a class II malocclusion is present and third molars are developing, the whole upper dentition can be shifted forwards through the use of skeletal anchorage, thus avoiding the need for implant replacement at the end of growth (Figure 5.4.3). The space closure through mesialisation of adjacent teeth is a solution that achieves a better aesthetic result in the upper anterior region during adolescence and therefore minimises self-esteem issues during this sensitive phase of psychosocial development (Anweigi et al., 2013).

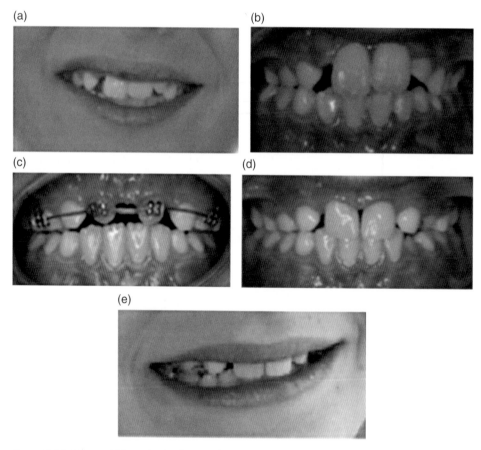

(a) (b) (c) (d) (e)

Figure 5.4.1 9-year-old boy who has lost teeth 21 and 11 due to ankylosis (a and b). Initially with the aid of a removable appliance and thereafter through the use of fixed mechanics, teeth 12 and 22 were bodily moved in the extraction space (c). The periodontal ligament brought the bone with the roots, and after 1 year of treatment the teeth were temporarily reconstructed and the permanent canines erupted at the place of the displaced lateral incisors. The aesthetic and functional impairment of the patient are now solved and a new evaluation will be made once all the permanent teeth have erupted (d and e). (Build-up by Dr Bühler.)

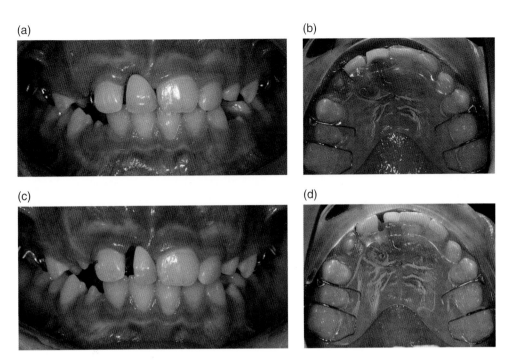

Figure 5.4.2 If tooth loss is monolateral, as in this 10-year-old boy (a and c), a removable appliance can be used to ensure the midline stability and mesial tip of the tooth adjacent to the tooth loss (b and d). The principle behind the treatment is to move the roots and the alveolar bone into an area that otherwise is at risk of becoming atrophic.

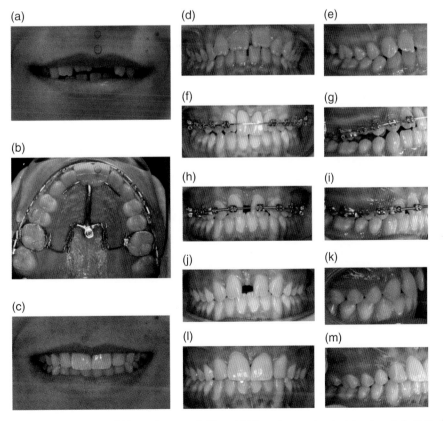

Figure 5.4.3 12-year-old boy whose teeth 11 and 21 have been extracted due to ankylosis (a, d and e) following dental trauma. With the help of a palatal implant (Straumann AG, Basel) (b), the whole posterior dentition was moved forward (d–j). A distal molar occlusion was obtained (e–m) and teeth 12 and 22 were displaced at the position of the extracted teeth 11 and 21 (j). The size discrepancy was then compensated by prosthetic reconstruction (c and l). (Prosthetics by Prof. Zitzmann.)

Early Loss Due to Pathologies

When the posterior teeth are lost prematurely, available space and facial growth have to be considered. The most critical situation is one of early loss of the second deciduous molars, since the mesial drift of the first permanent molar into the extraction space will shorten the arch length, thus voiding the potential space gain offered by the leeway space. Despite not supported by strong evidence, the mesialisation of the first permanent molar leads to space loss of approximately 2.5 mm for the lower deciduous molar and slightly less for the upper one in the initial weeks following extraction. If no space maintenance protocol is set, a borderline crowding case can easily be transformed into a clear extraction one. The use of a space maintainer in the case of second deciduous molar loss has to be evaluated by taking into consideration factors relating to the compliance of the patient, oral hygiene, the family situation and general health. The role of the orthodontist is crucial in the diagnostics with regard to space analysis, facial growth and the dental age. When spaces are present (i.e. the basal dental arch is adequate), a space maintainer can be avoided, especially in

brachiocephalic subjects with a tight posterior occlusal interdigitation (Splieth, 2011). In dolichocephalic patients, both upper and lower first molars drift mesially after early loss of the first deciduous molars, but in brachiocephalic types, this only occurs in the mandible (Alexander et al., 2015). Even in cases in which the extraction of a permanent tooth is foreseen, a space maintainer may still be indicated to manage the anchorage and avoid the development of dental asymmetries, which would make the future orthodontic treatment longer and more complicated, and therefore less acceptable to the patient. The presence of a distal or mesial molar relationship is a further reason to use a space maintainer, since the anchorage needs must be taken into account for the future correction of the sagittal discrepancy, as in Figure 5.4.4. The eruption sequence, the root development and the thickness of the bone overlying the second premolars are also factors to consider in the treatment plan.

The consequences on arch length of the early loss of a first deciduous molar are less clear than for a second deciduous molar. According to Tunison et al. (2008), there is evidence of a mean space loss in the mandible

(a)

(b)

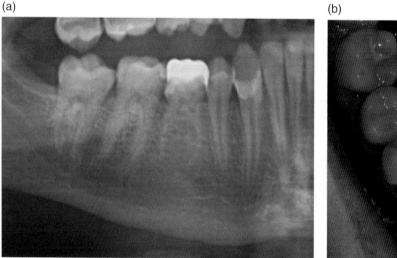
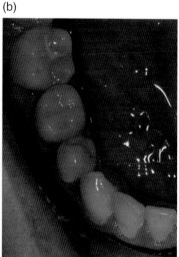

Figure 5.4.4 If the bone level between the deciduous molar and the adjacent permanent teeth is equal (a), occlusal contacts are ensured by composite reconstructions and the correction of the sagittal relation is facilitated by reducing the mesiodistal dimension (b).

of 1.5 mm per arch side and of 1 mm in the maxilla, but the clinical relevance of this has to be evaluated alongside the factors mentioned for the second deciduous molar. The pattern of tooth drift is different for the mandible and the maxilla. In the mandible, the deciduous canine moves distally into the extraction space, with consequences for the arch symmetry and the dental midline. In doliocephalic cases with additional crowding, a space maintainer is indicated, since the space loss becomes critical. In the maxilla, 1 mm of space loss is caused by mesial drift of the permanent molar (Splieth, 2011).

The early loss of first permanent molars is less common than that of deciduous molars. In cases where the extraction of a first molar is indicated, consultation with an orthodontist is essential due to the effects it will have on the patient's skeletal and dental development. Potential consequences include a decrease in the space post extraction, accelerated development and eruption of the second and third permanent molars, a decrease in caries or fillings on proximal surfaces of adjacent teeth, lingual tipping and retrusion of the incisors and counterclockwise rotation of the occlusal plane. Spontaneous space closure in the mandible is less likely than in the maxilla, and according to a recent meta-analysis, the optimal timing for the extraction of the first molar is set not by the chronological age of the patient but by the development of the furcation of the second molar (Saber et al., 2018). The decision to permit the mesial movement of the second molar depends on the space analysis and the presence of the third molars, but the sagittal relationship of the subject must also be taken into account. In some specific cases where the extraction of upper premolars is planned, their autotransplantation into the extraction site can be considered as a treatment option (Andreasen, 1992).

Tooth Loss Due to Crowding

During the early mixed dentition, intraalveolar crowding may lead to a lack of eruption of the lateral incisors. Once radiographic examination has confirmed the presence of the incisors, an orthodontic treatment must be initiated in order to allow their proper eruption. In cases of mild crowding in the maxilla, a non-extraction therapy has a good prognosis, since the leeway space can be used to gain space and transversal (skeletal/dental) or sagittal expansion may be possible. In the mandible, where there is less possibility of either transversal or sagittal expansion, each case has to be evaluated individually. A more serious situation is encountered when the deciduous canines are lost during the eruption of the lateral incisors. In this case, the probability of an extraction therapy is higher, especially if the affected jaw is the mandible. The decision on whether to aim for an extraction therapy depends generally on the soft-tissue balance, the inclination of the teeth in the mandible and the gingival biotype. In this situation, although the need for future extraction therapy is clear, a radiological evaluation is recommended in order to verify the position of the permanent canines and premolars, since the risk of retention or impaction is increased. There is no clear consensus concerning the management of a unilateral early dental loss due to crowding. In the case of early deciduous canine loss in the mandible, the orthodontist's main goal should be to avoid the creation of a dental asymmetry or midline shift. In cases with extreme crowding where the future extraction of permanent teeth has already been decided upon, the extraction of the contralateral deciduous canine may be indicated. When there is only a minor space deficit, a short but active orthodontic treatment to open up the space for the future eruption of the canine and avoid further asymmetry is ideal. The rationale behind this approach is that the extraction of the deciduous canine should be avoided because it will cause alveolar bone resorption in an area in which a permanent canine has to erupt.

Congenitally Missing Teeth

A common malformation observed in relation to the development of the masticatory system is known as tooth agenesis. The deciduous dentition is less affected than the permanent one, and although the prevalence has increased in recent decades, this is probably due to better diagnostics (Al-Ani et al., 2017a). Recent review papers report that the prevalence of subjects missing one or more permanent teeth ranges between 0.2 and 16.2 % (Rakhshan, 2015a).

Both environmental and genetic factors are involved in the aetiology of hypodontia, with the latter playing a more significant role (Al-Ani et al., 2017a, 2017b). Patients affected by hypodontia suffer from functional and aesthetic impairment, as well as psychosocial problems and the financial burden related to treatment (Nunn et al., 2003; Anweigi et al., 2013).

The role played by the orthodontist in the management of missing teeth differs according to the age of the patient and the number of teeth affected. The duration of treatment generally extends from the deciduous dentition to the termination of craniofacial development. A lifetime commitment is required from the patient following their initial diagnosis, extending past the completion of active treatment to incorporate the maintenance of retainers, implants and prostheses. The role of the orthodontist varies according to the severity of the condition. In the initial phase, functional and dentoalveolar development must be monitored. This is followed by interceptive treatment with removable appliances, and then by a more active phase where repositioning of the teeth follows a treatment plan agreed upon by an interdisciplinary team. The aim is to reach an optimal result at the end of craniofacial development. Patients suffering from hypodontia often present a significant clinical challenge for orthodontists, because in a number of cases the treatment time is prolonged and the outcome may be compromised.

The complexity of the treatment of patients with missing teeth lies in the fact that the severity of the functional and aesthetic aspects of the condition has clear psychological, social and financial consequences. The treatment approach has therefore to take into consideration the patient's (and their parents'/guardians') perception of the problem and the anticipation that long-term maintenance will be required, without forgetting the costs to both the patient and their family (Rakhshan, 2015a). Due to the complexity of the treatment plan, an experienced team of dental specialists should undertake these treatments.

The few studies available on the Oral Health-Related Quality of Life (OHRQoL) regarding hypodontia have confirmed that this condition may have a negative impact on quality of life (Meaney et al., 2012).

The perception of aesthetic impairment is related to the number and localisation of missing teeth, the craniofacial growth pattern, the age of the patient and the patient's psychological development and social interactions. The most extreme developmental dental anomaly of missing teeth is anodontia, where all teeth are absent. Oligodontia is the name given where six or more teeth are missing, whilst hypodontia involves the loss of fewer than six teeth (Nunn et al., 2003). Amongst patients suffering from hypodontia, the majority exhibit agenesis of the second lower premolars or upper lateral incisors, followed by the maxillary second premolar (Rakhshan, 2015b).

Whilst minor teeth irregularities can be accepted in the deciduous and early mixed dentition, they are less well accepted in the pre- and adolescent phases of psychosocial development. The patient's main concern directly relates to the number of teeth missing in the incisor region, and has mainly to do with spacing and poor aesthetics. In severe cases, an early establishment of an acceptable appearance may help socially, particularly at school. From this point of view, the orthodontist plays a pivot role in the interdisciplinary team, being able to move teeth in the aesthetic frontal area before the end of growth, ensuring a good basis for long-term solutions and reducing the burden on the patient (Schneider et al., 2016).

Patients suffering oligodontia often exhibit majora aesthetic impairment. In severe cases, there may also be anomalies of tooth shape and size. The facial changes are not related to a specific growth pattern, but to functional and dental adaptation resulting from the lack of teeth. The development and eruption of the teeth is the key factor in the development of the alveolar process. Normally, strain applied to the alveolar bone by the periodontal ligament on one side and the periosteum on the other is the key factor that keeps the bone in balance, as described by the mechanostat theory (Southard et al., 1992; Frost, 2003). Patients affected by tooth agenesis suffer from a lack of alveolar bone, the severity of which varies according to the number of teeth missing. Bone maintenance is a key factor in the treatment of patients with missing teeth, and efforts must be made to develop strategies to keep the bone height and width. The lack of alveolar development in the posterior segments may lead to an anterior rotation of the mandible and consequently a decreased lower anterior face height, a prominent chin, a class III tendency and "curled" and protruded lips (Ogaard and Krogstad, 1995). In conjunction with the deepening of the bite, missing posterior teeth may also result in overeruption of the opposing teeth and in nonworking interferences (Al-Ani et al., 2017a). According to Laing et al. (2010), patients with hypodontia claim they experience difficulty in chewing due to a small occlusal table. It has been hypothesised that hypodontia may pose functional limitations and affect well-being and quality of life, although a limited number of studies have been performed on this subject (Al-Ani et al., 2017a).

Through the application of orthopaedic and orthodontic force systems, the orthodontist can influence both bone modelling and bone remodelling (Lindskog-Stokland et al., 1993; Ruf and Pancherz, 1999). Tooth movement is not only crucial for the optimal positioning of prosthetic abutments, but may also serve as the means for developing a defective alveolar process (Diedrich et al., 1996) in the site of a missing tooth. The temporary skeletal anchorage devices (TADs) used to facilitate tooth movement have been shown to be able to maintain bone (Melsen et al., 2015a). The advantage of being able to maintain bone height is that the prognosis for future prosthetic replacement of a missing tooth is improved, as the need to graft an atrophic alveolar process before inserting an implant is reduced or eliminated.

The following variables must be taken into consideration: the number of missing teeth (multiple aplasia, between four and six teeth or single-tooth aplasia), the dentofacial growth phase (deciduous, mixed or permanent dentition) and the affected area (anterior or posterior).

Anodontia

Anodontia may occur as part of a syndrome, especially one of the numerous types of ectodermal dysplasia, but also in an isolated form, although it is mainly genetically determined (Mostowska et al., 2003). In spite of a total lack of permanent teeth, patients with anodontia mostly have normal eruption of deciduous teeth. Only 1% of patients with missing permanent teeth also have a lack of deciduous teeth (Yonezu et al., 1997; Al-Ani et al., 2017a). As the lower face height is completely dependent on the vertical development of the alveolar process as teeth erupt, it is crucial to maintain the deciduous dentition as long as possible and to avoid the normal wear of deciduous teeth. This can best be achieved by providing children with a bite plate with contact only on an anterior bite plane as early as possible. In doing so, the maximum activity of the masseter and the temporalis muscles are reduced and the passive eruption of the lateral teeth can be

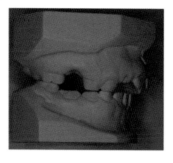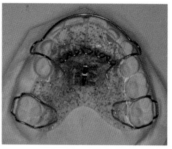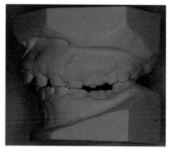

Figure 5.4.5 7.2-year-old girl whose tooth 55 was prematurely lost. Due to the distal molar relationship, the space maintainer is mandatory.

enhanced. If teeth have been lost, a soft tissue-borne activator with a construction bite greater than the freeway space should be inserted and worn at night, whilst transcortical implants may be necessary to prevent overclosure during the day (Figure 5.4.5).

Oligodontia and Hypodontia in the Posterior Region

In relation to oligodontia, a treatment has to be planned as soon as the condition is detected. It is important to foresee where a replacement with an implant or fixed prosthesis can be performed. In cases where replacement teeth are to be inserted later, it is always important to avoid overloading of the deciduous teeth in order to reduce root resorption and preserve the deciduous teeth for as long as possible. As in the case of anodontia, an anterior bite plate can be used to reduce occlusal loadings.

Where space closure is foreseen, it is recommended to first slenderise the deciduous molars either mesially and distally or on one side only, depending on the type of space closure planned. The role of the orthodontist in this mixed-dentition phase is therefore to allow the vertical development of the alveolus and allow dental drifting by monitoring radiologically the root status of the deciduous teeth without successors and strategically slenderising the desired areas. When a patient presents with a sagittal discrepancy, a removable appliance such as an activator can be used, keeping in mind that

the acrylic must be trimmed to allow the eruption of the permanent teeth and to distribute the occlusal load evenly over the existing deciduous teeth.

Once the permanent teeth have erupted, the active movement of the available teeth can start. In patients with class I or II malocclusions and lower premolar aplasia, a planned space closure should start in the lower arch with the removal of the distal root of the deciduous teeth, using the mesial root as anchorage (Figure 5.4.6). It has been suggested that the root be moved first in order to avoid collapse of the alveolar ridge following the extraction, and it has been shown that teeth can be moved into areas where the alveolar ridge is reduced (Lindskog-Stokland et al., 1993); this also limits the root resorption often observed when teeth are moved through atrophic alveolar process. Once the space closure with respect to the mesial root is completed, the mesial root can be extracted and a TAD – ideally with a bracket-head – placed distal to the canine, to serve as either a direct or an indirect anchorage (Figure 5.4.6).

In the situation where there is aplasia of the upper posterior teeth, deciduous tooth slenderising can also be performed, but the removal of a distal deciduous root is more complicated, and therefore is not indicated.

In the case of agenesis of all lower premolars, the second deciduous molar should be replaced by moving the posterior teeth mesially and the first deciduous molar can be used as anchorage for the initial part of the

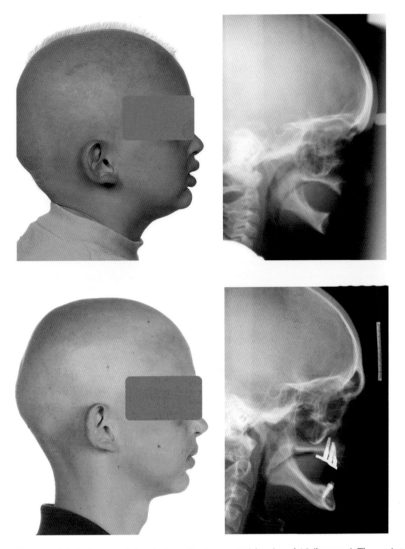

Figure 5.4.6 Ectodermal dysplasia patient at ages 6 (top) and 18 (bottom). The maintenance of a proper vertical dimension has been ensured by the use of early implants. *Source:* Courtesy of Dr. H. Gjorup, University Hospital, Aarhus University, Denmark.

movement. Space closure in the absence of upper third molars is generally avoided because of the loss of an antagonist for the upper second molar. The advantage of space closure is that it reduces the number of implants required, improves the long-term prognosis and decreases the financial burden for the patient.

When there is ankylosis of the deciduous molar with infraocclusion to a degree that it influences the marginal bone height of the adjacent teeth, the deciduous tooth has to be surgically loosened and, if there is no favourable response, removed. If the deciduous ankylosed molar is kept, a progressive infraocclusion will make the extraction more invasive, necessitating a flap and bone removal. This will lead to an alveolar bone defect in an area where bone maintenance is crucial for future implants. It is therefore important to extract the deciduous molar at the first sign of reduced ridge height and tipping of the adjacent teeth towards the ankylosed tooth. If the vertical position of the bone margin of the deciduous molar is level with the adjacent teeth, it can be kept for as long as possible, although interproximal reduction will still be necessary in order to mirror its mesiodistal dimension (Figure 5.4.7).

The ideal time for orthodontic treatment in the case of aplasia of the mandibular second premolars is usually early adolescence, since most of the remaining developing permanent teeth are erupting and most facial growth has already occurred.

Oligodontia and Hypodontia in the Anterior Region

When teeth are missing in the anterior region, the patient's (and parents'/guardians') chief complaints are focused on aesthetics and speech disturbances. This is particularly the case where both the upper and the lower jaws are affected, since the lack of an anterior stop for the tongue (Figure 5.4.8) increases the occurrence of articulation anomalies, and psychosocial problems may occur. As long as the transversal sutural growth is still present, it is of the utmost importance to avoid any prosthetic replacement that will limit the natural transversal maxillary growth. If a plate is used, an expansion screw has to be incorporated to replicate the natural increase in the transversal dimension. If a fixed temporary replacement is foreseen, a trans-sutural connection should be avoided (Figure 5.4.9).

In patients where the oligodontia affects the lower incisors, the therapeutic choice is primarily aimed at bone maintenance, since the collapse of the anterior lower alveolar ridge occurs in both vertical and buccolingual dimensions (Carlsson et al., 1967; Tallgren, 1972) and decreases the possibility of replacing the missing teeth with an implant or fixed prosthesis. An additional limiting factor is that the prognosis for bone grafting in the lower incisor region is considered poor. It is therefore advisable to move the available

incisors towards the midline, leaving the empty spaces mesial to the canines, or aim for a total space closure (Figures 5.4.10 and 5.4.11). The insertion of a short transcortical screw 2–3 mm below the marginal ridge may reduce bone atrophy. A bonded bridge in these cases is the least invasive solution, but since the vertical development of the alveolus occurs throughout life (Fudalej et al., 2007) it is advisable to move the permanent teeth anteriorly without fully closing the space. Depending on the needs of the patient, the final tooth movement to close the spaces orthodontically or with bridges should be carried out after the growth spurt. Substitution of the lower incisors with canines and premolars has been suggested, but this is rarely an acceptable solution as there is a poor morphological similarity between the three. The absence of lower incisors is often linked to missing premolars, and in this case space closure of the incisors is not indicated due to the significant amount of excess space and the risk of retracting the lower anterior segment.

In the case of aplasia of the upper lateral incisors, several points must be considered when deciding whether to close the space, allowing canine mesialisation (so-called canine substitution), or to open the space for final prosthetic or implant solutions. As always, the patient must be evaluated as a whole. When spacing occurs alongside a neutral or class III malocclusion and a large canine, space opening for future implants or an adhesive bridge is indicated. Such opening is indicated in cases of a significant space deficit, a retrognathic maxilla or a mild skeletal class III. Substitution of the permanent canine with the first premolar may be impossible when the first premolar is biradicular, since the risk of root fenestration increases with mesialisation of the tooth. Moreover, the colour of the canine may be relevant, although modern bleaching techniques achieve an acceptable camouflage. Aplasia of a single incisor brings with it the problem of a difference in size and colour between the canine and the lateral

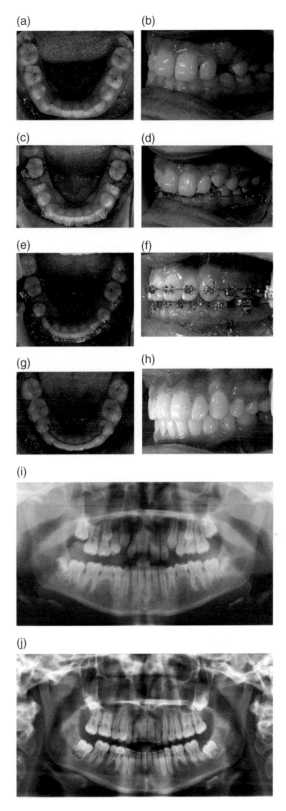

Figure 5.4.7 Extraction of teeth 75 and 85, due to their short roots and posterior crowding (a, b and i). The distal root was first extracted (c and d), and the first molars were mesialised with the help of mini-implants (c, d, e and f). The final occlusion consisted in extreme mesial occlusion and the posterior crowding was solved (g, h and j). *Source:* Melsen et al. (2015b).

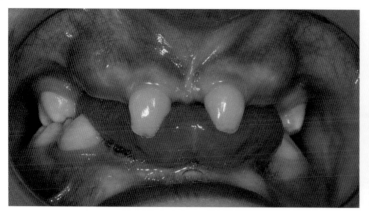
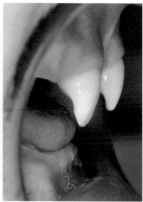

Figure 5.4.8 5-year-old boy affected by ectodermal dysplasia. The absence of teeth in the front region reduces the anterior stop of the tongue during speech and swallowing.

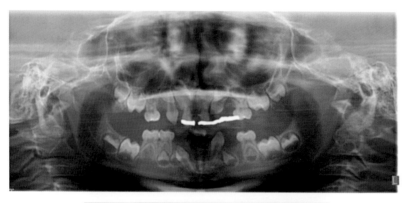

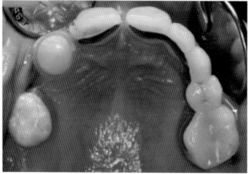

Figure 5.4.9 To ensure an anterior limit for the tongue and improve aesthetics, fixed reconstructions can be applied. An attempt should be made not to connect the two hemimaxillae, in order to allow the natural transversal growth.

incisor, and may create an inharmonious smile line. The space-opening option, on the other hand, condemns the growing adolescent to a temporary prosthetic solution that will become definitive only once the growth velocity has slowed substantially. The optimal age for replacement of incisors by implants has not yet been defined, as the alveolar process may never stop growing completely.

(a)

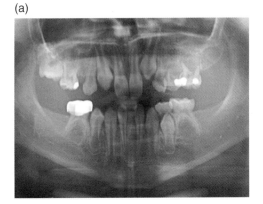

(b)

(c)

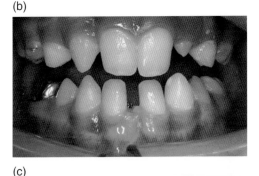

(d)

Figure 5.4.10 Root and tooth movement maintains the height and width of the alveolar bone (a–d). The roots of the incisors are moved first, and then the canines are moved forward (c and d). The small bite blocks on the premolars allow for a gradual extrusion of the posterior teeth, thus keeping the vertical dimension.

Space closure through canine mesialisation does, however, provide a complete solution. Once the orthodontic treatment is finished and the prosthetic camouflage of the front teeth has been carried out, the patient's continued role is to maintain the result, and no further active treatment is needed. In the case of protruded upper jaw, the overjet may be reduced by using the space given by the aplasia of the upper lateral incisors; the canines will substitute the lateral incisors and the molars will end up in a distal relationship (Kokich, 2005).

Zachrisson and coworkers described a series of cases and offered finishing tips that could be used to obtain a natural smile with canine substitution (Figure 5.4.12) (Rosa and Zachrisson, 2010; Rosa et al., 2016). They also showed that the results were stable after 10 years and the periodontium was healthy. However, a recent investigation comparing the attractiveness of canine substitution and implant replacement assessed by dentists and laypeople revealed that dentists did not have a special preference for space closure over an implant but laypeople preferred the canine substitution solution (Schneider et al., 2016).

A key consideration with space closure is the length of the treatment. Although the use of TADs allows for the application of consistent force systems (Kanavakis et al., 2014), the duration of treatment is still long, and therefore is associated with a higher risk of root resorption. A major concern in patients with space opening is the retention strategy to employ until the time is right for implant insertion, as it has been repeatedly shown that early implant placement will lead to implant infraocclusion, which leads in turn to detrimental aesthetic and biological effects (Thilander et al., 2001; Fudalej et al., 2007). Another concern is related to the risk of alveolar ridge resorption once the space is opened. However, according to Kokich, the alveolar ridge obtained through orthodontic tooth movement is more stable, due to the residual loading exerted by the supracrestal fibres (Southard et al., 1992; Kokich, 2005).

(a)

(b)

(c)

(d)

(e)

(f)

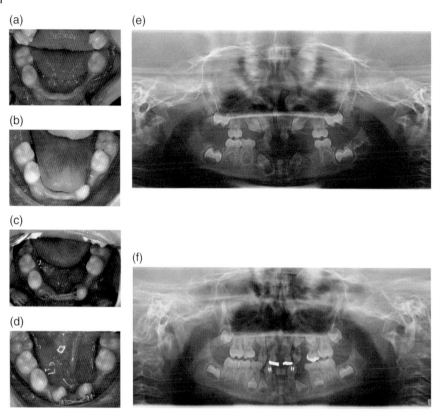

Figure 5.4.11 Boy with ectodermal dysplasia (a and b) at ages 5 and 7 (e and f). After being surgically exposed, tooth 43 has been moved into the arch (c), preserving the width and height of the alveolar bone in the anterior region (d and f).

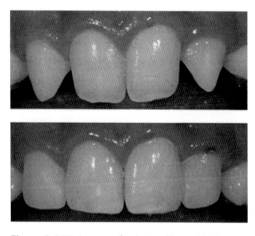

Figure 5.4.12 In case of aplasia of lateral incisors, the canine can be shifted mesially and the final camouflage will be reached by composite reconstruction (lower picture) or veneers, according to the gingival exposure. *Source: Courtesy of Prof. Zitzmann.*

Bone-maintaining properties have been demonstrated in mini-implants (Melsen et al., 2015a) when a horizontally placed TAD used to mesialise the posterior teeth was left in place after the end of treatment and contributed to the maintenance of the bone density, as well as both the height and width of the alveolar process. Based on these observations, Ciarlantini and Melsen (2017) have described a temporary solution to the space-maintenance problem using a pontic fixed to a horizontally placed TAD inserted from the lingual aspect in the upper lateral region. The bracket head allows for the insertion of a full-size wire that carries the pontic (Figure 5.4.13).

The literature regarding the optimal treatment of patients suffering from agenesis or hypodontia does not offer an evidence-based solution. A consensus paper concluded that

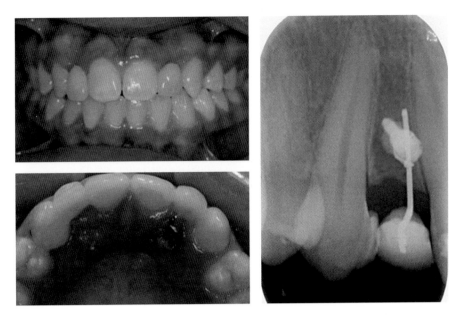

Figure 5.4.13 In case of missing lateral incisors at the end of orthodontic treatment for space opening, the alveolar bone has to be kept until final reconstruction is made. A mini-implant containing a full-size stainless-steel arm carrying an artificial tooth can be used. The advantages are twofold: it provides bone maintenance and doesn't require preparation of the adjacent teeth. Courtesy of Dr Ciarlantini.

the care of patients with congenitally missing lateral incisors is best achieved through a structured multidisciplinary approach (Johal et al., 2013). The number of options is considerable, including space closure, canine substitution with another tooth and implant-supported restoration. The decision must be made for each patient individually, taking into consideration the long-term maintenance demands, psychosociological factors and the financial burden for the patient and their family.

References

Al-Ani, A. H., Antoun, J. S., Thomson, W. M., Merriman, T. R., Farella, M. 2017a. Hypodontia: an update on its etiology, classification, and clinical management. *BioMed Research International*, **2017**, 9378325.

Al-Ani, A. H., Antoun, J. S., Thomson, W. M., Merriman, T. R., Farella, M. 2017b. Maternal smoking during pregnancy is associated with offspring hypodontia. *Journal of Dental Research*, **96**, 1014–19.

Alexander, S. A., Askari, M., Lewis, P. 2015. The premature loss of primary first molars: space loss to molar occlusal relationships and facial patterns. *The Angle Orthodontist*, **85**, 218–23.

Andreasen, J. O. 1992. *Atlas of Replantation and Transplantation of Teeth*. Fribourg: Mediglobe.

Anweigi, L., Allen, P. F., Ziada, H. 2013. The use of the Oral Health Impact Profile to measure the impact of mild, moderate and severe hypodontia on oral health-related quality of life in young adults. *Journal of Oral Rehabilitation*, **40**, 603–8.

Carlsson, G. E., Bergman, B., Hedegard, B. 1967. Changes in contour of the maxillary alveolar process under immediate dentures. A longitudinal clinical and x-ray cephalometric study covering 5 years. *Acta Odontologica Scandinavica*, **25**, 45–75.

Ciarlantini, R., Melsen, B. 2017. Semipermanent replacement of missing maxillary lateral incisors by mini-implant retained pontics: a follow-up study. *American Journal of Orthodontics and Dentofacial Orthopedics*, **151**, 989–94.

Diedrich, P. R., Fuhrmann, R. A., Wehrbein, H., Erpenstein, H. 1996. Distal movement of premolars to provide posterior abutments for missing molars. *American Journal of Orthodontics and Dentofacial Orthopedics*, **109**, 355–60.

Duggal, M. S., Cameron, A. C., and Toumba, J. 2013. *Paediatric Dentistry at a Glance*. Chichester: Wiley-Blackwell.

Frost, H. M. 2003. Bone's mechanostat: a 2003 update. *The Anatomical Record. Part A, Discoveries in Molecular, Cellular, and Evolutionary Biology*, **275**, 1081–101.

Fudalej, P., Kokich, V. G., Leroux, B. 2007. Determining the cessation of vertical growth of the craniofacial structures to facilitate placement of single-tooth implants. *American Journal of Orthodontics and Dentofacial Orthopedics*, **131**, S59–67.

Johal, A., Katsaros, C., Kuijpers-Jagtman, A. M., Angle Society of Europe Membership. 2013. State of the science on controversial topics: missing maxillary lateral incisors – a report of the Angle Society of Europe 2012 meeting. *Progress in Orthodontics*, **14**, 20.

Kanavakis, G., Ludwig, B., Rosa, M., Zachrisson, B., Hourfar, J. 2014. Clinical outcomes of cases with missing lateral incisors treated with the "T"-Mesialslider. *Journal of Orthodontics*, **41**(Suppl. 1), S33–8.

Kokich, V. 2005. Early management of congenitally missing teeth. *Seminars in Orthodontics*, **11**, 146–51.

Laing, E., Cunningham, S. J., Jones, S., Moles, D., Gill, D. 2010. Psychosocial impact of hypodontia in children. *American Journal of Orthodontics and Dentofacial Orthopedics*, **137**, 35–41.

Lindskog-Stokland, B., Wennstrom, J. L., Nyman, S., Thilander, B. 1993. Orthodontic tooth movement into edentulous areas with reduced bone height. An experimental study in the dog. *European Journal of Orthodontics*, **15**, 89–96.

Meaney, S., Anweigi, L., Ziada, H., Allen, F. 2012. The impact of hypodontia: a qualitative study on the experiences of patients. *European Journal of Orthodontics*, **34**, 547–52.

Melsen, B., Huja, S. S., Chien, H. H., Dalstra, M. 2015a. Alveolar bone preservation subsequent to miniscrew implant placement in a canine model. *Orthodontics & Craniofacial Research*, **18**, 77–85.

Melsen, B., Verna, C., Luzi, C. 2015b. *Mini-Implants and their Clinical Applications: The Aarhus Experience*. Bologna: Edizioni Martina.

Mostowska, A., Kobielak, A., Trzeciak, W. H. 2003. Molecular basis of non-syndromic tooth agenesis: mutations of MSX1 and PAX9 reflect their role in patterning human dentition. *European Journal of Oral Sciences*, **111**, 365–70.

Nunn, J. H., Carter, N. E., Gillgrass, T. J., Hobson, R. S., Jepson, N. J., Meechan, J. G., Nohl, F. S. 2003. The interdisciplinary management of hypodontia: background and role of paediatric dentistry. *British Dental Journal*, **194**, 245–51.

Ogaard, B., Krogstad, O. 1995. Craniofacial structure and soft tissue profile in patients with severe hypodontia. *American Journal of Orthodontics and Dentofacial Orthopedics*, **108**, 472–7.

Ostler, M. S., Kokich, V. G. 1994. Alveolar ridge changes in patients congenitally missing mandibular second premolars. *Journal of Prosthetic Dentistry*, **71**, 144–9.

Rakhshan, V. 2015a. Congenitally missing teeth (hypodontia): a review of the literature concerning the etiology, prevalence, risk factors, patterns and treatment. *Dental Research Journal*, **12**, 1–13.

Rakhshan, V. 2015b. Meta-analysis of observational studies on the most commonly missing permanent dentition (excluding the third molars) in non-syndromic dental patients or randomly-selected subjects, and the factors affecting the observed rates. *Journal of Clinical Pediatric Dentistry*, **39**, 199–207.

Rosa, M., Zachrisson, B. U. 2010. The space-closure alternative for missing maxillary lateral incisors: an update. *Journal of Clinical Orthodontics*, **44**, 540–9, quiz 561.

Rosa, M., Lucchi, P., Ferrari, S., Zachrisson, B. U., Caprioglio, A. 2016. Congenitally missing maxillary lateral incisors: long-term periodontal and functional evaluation after orthodontic space closure with first premolar intrusion and canine extrusion. *American Journal of Orthodontics and Dentofacial Orthopedics*, **149**, 339–48.

Ruf, S., Pancherz, H. 1999. Temporomandibular joint remodeling in adolescents and young adults during Herbst treatment: a prospective longitudinal magnetic resonance imaging and cephalometric radiographic investigation. *American Journal of Orthodontics and Dentofacial Orthopedics*, **115**, 607–18.

Saber, A. M., Altoukhi, D. H., Horaib, M. F., El-Housseiny, A. A., Alamoudi, N. M., Sabbagh, H. J. 2018. Consequences of early extraction of compromised first permanent molar: a systematic review. *BMC Oral Health*, **18**, 59.

Schneider, U., Moser, L., Fornasetti, M., Piattella, M., Siciliani, G. 2016. Esthetic evaluation of implants vs canine substitution in patients with congenitally missing maxillary lateral incisors: are there any new insights? *American Journal of Orthodontics and Dentofacial Orthopedics*, **150**, 416–24.

Southard, T. E., Southard, K. A., Tolley, E. A. 1992. Periodontal force: a potential cause of relapse. *American Journal of Orthodontics and Dentofacial Orthopedics*, **101**, 221–7.

Splieth, C. 2011. *Revolutions in Pediatric Dentistry*. London: Quintessence.

Tallgren, A. 1972. The continuing reduction of the residual alveolar ridges in complete denture wearers: a mixed-longitudinal study covering 25 years. *Journal of Prosthetic Dentistry*, **27**, 120–32.

Thilander, B., Odman, J., Lekholm, U. 2001. Orthodontic aspects of the use of oral implants in adolescents: a 10-year follow-up study. *European Journal of Orthodontics*, **23**, 715–31.

Tunison, W., Flores-Mir, C., Elbadrawy, H., Nassar, U., El-Bialy, T. 2008. Dental arch space changes following premature loss of primary first molars: a systematic review. *Pediatric Dentistry*, **30**, 297–302.

Yonezu, T., Hayashi, Y., Sasaki, J., Machida, Y. 1997. Prevalence of congenital dental anomalies of the deciduous dentition in Japanese children. *Bulletin of Tokyo Dental College*, **38**, 27–32.

Unit 6

Management of Oral Health Conditions

6.1

Viral Causes Affecting the Oral Mucosa

Michael M. Bornstein[1], Cynthia K. Y. Yiu[2] and Valerie G. A. Suter[3]

[1] *Oral and Maxillofacial Radiology, Applied Oral Sciences, Faculty of Dentistry, The University of Hong Kong, Hong Kong, China*
[2] *Paediatric Dentistry, Faculty of Dentistry, The University of Hong Kong, Hong Kong, China*
[3] *Department of Oral Surgery and Stomatology, School of Dental Medicine, University of Bern, Bern, Switzerland*

Introduction

The primary aim of the dental practitioner when examining children affected by alterations of the oral mucosa is to make a correct diagnosis and choose the appropriate treatment modality. When failing to detect a mucosal lesion or being unable to obtain a tentative diagnosis, including potential differential diagnoses, important diseases might be overlooked and inappropriate treatment forms selected (Rioboo-Crespo et al., 2005). This is of special relevance for viral infections, as the sequelae may vary from the inconsequential to the potentially fatal and can differ from person to person (Lynch, 2000). Furthermore, children who have medical risk factors tend to be affected more frequently and more severely by viral infections. In general, children differ from adults regarding the effects of viral infections, as they serve as highly effective incubators for viral replication and infectious spread (Sällberg, 2009). This is due to the fact that in the neonate or child, the specific immunity is still immature. Furthermore, children tend to exchange infected fluids more readily than adults because of a lack of hygiene.

Viral diseases of the oral mucosa and the perioral region are frequently encountered in dental practice, but have unfortunately only received limited research interest (Slots, 2000). Unlike epidemiological studies on the prevalence of caries and periodontal disease, studies on the incidence, various manifestations and treatement concepts of viral infections in children are scarce (Rioboo-Crespo et al., 2005). Viruses are known to be important ulcerogenic and tumorigenic agents of the human mouth, and they either produce symptoms directly in the oral cavity or are spread during treatment of the oral cavity, resulting in systemic manifestations. This chapter will focus on the most common viral infections in children, and will also address oral diseases associated with viruses that might be transmitted through dental treatments.

Common Viral Infections in Children that Affect the Oral Mucosa

The soft tissues of the mouth, oropharynx and salivary glands are particularly susceptible to various viral infections, some of which are site-specific. The most common viral agents affecting children are the herpesviruses, papillomaviruses and coxsackieviruses.

Management of Dental Emergencies in Children and Adolescents, First Edition.
Edited by Klaus W. Neuhaus and Adrian Lussi.
© 2019 John Wiley & Sons Ltd. Published 2019 by John Wiley & Sons Ltd.
Companion website: www.wiley.com/go/neuhaus/dental_emergencies

Herpesviruses

Eight members of the Herpesviridae family (also known as the human herpesviruses, HHVs) commonly infect humans (Dreyfus, 2013), and close to 100% of the adult population is infected with at least one of these (Grinde, 2013). The five that cause the most health concerns are herpes simplex virus types 1 and 2 (HSV-1 and HSV-2), varicella zoster virus (VZV), Epstein–Barr virus (EBV) and cytomegalovirus (CMV).

Herpes Simplex Virus

HSV-1 (also known as HHV-1) classically causes infection above the waist and localised to the mouth and oropharynx, whereas HSV-2 (HHV-2) usually causes genital infections. HSV-1 of the perioral region can be grouped into two forms of mucocutaneous lesion: (i) a primary form, which typically is seen in younger patients as herpetiform gingivostomatitis, but which often remains asymptomatic; and (ii) a secondary form that results from reactivation of the virus and which manifests itself as recurrent herpes labialis (fever blisters or cold sores).

Primary herpetic gingivostomatitis is the most common clinical presentation of a primary HSV-1 infection, occurring in 15% of children in the first 9 years of life (Faden, 2006). It is seen most often in preschoolers aged between 1 and 4 years, and the severity of the disease is highly variable. Oral lesions appear on the first day of illness in 85% of affected children and may persist for a period of 7–18 days. Oral lesions typically affect the lips, tongue, gingivae (Figure 6.1.1), buccal mucosa and hard and soft palates. Unlike recurrent herpetic lesions, which are limited to the keratinised mucosa, the primary HSV-1 infection affects both the keratinised and nonkeratinised oral mucosa. The oral mucosal lesions present as small, 1–2 mm blisters that break down rather quickly and coalesce to form shallow, painful ulcers covered by a yellowish-grey pseudomembrane and surrounded by an erythematous halo (Figure 6.1.2). These ulcers heal gradually in 10–14 days, without scarring. The oral mucosal features are usually accompanied by pyrexia, lethargy, loss of appetite, fractiousness and hypersalivation (Arduino and Porter, 2008). Following infection and local replication at the mucosal surfaces, HSV-1 enters sensory nerve endings and is transported by retrograde axonal transport to the neuronal cell bodies, culminating in a latent infection of these neurones. The trigeminal ganglion is the primary site of latency, in which the virus remains present lifelong, and serves as a reservoir for later recurrent herpetic infection (Nicoll et al., 2012).

Reactivation of HSV-1 in the sensory ganglion causes cutaneous and mucocutaneous recurrent herpetic infection. Reactivation

(a)

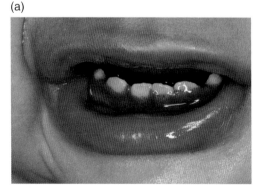

(b)

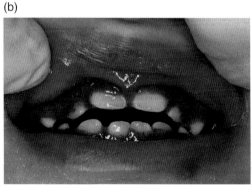

Figure 6.1.1 20-month-old boy with a primary herpetic gingivostomatitis exhibiting characteristic widespread inflammation of the gingiva in the (a) upper and (b) lower jaws, which appears pinkish-red and distinctly swollen.

(a)

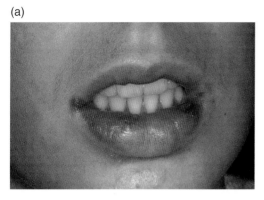

(b)

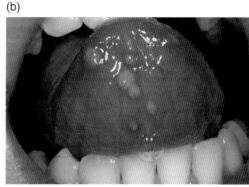

Figure 6.1.2 16-year-old girl with a primary herpetic gingivostomatitis exhibiting characteristic 1–2 mm blisters that break down rather quickly and coalesce to form shallow, painful ulcers covered by a yellowish-grey pseudomembrane, and surrounded by an erythematous halo on the (a) lips and (b) tongue.

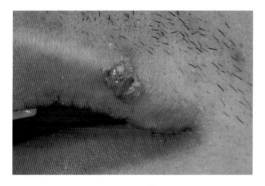

Figure 6.1.3 Reactivation of an HSV-1 infection presenting as herpes labialis with typical vesicular lesions on the upper left lip in a 20-year-old patient. These lesions are highly infective at this stage.

can be spontaneous, or it can be triggered by a number of factors, such as fever, ultraviolet light exposure, common cold, emotional stress, fatigue, trauma, immunosuppression, chemotherapy and menstruation (Arduino and Porter, 2008). The lesions typically occur on the mucocutaneous junction of the face, usually on the lips (Figure 6.1.3). Prodromal symptoms are frequently reported, and include paraesthesia, tenderness, pain, burning sensation and itching sensation at the site of reactivation. The lesions of the recurrent infection are usually red macules that rapidly become vesicular, being highly infective at this stage. Later, these lesions form pustular scabs and ulcers, which usually heal within 7–10 days (Leung and Barankin, 2017).

HSV-1 is shed in high numbers from active herpes labialis lesions, particularly during the blister and ulcer stages. The risk to the dental health-care provider of acquiring an HSV-1-based infection from a patient is greatest at these times, although transmission is also possible at the crust stage. Primary inoculation from a patient resulting in herpetic gingivostomatitis is unlikely, but there is an occupationally relevant risk of acquiring herpetic whitlow or ocular herpetic infections (Lewis, 2004). Herpetic whitlow (also known as herpetic paronychia) presents with prodromal features of local pain, tingling or a burning sensation, followed by an acute vesicular eruption, affecting the distal phalanx of one or more fingers. Ocular HSV-1 infections cause multiple pathologies, with perhaps the most destructive being herpes stromal keratitis (HSK). HSK lesions can recur throughout life and often cause progressive corneal scarring, resulting in visual impairment (Rowe et al., 2013). The aerosols generated by dental high-speed handpieces and ultrasonic instruments represent important routes of transmission of HSV-1 for the dental team. Thus, wearing gloves, masks and eye protection during treatment of all patients is essential, and it is advisable to postpone treatment in patients with active HSV-1 lesions. By the same token, dentists or hygienists should not provide treatment whilst themselves having an active HSV-1 infection (Scott et al., 1997).

Aciclovir is the first-line drug for the management of HSV and VZV infections (Piret and Boivin, 2016), but other nucleoside analogues such as valacyclovir and famciclovir have also been discussed. Depending on the manifestation of the disease and the status of the patient (immunocompetent versus immunocompromised), topical, oral or intravanous routes of application have been proposed (Levin et al., 2016). Long-term administration of aciclovir for the treatment of severe infections in immunocompromised patients can lead to the development of drug resistance. New categories of potential HSV antivirals, such as lipid-conjugated nucleotide analogues (brincidofovir) and helicase–primase inhibitors, are under investigation.

Varicella Zoster Virus

VZV (also known as HHV-3) shares many similarities with HSV, as it is also associated with vesicular lesions, infection of neuronal tissue and latent infection of ganglia, and the primary infection occurs at mucosal surfaces. However, VZV transmission does not require intimate, skin-to-skin contact like that of HSV, but occurs more commonly via an aerosol route (Schleiss, 2009). The most common clinical manifestation of VZV infection is chickenpox, followed by herpes zoster (shingles). Chickenpox occurs more commonly in children, and typically reactivates as shingles in adults.

Chickenpox is characterised by a prodromal illness period followed by oral vesicles and ulcers typically located on the lips, palate and buccal mucosa (Pinto and Hong, 2013). Oral vesicles rupture, leaving shallow round ulcerations surrounded by an erythematous halo. The subsequent skin rash is typically pruritic and maculopapular, with formation of vesicles and pustules that rupture, leaving hard, brown-crusted lesions. The crusts eventually exfoliate, leaving mild to moderate scarring (Pinto, 2005). The disease is self-limiting, lasting 5–10 days. However, immunocompromised patients risk involvement of the central nervous and pulmonary systems, resulting in a higher mortality rate in this group (Clarkson et al., 2017). The management of a primary VZV infection is symptomatic only, but a vaccine against VZV is readily available and is given to infants starting from 11–24 months of age.

Shingles is the secondary infection of VZV and tends to occur only in middle to late life, via viral reactivation. Certain conditions characterised by immunosuppression predispose individuals to develop shingles, such as hematopoietic or lymphoid malignancies, human immunodeficiency virus (HIV) seropositivity, chemotherapy and transplantation (Lynch, 2000). Typically, lesions occur in a dermatomal distribution on the thorax, but when present in the orofacial region, they can appear following the divisions of the trigeminal nerve. When they occur on the oral mucosa, clinical features are unilateral vesicles and ulcers (Figure 6.1.4). Postherpetic neuralgia (PHN) occurs in approximately 30% of

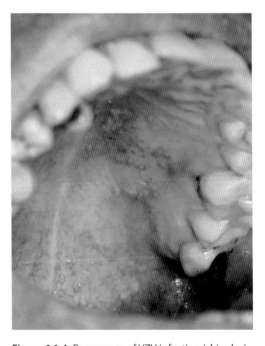

Figure 6.1.4 Recurrence of VZV infection (shingles) exhibiting unilateral vesicles and ulcers on the left hard palate in a 55-year-old man following the divisions of the trigeminal nerve (V2, left).

patients with shingles and is characterised by a localised, very acute, sharp pain (McCullough and Savage, 2005). It is usually seen in elderly and immunocompromised persons, can induce psychosocial dysfunction and can have a negative impact on quality of life (Feller et al., 2017).

VZV represents the most widespread vaccine-preventable childhood infectious disease in industrialised countries. Due to its relevant burden on health-care resources, several countries have introduced VZV vaccination into their recommended routine childhood national immunisation schedule (Gabutti et al., 2016). The United States was the first country to recommend universal vaccination. In the European Union, the use of varicella vaccine is still heterogeneous, with some countries recommending universal vaccination in children at a national or regional level, others recommending it only in high-risk groups and others having no recommendation at all (Carrillo-Santisteve and Lopalco, 2014).

Epstein–Barr Virus

EBV (also known as HHV-4) is the causative agent of infectious mononucleosis, but it is also associated with neoplastic processes such as Burkitt's lymphoma, nasopharyngeal carcinoma and oral hairy leukoplakia (HL) (Gondivkar et al., 2012).

Infectious mononucleosis (also known as "kissing disease") is primarily transmitted through close contact (sharing of straws, kissing and other forms of saliva exchange). Most children affected by a primary infection remain asymptomatic. However, in young adults, oral and systemic symptoms may be seen. Oral lesions of infectious mononucleosis characteristically consist of pharyngitis and petechial hemorrhages of the soft palate and oral pharynx with concomitant fever and cervical lymphadenopathy (Lynch, 2000). The common oral-pharyngeal lesions of infectious mononucleosis require no treatment and resolve spontaneously. Nevertheless, symptoms can be more severe in adults. Infectious mononucleosis is in most cases a benign, acute and self-limiting disease, but chronic forms of EBV infection may result very rarely in severe or even fatal conditions (Okano and Gross, 2012).

Cytomegalovirus

Most infections with CMV (also known as HHV-5) remain asymptomatic, but less than 10% of patients present with flu-like symptoms. CMV can be frequently found in cases with mucosal ulcers as the only ulcerogenic viral agent in acquired immune deficiency syndrome (AIDS) patients (Itin and Lautenschlager, 1997). When a baby is born with CMV, it is called congenital CMV infection. CMV is the most common cause of congenital infection in the world. Symptomatic infants are at increased risk of developing permanent sequelae, including sensorineural hearing loss and neurodevelopmental delay (James and Kimberlin, 2016).

Human Herpesvirus 8

The emergence of HIV/AIDS almost 4 decades ago led to an increased incidence of diseases caused by HHV-8 coinfection, particularly Kaposi sarcoma and multicentric Castleman disease. Over time, the development of highly effective AIDS therapies has resulted in a decreased incidence of HHV-8-associated entities, which are now more commonly found in patients with undiagnosed or untreated AIDS. Due to their rarity, some of these diseases may be difficult to recognise without appropriate clinical information (Auten et al., 2017).

Papillomaviruses

Human papillomavirus (HPV) is a small double-stranded DNA virus that is known to be the most common sexually transmitted disease worldwide. There are more than 100 types of HPV, and varying degrees of risk are linked with infection by each. Many infections are only short-lived and clinically relatively unimportant, but repeated infection with particular types can cause a considerable burden in both men and women, resulting in HPV-related malignancies (Pringle, 2014). Clinical infections with low-risk genotypes manifest as oral squamous papilloma, verruca vulgaris (common wart), condyloma acuminatum or focal/multifocal epithelial hyperplasia (Heck's disease). Clinically manifest infections with HPV apprear in children younger than 1 year, presumably as a result of vertical transmission from the mother, and in adolescents at the time of sexual debut.

Oral Squamous Papilloma

Papilloma occurs over a wide age range and presents as an exophytic, sessile or peduncu-lated growth of squamous epithelium, with papillary projections. The lesion can appear pink or white, depending on the degree of keratinisation. It is commonly found on the hard and soft palates (Figures 6.1.5 and 6.1.6), uvula and lips (Clarkson et al., 2017). With its broad range of features, oral squamous papil-loma is clinically and pathologically chal-lenging to distinguish from condyloma acuminatum or verruca vulgaris. The squa-mous papilloma is presumed to be caused by low-risk types of HPV, and genotypes 6 and 11 have often been detected (Pringle, 2014).

Verruca Vulgaris (Common Wart)

Warts are caused mainly by HPV types 2 and 4. Verruca vulgaris is similar in appearance to squamous papillomas and tends to involve mucosal areas in which keratinisation of the epithelium resembles that of the skin, such as the gingivae and hard palate. In children, warts on the skin are most commonly observed on the hands and fingers (Figure 6.1.7), but are also found on the lips (Figure 6.1.8) and less commonly in the mouth. Oral warts are usually asymptomatic, but they may be persistent and should be treated to avoid self-contamination or spread of the virus to other children. Uncommonly, warts regress spontaneously (Feller et al., 2017). Usually, intraoral warts result from self-contamination. It has been emphasised that the diagnosis of oral verruca should be preserved for lesions showing histological

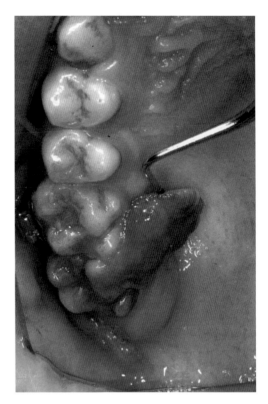

Figure 6.1.5 Characteristic oral squamous papilloma in a 15-year-old boy presenting as an exophytic, pedunculated, pinkish growth in the right palate in the region of the second molar.

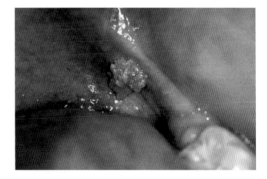

Figure 6.1.6 Characteristic oral squamous papilloma in a 12-year-old girl presenting as an exophytic, pedunculated, pinkish growth with papillary projections located on the left palatoglossal fold.

characteristics of verruca vulgaris of the skin. On clinical examination, a verruca is often indistinguishable from a squamous papilloma or condyloma (Syrjänen, 2002).

(a)   (b)

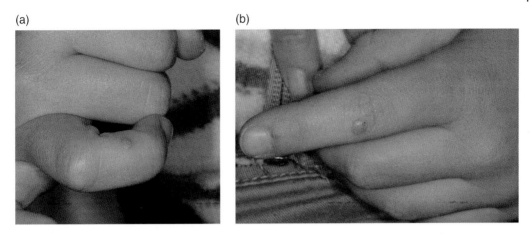

Figure 6.1.7 7.5-year-old girl with common warts on (a) the right ring finger and (b) the left index finger.

(a)   (b)

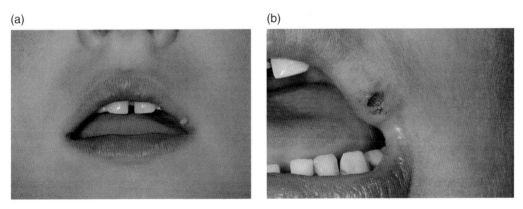

Figure 6.1.8 5-year old girl with a common wart on the upper left lip, confirmed by histopathology to be verruca vulgaris. (a) Initial manifestation. (b) After excision with a CO_2 laser.

Condyloma Accuminatum (Venereal Wart)

Condyloma acuminatum is generally regarded as a sexually transmitted disease, affecting the skin and mucous membranes of the anogenital tract. When diagnosed in children, it may indicate sexual abuse. Intraorally, condyloma commonly presents as a group of multiple pink nodules on the labial mucosa, soft palate and lingual frenum.

Epithelial Hyperplasia (Heck's Disease)

Focal epithelial hyperplasia is an asymptomatic benign mucosal disease that is mostly observed in specific groups in certain geographical regions. It is usually a disease of childhood and adolescence. Clinically, epithelial hyperplasia is typically characterised by multiple painless soft sessile papules, plaques or nodules, which may coalesce to give rise to larger lesions (Figure 6.1.9). HPV genotypes 13 and 32 have been associated and detected in the majority of lesions. Epithelial hyperplasia sometimes resolves spontaneously, but treatment is often indicated as a consequence of aesthetic impairments or even interference with occlusion (Said et al., 2013).

Potentially Malignant and Malignant Disorders

About 5% of all cancers worldwide are attributable mainly to the so-called "high-risk HPVs", including HPV types 16, 18, 31,

(a)

(b)

(c)

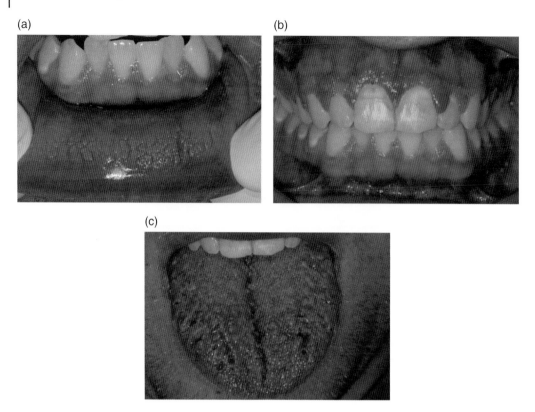

Figure 6.1.9 Epithelial hyperplasia in a 21-year old man, characterised by multiple painless soft sessile papules and nodular exophytic lesions, which coalesce to give rise to even larger manifestations on the (a) lips, (b) gingivae and (c) tongue.

33, 35, 39, 45, 51, 52, 56, 58 and 59 (de Sanjosé et al., 2018). These high-risk types are associated with squamous cell carcinomas (SCCs) of the anogenital and oropharyngeal tracts. SCC of the oropharynx is increasing in incidence, supposedly due to an increase in HPV-related SCC, particularly amongst middle-aged white men; sexual behavior is a risk factor (Pytynia et al., 2014).

The significance of HPV infection in the malignant progression of oral potentially malignant disorders is a major concern. Whether the risk of malignant progression is related to viral loads remains unclear. Common high- and low-risk HPV DNAs have been investigated in oral lichen planus, oral leukoplakia and controls, and higher HPV-16/18 DNA loads have been reported in patients in comparison to controls. Nevertheless, the clinical significance of

high-risk HPV loads in the malignant progression of oral potentially malignant disorders needs to be clarified (Chen and Zhao, 2017).

With pimary prevention through vaccination, there is actually an effective solution to the cancer-related burden of HPV. HPV vaccines are now included in immunisation programmes in many countries. Unfortunately, uptake has been impacted by a reduced confidence in the safety of the HPV vaccine. Nevertheless, recent findings have not demonstrated an increased risk of severe adverse events, and the risk–benefit profile for HPV vaccines remains highly favourable (Phillips et al., 2018). Furthermore, only a few countries have implemented a universal HPV vaccination programme for adolescent boys and girls. Many are arguing that female-only vaccination programmes protect males via

(a)

(b)

(c)

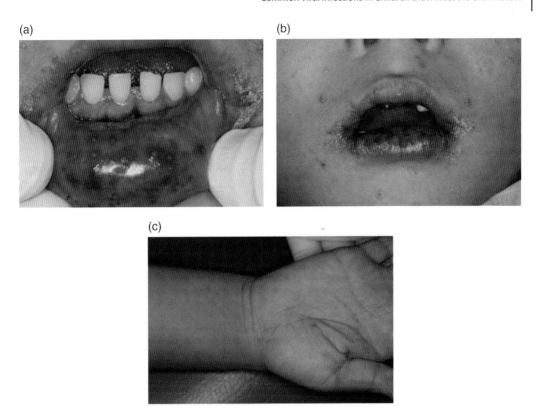

Figure 6.1.10 (a) 5-year old boy with hand-foot-and-mouth disease exhibiting multiple superficial erosions and small vesicular lesions surrounded by an erythematous halo on the lower vestibular mucosa. (b) The gingiva is normal and unaffected, unlike in lesions originating from HSV-1 infection in gingivostomatitis herpetica. Lesions on the lips and cutaneous manifestations surrounding the lips can rupture and form erosions and crusts. (c) On the palm, the vesicular lesions are small and discrete, and usually do not rupture.

herd immunity and that men who have sex with men can be protected via targeted vaccination programmes. Oppsing this notion, experts in the field have stated that the most effective, practical, ethical and potentially cost-effective solution is universal HPV vaccination, which might lead to control of HPV-related diseases in men and women alike (Prue et al., 2017).

Coxsackieviruses

The coxsackieviruses cause primarily two clinically relevant conditions involving the oral mucosa: (i) hand-foot-and-mouth disease and (ii) herpangina. Hand-foot-and-mouth disease is common in infants and young children. It usually causes fever, small vesicles that

result in painful shallow ulcerations in the mouth and vesicular lesions surrounded by an erythematous halo on the hands and feet (Figure 6.1.10), mostly the lateral and dorsal areas of the fingers and toes, palms and soles (Pinto, 2005). The cutaneous lesions eventually rupture, and the resulting ulcers become encrusted (Lynch, 2000).

Most infected children recover in a week or two. The most common cause of hand-foot-and-mouth disease is infection with coxsackievirus A16. Coxsackievirus belongs to a group of viruses called nonpolio enteroviruses in the Picornaviridae family, and other types of enterovirus can sometimes also cause hand-foot-and-mouth disease. People infected with hand-foot-and-mouth disease can spread the infection through coughing or sneezing, as well as through direct contact with their blister fluid or faeces (Lynch, 2000). Hand-foot-and-mouth disease is often confused with foot-and-mouth disease (also known hoof-and-mouth disease), which affects cattle, sheep and swine. However, the two diseases are caused by different viruses and are not related. Humans do not get the animal disease, and animals do not get the human disease.

Herpangina is caused by coxsackievirus type A, and like hand-foot-and-mouth disease, infections are transmitted through contaminated droplets of saliva or a faecal–oral route. Herpangina occurs more frequently in children than in adults. Following exposure, infected individuals have a brief, nonspecific prodrome of fever and malaise, followed by an erythematous pharyngitis and dysphagia. These symptoms are followed by the appearance of a vesicular eruption involving the soft palate, tonsillar pillars and fauces. The vesicles rapidly rupture to form shallow ulcers covered by pseudomembrane and are surrounded by an erythematous halo, mimicking recurrent aphthous ulcers. The lesions resolve within 1 week without any significant additional symptoms (Lynch, 2000).

Viral Infections in Children that Less Frequently or Only Indirectly Affect the Oral Mucosa

Mumps Virus

Mumps is a common childhood infection caused by the mumps virus, a member of the Paramyxoviridae family. The defining feature of classical mumps is swelling of the parotid gland. However, the mumps virus doesn't affect only the salivary glands but also other glands including the pancreas and reproductive glands, which may result in male infertility (Sällberg, 2009). It is highly neurotropic, and can cause central nervous system infection, leading to aseptic meningitis and viral encephalitis. Mumps is vaccine-preventable,

and routine vaccination has proven highly effective in reducing its incidence. This approach is presently used by most developed countries. Since the introduction of the mumps vaccine, the age of appearance of mumps infection has shifted from childhood to adolescence and young adulthood: ages with a higher incidence of disease complications and sequelae. Even though the vaccine has drastically reduced mumps cases, outbreaks continue to occur. These have most commonly been seen where people have had prolonged, close contact with a person who has mumps, such as attending the same class, playing on the same sports team or living in the same dormitory (Scully and Samaranayake, 2016).

Measles (Rubeola)

Measles is a very contagious disease caused by the measles virus, a member of the Paromyxoviridae family. It spreads through the air when an infected person coughs or sneezes. Measles starts with fever, then produces a cough, runny nose and red eyes, and finally a rash of tiny, red spots (maculopapular rash) breaks out. It begins at the head and spreads to the rest of the body, and often causes itching. Oral mucosal manifestations known as Koplik's spots preceed the cutanueous lesions and are considered pathognomonic for measles, but these are temporary and therefore rarely seen. Recognising these spots before a person reaches their maximum infectiousness can help physicians reduce the spread of the disease (Clarkson et al., 2017).

Measles can be prevented with a triple vaccine against measles, mumps, and rubella (German measles), known as the MMR vaccine. The US Centers for Disease Control and Prevention (CDC) recommends children get two doses of the MMR vaccine, the first at 12–15 months and the second 4–6 years. Teens and adults should keep up to date on their MMR vaccination. The MMR vaccine is very safe and effective (CDC, n.d.-b). Unfortunately, vaccination programs are not standardised internationally, and even in highly developed countires the vaccine need only be taken on a voluntary basis. Underlining the critical problems involved in battling preventable diseases, there were 21 315 cases of measles and 35 measles-related deaths recorded in Europe in 2017 (Kmietowicz, 2018).

Human Immunodeficiency Virus

AIDS is the most serious expression of disease resulting from infection with HIV. CD4 cells, the major cells targeted by HIV, are killed and replaced in large numbers during the course of the infection, until the capacity of the immune system to respond further is exhausted, resulting in severe immunodeficiency. People with HIV who do not receive treatment will typically progress through three stages of disease. Stage 1 is the acute HIV infection, where patients experience a flu-like illness that may last for a few weeks. People with an acute HIV infection usually have a large amount of virus in their blood, and are highly contagious. Stage 2 is the clinical latency phase, where the HIV is characterised by its inactivity or dormancy. During this phase, the HIV is still active, but it reproduces at very low levels, and patients may not have any symptoms or feel sick. Without treatment, this period can last a decade or longer, but some patients progress through it much faster. At the end of this phase, the viral load of affected patients starts to go up, and the CD4 cell count begins to go down. Thus, the patient moves into Stage 3, the AIDS phase (CDC, n.d.-a).

A diagnosis of AIDS implies that there has been some damage to the immune system resulting in opportunistic infections or secondary cancers (McCullough and Savage, 2005). Several oral lesions associated with HIV infection have been identified to have a viral aetiology. The early stages of AIDS include oral and vulvovaginal candidiasis, pneumococcal infections, tuberculosis and reactivation of HSV and VZV. Hairy leukoplakia (HL), an EBV-induced epithelial

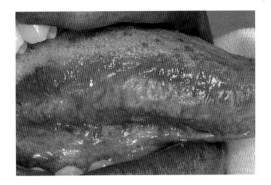

Figure 6.1.11 HL in a 29-year-old man recently diagnosed with HIV, exhibiting a whitish, curdoroy-like pattern on the right lateral border of the tongue.

hyperplasia affecting the borders of the tongue, is a prominent oral manifestation of HIV infection (Braz-Silva et al., 2017). It is an oral epithelial white lesion, and was not described before the AIDS epidemic (Figure 6.1.11). It shows characteristic histopathology. Whilst initially associated with HIV, immunosuppression and progression to AIDS, HL is seen also in association with other forms of immunosuppression, such as organ-transplant patients, those with lymphoproliferative disease and those who use steroid inhalers. It has also been described rarely in apparently immunocompetent individuals (Greenspan et al., 2016). Malignancies in patients with AIDS are generally virally related and include EBV lymphomas, Kaposi's sarcoma associated with HHV-8 and cervical and anal carcinomas originating from papillomavirus.

Due to a combination of tailored antiretroviral therapy applied to HIV-positive mothers and their infants and avoidance of breastfeeding in this population, HIV infection has mainly been eliminated in first-world countries in newborns. Nevertheless, HIV-exposed uninfected children seem to be more susceptible to infection. It is unclear whether this is due to environmental exposure to their HIV-positive mother and maternally derived pathogens or an immunological consequence of the exposure to HIV in utero (Afran et al., 2014).

Conclusion

Viral infections relevant to oral health mainly result in oral ulcerations or oral tumours and may be limited to acute infections, but recurrences and even malignancies on the basis of viral infections can be seen. The acute phases of infection are typically painful, and are thus of clinical relevance in children and infants due to the inadequate nutrition that can result from a lack of enthusiasm for eating. The dental health-care provider should be familiar with the common soft-tissue lesions seen in children so that they can provide appropriate diagnosis, management and referral – ideally to a family physician or paediatrician who is already familiar with the patient's past medical history. Furthermore, vaccination programmes are increasingly preventing many severe viral childhood infections. This has certainly changed the panorama of viral infections affecting children around the world, but childhood viral infections are still a serious health problem in developing countries, and outbreaks of specific viral diseases in highly developed countries are frequently reported.

References

Afran, L., Garcia Knight, M., Nduati, E., Urban, B. C., Heyderman, R. S., Rowland-Jones, S. L. 2014. HIV-exposed uninfected children: a growing population with a vulnerable immune system? *Clinical & Experimental Immunology*, **176**, 11–22.

Arduino, P. G., Porter, S. R. 2008. Herpes simplex virus type 1 infection: overview on relevant clinico-pathological features. *Journal of Oral Pathology and Medicine*, **37**, 107–21.

Auten, M., Kim, A. S., Bradley, K. T., Rosado, F. G. 2017. Human herpesvirus 8-related diseases: histopathologic diagnosis and disease mechanisms. *Seminars in Diagnostic Pathology*, **34**, 371–6.

Braz-Silva, P. H., Schussel, J. L., López Ortega, K., Gallottini, M. 2017. Oral lesions as an important marker for HIV progression. *Dermatology Online Journal*, **23**(9), pii: 13030/qt9t26m7n3.

Carrillo-Santisteve, P., Lopalco, P. L. 2014. Varicella vaccination: a laboured take-off. *Clinical Microbiology and Infection*, **20**(Suppl. 5), 86–91.

Centers for Disease Control and Prevention (CDC). n.d.-a HIV/AIDS. Available from: https://www.cdc.gov/hiv/ (last accessed 30 January 2019).

Centers for Disease Control and Prevention (CDC). n.d.-b Measles (rubeola). Available from: https://www.cdc.gov/measles/index.html (last accessed 30 January 2019).

Chen, X., Zhao, Y. 2017. Human papillomavirus infection in oral potentially malignant disorders and cancer. *Archives of Oral Biology*, **83**, 334–9.

Clarkson, E., Mashkoor, F., Abdulateef, S. 2017. Oral viral infections: diagnosis and management. *Dental Clinics of North America*, **61**, 351–63.

de Sanjosé, S., Brotons, M., Pavón, M. A. 2018. The natural history of human papillomavirus infection. *Best Practice & Research: Clinical Obstetrics and Gynaecology*, **47**, 2–13.

Dreyfus, D. H. 2013. Herpesviruses and the microbiome. *Journal of Allergy and Clinical Immunology*, **132**, 1278–86.

Faden, H. 2006. Management of primary herpetic gingivostomatitis in young children. *Pediatric Emergency Care*, **22**, 268–9.

Feller, L., Khammissa, R. A. G., Fourie, J., Bouckaert, M., Lemmer, J. 2017. Postherpetic neuralgia and trigeminal neuralgia. *Pain Research and Treatment*, **2017**, 1681765.

Gabutti, G., Franchi, M., Maniscalco, L., Stefanati, A. 2016. Varicella-zoster virus: pathogenesis, incidence patterns and vaccination programs. *Minerva Pediatrics*, **68**, 213–25.

Gondivkar, S. M., Parikh, R. V., Gadbail, A. R., Solanke, V., Chole, R., Mankar, M., Balsaraf, S. 2012. Involvement of viral factors with head and neck cancers. *Oral Oncology*, **48**, 195–9.

Greenspan, J. S., Greenspan, D., Webster-Cyriaque, J. 2016. Hairy leukoplakia; lessons learned: 30-plus years. *Oral Diseases*, **22**(Suppl. 1), 120–7.

Grinde, B. 2013. Herpesviruses: latency and reactivation – viral strategies and host response. *Journal of Oral Microbiology*, **5**, doi: 10.3402/jom.v5i0.22766.

Itin, P. H., Lautenschlager, S. 1997. Viral lesions of the mouth in HIV-infected patients. *Dermatology*, **194**, 1–7.

James, S. H., Kimberlin, D. W. 2016. Advances in the prevention and treatment of congenital cytomegalovirus infection. *Current Opinions in Pediatrics*, **28**, 81–5.

Kmietowicz, Z. 2018. "Tragedy" of 35 deaths from measles in Europe last year is unacceptable, says WHO. *British Medical Journal*, **360**, k795.

Leung, A. K. C., Barankin, B. 2017. Herpes labialis: an update. *Recent Patents on Inflammation & Allergy Drug Discovery*, **11**, 107–13.

Levin, M. J., Weinberg, A., Schmid, D. S. 2016. Herpes simplex virus and varicella-zoster virus. *Microbioloy Spectrum*, **4**(3), doi: 10.1128/microbiolspec.DMIH2-0017-2015.

Lewis, M. A. 2004. Herpes simplex virus: an occupational hazard in dentistry. *International Dental Journal*, **54**, 103–11.

Lynch, D. P. 2000. Oral viral infections. *Clinical Dermatology*, **18**, 619–28.

McCullough, M. J., Savage, N. W. 2005. Oral viral infections and the therapeutic use of antiviral agents in dentistry. *Australian Dental Journal*, **50**(Suppl. 2), S31–5.

Nicoll, M. P., Proença, J. T., Efstathiou, S. 2012. The molecular basis of herpes simplex virus latency. *FEMS Microbiology Reviews*, **36**, 684–705.

Okano, M., Gross, T. G. 2012. Acute or chronic life-threatening diseases associated with Epstein-Barr virus infection. *American Journal of the Medical Sciences*, **343**, 483–9.

Phillips, A., Patel, C., Pillsbury, A., Brotherton, J., Macartney, K. 2018. Safety of human papillomavirus vaccines: an updated review. *Drug Safety*, **41**(4), 329–46.

Pinto, A. 2005. Pediatric soft tissue lesions. *Dental Clinics of North Amercia*, **49**, 241–58.

Pinto, A., Hong, C. H. 2013. Orofacial manifestations of bacterial and viral infections in children. *Journal of the Californian Dental Association*, **41**, 271–9.

Piret, J., Boivin, G. 2016. Antiviral resistance in herpes simplex virus and varicella-zoster virus infections: diagnosis and management. *Current Opinion in Infectious Diseases*, **29**(6), 654–62.

Pringle, G. A. 2014. The role of human papillomavirus in oral disease. *Dental Clinics of North America*, **58**, 385–99.

Prue, G., Lawler, M., Baker P., Warnakulasuriya, S. 2017. Human papillomavirus (HPV): making the case for "Immunisation for All". *Oral Diseases*, **23**, 726–30.

Pytynia, K. B., Dahlstrom, K. R., Sturgis, E. M. 2014. Epidemiology of HPV-associated oropharyngeal cancer. *Oral Oncology*, **50**, 380–6.

Rioboo-Crespo, M. R., Planells-del Pozo, P., Rioboo-García, R. 2005. Epidemiology of the most common oral mucosal diseases in children. *Medicina Oral Patologia Oral y Cirugia Bucal*, **10**, 376–87.

Rowe, A. M., St Leger, A. J., Jeon, S., Dhaliwal, D. K., Knickelbein, J. E., Hendricks, R. L. 2013. Herpes keratitis. *Progress in Retinal and Eye Research*, **32**, 88–101.

Said, A. K., Leao, J. C., Fedele, S., Porter, S. R. 2013. Focal epithelial hyperplasia – an update. *Journal of Oral Pathology and Medicine*, **42**, 435–42.

Sällberg, M. 2009. Oral viral infections of children. *Periodontology* **2000**, 49, 87–95.

Schleiss, M. R. 2009. Persistent and recurring viral infections: the human herpesviruses. *Current Probems in Pediatric and Adolescent Health Care*, **39**, 7–23.

Scott, D. A, Coulter, W. A., Lamey, P. J. 1997. Oral shedding of herpes simplex virus type 1: a review. *Journal of Oral Pathology and Medicine*, **26**, 441–7.

Scully, C., Samaranayake, L. P. 2016. Emerging and changing viral diseases in the new millennium. *Oral Diseases*, **22**, 171–9.

Slots, J. 2000. Oral viral infections of adults. *Periodontology* **2000**, 49, 60–86.

Syrjänen, S. 2002. Human papillomavirus infections and oral tumors. *Medical Microbiology and Immunology*, **192**, 123–8.

6.2

Non-infective Swellings: Cysts, Tumours and Ranulas

Valerie G. A. Suter[1] and Michael M. Bornstein[2]

[1] *Department of Oral Surgery and Stomatology, School of Dental Medicine, University of Bern, Bern, Switzerland*
[2] *Oral and Maxillofacial Radiology, Applied Oral Sciences, Faculty of Dentistry, The University of Hong Kong, Hong Kong, China*

Introduction

Swellings can appear extraorally, intraorally or in combination. If infectious origins have been excluded, non-infectious swellings can be caused by either benign or malign processes. Benign processes are far more common in children, but it is important to identify the rare malignant entities without delay. Besides a structured clinical examination, further diagnostic tools can be applied, and clinicians have to decide which are the most appropriate for the situation at hand. Radiographic imaging representing hard or soft tissues can help identify the origin and nature of a swelling. Probe aspiration may help identify the fluid content and differentiate a swelling from a solid tumour. Incisional or excisional biopsies are further options for diagnosis and treatment planning, and may even be performed simultaneously with therapy.

Tumours, Cysts and Extravasation or Retention Phenomena in the Soft Tissues

Mucocele is a general term often used to describe extravasation and retention phenomena. The size can vary from a few millimetres to more than two centimetres (Wu et al., 2011; Bezerra et al., 2016). Pain is not typically associated with an extravasation phenomenon, but the swelling can be functionally disturbing when eating or speaking. This is often the reason for initial consultation.

Mucus extravasation phenomena often affect children. They result from an injured duct of a small salivary gland, causing saliva not to be drained correctly to the oral cavity, and to accumulate in the surrounding soft tissues, leading to a localised swelling (Figure 6.2.1a). Upon clinical examination, the swelling is submucosal and well demarcated. It can usually be displaced by digital inspection. Often, a bluish colour is seen shining through the normal overlying mucosa (Figure 6.2.1b), or else an inconspicuous pink mucosal colour can be present. Sometimes, a white patch on or besides the swelling is observed because of tissue hyperkeratosis induced by mechanical irritation. A local trauma, often caused by a bite injury, is a well-known aetiology responsible for the formation of an extravasation phenomenon. This is also why extravasation phenomena occur most often on the lower lip (Martins-Filho et al., 2011; Wu et al., 2011; Bezerra et al., 2016). In children, chronic lip biting, habits of sucking and parafunction are

Management of Dental Emergencies in Children and Adolescents, First Edition.
Edited by Klaus W. Neuhaus and Adrian Lussi.
© 2019 John Wiley & Sons Ltd. Published 2019 by John Wiley & Sons Ltd.
Companion website: www.wiley.com/go/neuhaus/dental_emergencies

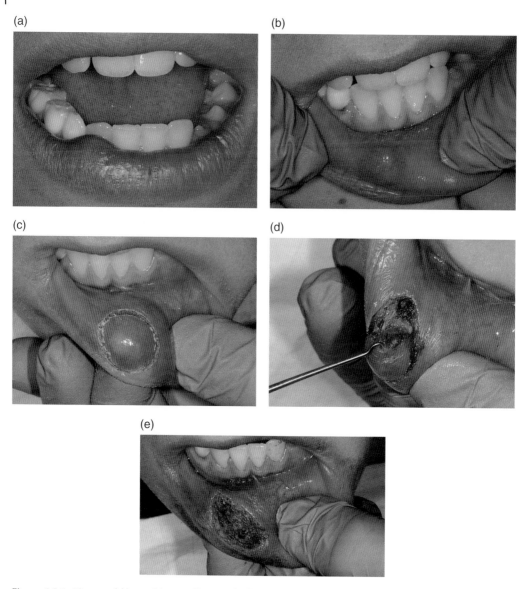

Figure 6.2.1 13-year-old boy with a swelling on the lower right lip. (a) Extraoral view. (b) Bluish shining submucosal swelling. (c) Demarcation of the lesion with CO_2 laser for excisional biopsy. (d) Ongoing excisional biopsy with CO_2 laser without any bleeding. (e) Wound left to open granulation after excisional biopsy. The specimen was sent to histopathological examination and has been confirmed as an extravasation cyst of a small salivary gland of the lower lip.

common, which may explain why mucus extravasation phenomena have the highest prevalence in this population (Martins-Filho et al., 2011). They are also infrequently seen on the tongue, buccal mucosa and palate (Yagüe-García et al., 2009; Martins-Filho et al., 2011; Wu et al., 2011; Bezerra et al., 2016). When localised on the ventrum of the tongue, they are called Blandin–Nuhn mucoceles, corresponding to the name of the seromucous salivary glands found there.

If the clinical features are compatible with an extravasation phenomenon, an excisional biopsy can be performed (Figure 6.2.1c–e). It is, however, important to complete the treatment with a histopathologic analysis to confirm the diagnosis and exclude any other benign or malignant pathology. A few rare cases of mucosa-associated lymphoid tissue (MALT) lymphoma in relation to minor salivary glands and with a clinical presentation similar to a mucocele have been described in the literature (Ryu et al., 2009; Bombeccari et al., 2011). Usually, adjacent salivary glands are also excised to minimise the risk of recurrence. Typical instruments used for excision are the scalpel, the electrotome and the laser (CO_2 laser, diode laser, KTP, Er,Cr:YSGG) (Yagüe-García et al., 2009; Wu et al., 2011; Romeo et al., 2013). Alternative techniques include cryosurgery (Moraes et al., 2012) and micromarsupialisation (Giraddi and Saifi, 2016). Micromarsupialisation involves passing a suture through the lesion. The lesion is compressed to extravasate the fluid and the suture is knotted and kept for 10 days. This minimally invasive technique is well tolerated by children, but has an increased risk of recurrence and does not provide a proper histopathological diagnosis. Only very small and superficial extravasation phenomena may resolve without any further treatment.

If a salivary duct is obstructed, mucus will be retained and the duct will be dilated, leading to a retention phenomenon. The typical localisation is the floor of the mouth (Figure 6.2.2). Mucoceles in this location are called ranulas, because they look similar to a froglet (*ranula* = "little frog" in Latin) (Figure 6.2.3). Those restricted to the floor of the mouth are known as simple mucoceles, in

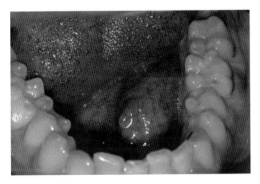

Figure 6.2.2 Retention phenomenon on the left floor of the mouth.

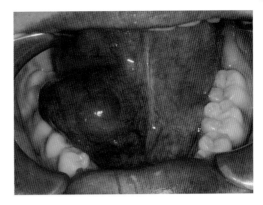

Figure 6.2.3 Ranula on the right floor of the mouth in a 13-year-old boy.

contrast to the more expanded plunging ranulas extending in adjacent spaces. Ranulas above the mylohyoid muscle are excised intraorally, whereas those below need both an intra- and an extraoral approach. However, plunging ranulas do not need to be excised totally. For this reason, it is essential to differentiate ranulas from tumours or cysts before surgical intervention. Additional radiographic examination with computed tomography (CT), magnetic resonance imaging (MRI) or ultrasound may be helpful. Because of their low radiation dose, ultrasound and MRI are favoured in children (Kurabayashi et al., 2000; Brown and Harave, 2016). The radiologic identification of a cyst like lesion in the submandibular space and the typical "tail sign" to the sublingual space are highly suggestive for a plunging ranula (La'porte et al., 2011; Brown and Harave, 2016).

Cysts from remnants of the thyroglossal duct can arise along the migratory pathway from the foramen cecum of the tongue to the infrahyoid region. They usually present as a firm mass in the midline of the neck, rarely lateral, with about one-quarter being in the suprahyoidal position. There is a predominance in children (Thompson et al., 2016).

Malignant tumours are rare in the head and neck region of children (1.5 cases per 1 million). Soft-tissue malignancies include lymphomas, neuroectodermal tumours, thyroid malignancies and soft-tissue sarcoma (Qaisi and Eid, 2016). Nevertheless, any inconclusive swelling or lump in children should be investigated with adequate radiological techniques or tissue biopsy with subsequent histopathological or cytological analysis, depending on the sampling technique. Furthermore, every excisional soft-tissue biopsy intended as treatment of a lesion should also be analysed by histopathology, as clinical signs and symptoms are not always conclusive, and malignancy might otherwise be missed.

Jaw Cysts, Odontogenic Tumours and Treatment in Children

Cysts are fluid-filled cavities lined by an epithelial membrane. Jaw cysts originate from odontogenic or nonodontogenic epithelial remnants. They often grow slowly, and remain asymptomatic as long as they are contained within the jaw bone. When the cortical bone plate is perforated, a swelling can appear. It is not uncommon that a cyst is only detected in an advanced stage. In contrast to an abscess, which is typically fluctuating, a cyst that has perforated the cortical bone is more firm on palpation. To determine the origin of the swelling, radiographic imaging is necessary. When a jaw cyst is suspected, panoramic radiograph is the standard imaging, except in the anterior maxilla, where an occlusal radiograph may be advantageous. In some situations, a periapical radiograph is helpful, but because of its restricted size, it often cannot fully represent a jaw cyst. Three-dimensional radiographic imaging using cone-beam computed tomography (CBCT) is helpful in identifying the relationship of a cyst to vital anatomical structures like the inferior alveolar nerve, the sinus or adjacent teeth. This is indicative for a precise and individualised treatment plan, and to avoid complications upon surgery. Different CBCT devices now allow high-speed or low-dose protocols that can reduce the ionising radiation dose, especially for children (Oenning

et al., 2018); low-dose protocols for paediatric CBCT applications can achieve as much as a 50% dose reduction compared with manufacturers' recommendations (Hidalgo Rivas et al., 2015).

Radicular Cysts

Overall, radicular cysts are the most frequently encountered cyst type. In paediatric populations, their prevalence varies according to geographic location: in some areas, they are the most common cyst in children (Jones et al., 2006; Soluk Tekkesin et al., 2016), whilst in others, the dentigerous cyst is more prevalent (Ochsenius et al., 2007; de Souza et al., 2010; Lo Muzio et al., 2017). They are most common in countries with high caries prevalence and a low socioeconomic status (Lo Muzio et al., 2017). Children aged between 13 and 17 years are the most affected (Figure 6.2.4) (Soluk Tekkesin et al., 2016).

Radicular cysts are predominately found in the anterior maxilla in children's permanent dentition (Soluk Tekkesin et al., 2016). This is probably because dental traumas most commonly affect anterior incisors (Figure 6.2.4). If a tooth with pulpa necrosis is not properly treated at an early stage, the inflammation can trigger the development of a radicular cyst. To treat a radicular cyst, the causative tooth has to be treated by conservative endodontic treatment or, in rarer cases – when it is deemed unworthy of preservation – extracted. Following root canal treatment, the radicular cyst is enucleated; in cases of expanded cyst, a decompression can be performed first (Allon et al., 2015). Histopathological analysis is mandatory in any case to confirm the diagnosis.

Dentigerous Cysts

A considerable majority of dentigerous cysts are related to lower third molars in the young-adult population. The second most affected tooth is the upper canine (Figure 6.2.5), followed by the mandibular premolars. Thus, in paediatric populations,

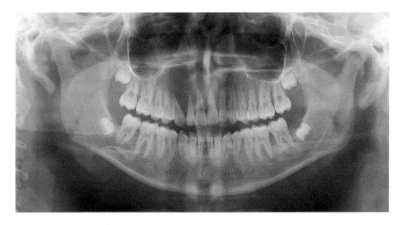

Figure 6.2.4 Panoramic radiograph with a well-demarcated osteolysis in the right maxilla involving the apices of teeth 11, 12, 13, 14 and 15 and displacement of the right sinus floor. The patient, a 13-year-old girl, has a known history of dental trauma.

(a)

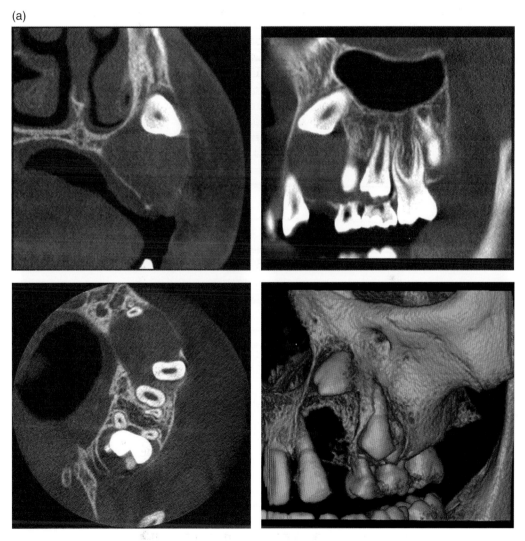

Figure 6.2.5 CBCT (3D Accuitomo 170, Morita Corp., Kyoto, Japan; field of view 6 × 5 cm, voxel size 125 μm) exhibiting an osteolytic, well-demarcated lesion in the left lateral maxilla and displacement of tooth 23 in a 10-year-old girl. Histopathological examination after cystectomy confirmed a dentigerous cyst. The girl was monitored and tooth 23 showed a sponatenous eruption 1.5 years after surgery. (a) CBCT finding of the initial osteolysis. (b) Representation of the displaced tooth 23.

(b)

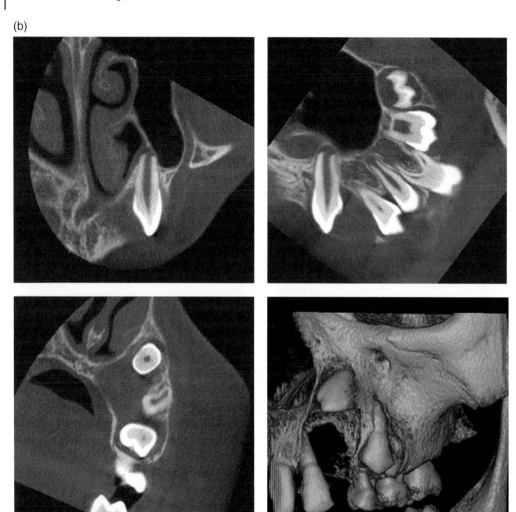

Figure 6.2.5 (Continued)

the mixed dentition is mostly affected by dentigerous cysts (Soluk Tekkesin et al., 2016). Dentigerous cysts can also be related to supernumerary teeth or odontoma (Kaugars et al., 1989; Lin et al., 2013; Mossaz et al., 2014). Treatment is normally enucleation of the cyst and subsequent histopathological analysis. Expect for third molars, teeth are usually worth maintaining in children. After removal of the cyst, spontaneous eruption of the tooth is possible; in other cases, orthodontic treatment is indicated.

Eruption Cysts

Another group of cysts previously classified as a subgroup of dentigerous cysts but now recognised as a separate entity is the eruption cysts. These present as soft translucent lesions filled with blood or fluid and overlying a tooth in eruption (Figure 6.2.6). They often have a dark bluish-purple colour. They are typically found in children, associated with both deciduous and permanent teeth. In a series of 66 cases, the maxillary first molar

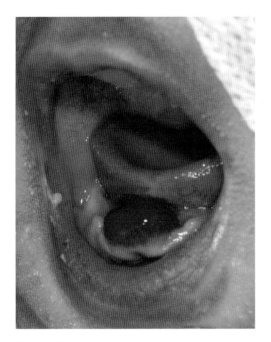

Figure 6.2.6 Eruption cyst on the anterior lower jaw in a neonate.

was most often affected in the deciduous dentition and the upper central incisor in the permanent (Şen-Tunç et al., 2017). The aetiology remains unknown, and there are controversial discussions in the literature over whether eruption cysts are favoured by early caries, trauma, a lack of space or infection. Most are asymptomatic, in which case informing the parents and monitoring the child until tooth eruption is sufficient. Normally, the cyst resolves simultaneous to the eruption of the tooth. If there is discomfort on mastication or an esthetic concern, the eruption cyst can be treated by incision and drainage of the content or excision with exposure of the crown.

Odontogenic Keratocysts

The odontogenic keratocyst has characteristics of both a cyst and a tumour. It is a benign and fluid-filled cavity within the jaw bone with properties of a cyst, and the treatment modalities are similar to those for other cysts, but it has a neoplastic nature with an aggressive, sometimes destructive growth pattern, and it often recurs after surgery. In 2005, a consensus panel of the World Health Organization (WHO) reclassified the keratocyst as a keratocystic odontogenic tumour, because of its neoplastic nature and a mutation in the PTCH gene (Philipsen, 2005; Wright and Vered, 2017). With the fourth edition of the WHO classification of head and neck tumours, however, it was reverted to a cyst, as the odontogenic keratocyst (El-Naggar et al., 2017). Note that this does not mean the consensus panel is saying the odontogenic keratocyst does not have neoplastic propreties (Wright and Vered, 2017).

The odontogenic keratocyst has its origin in epithelial cells derived from the dental lamina or from the basal cells of the oral epithelium and is histopathologically characterised by a lining parakeratinised epithelium. A considerable number of odontogenic keratocysts are diagnosed between the ages of 10 and 20 years (Figure 6.2.7), and individual cases are seen in children under 10 years (Shear and Speight, 2007). Possible signs and symptoms are swelling, pain and paresthesia, but they often remain asymptomatic until they have reached a large size. Before expansion, the odontogenic keratocyst usually grows into the marrow spaces of the jaw. The mandible, with predilection of the region of the angle, is most often involved. When an odontogenic keratocyst is diagnosed, it is very important to screen for other jaw lesions and clinical signs possibly associated with Gorlin–Goltz syndrome (Figure 6.2.8). This syndrome has an autosomal-dominant trait with mutation of the PTCH1 (patched1) gene, a tumour-suppressor gene on chromosome 9q22.3. It involves the presence of multiple naevoid basal cell carcinomas of the skin and multiple odontogenic keratocysts in the jaws before the age of 20 years. Characteristic skeletal abnormalities consist in a broad nasal root, frontal and parietal bossing of the head, bifid rips and unusual vertebrae. Intracranially, the falx cerebri may be calcified and the sella turcica has been described to exhibit an atypical shape. The

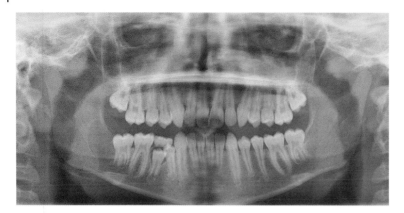

Figure 6.2.7 Panoramic radiograph of 14-year-old boy. Teeth 17, 27, 44, 45 and 47 are not fully erupted. In the right posterior mandible, a well-demarcated osteolysis was conspicuous. Histopathological analysis revealed the presence of an odontogenic keratocyst. There were no hints of Gorlin–Goltz syndrome.

(a)

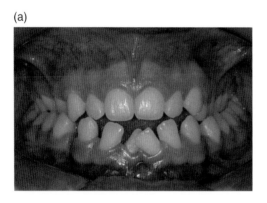

(b)

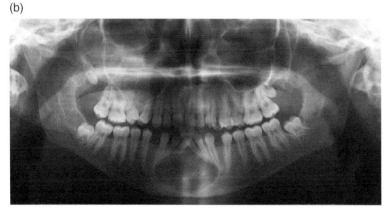

Figure 6.2.8 17-year-old girl with multiple osteolytic lesions and displacement of teeth. (a) Clinical intraoral view. (b) Panoramic radiograph with an osteolysis from region 13–18/right maxillary sinus and displacement of tooth 18; osteolysis in region 28/left maxillary sinus, retained tooth 28; osteolysis in the central anterior mandible with displacement of the roots of teeth 31, 32, 33, 41, 42 and 43; retained tooth 48 with an osteolysis posterior of the crown. All biopsies confirmed the presence of an odontogenic keratocyst. The patient and her mother were affected by Gorlin–Goltz syndrome.

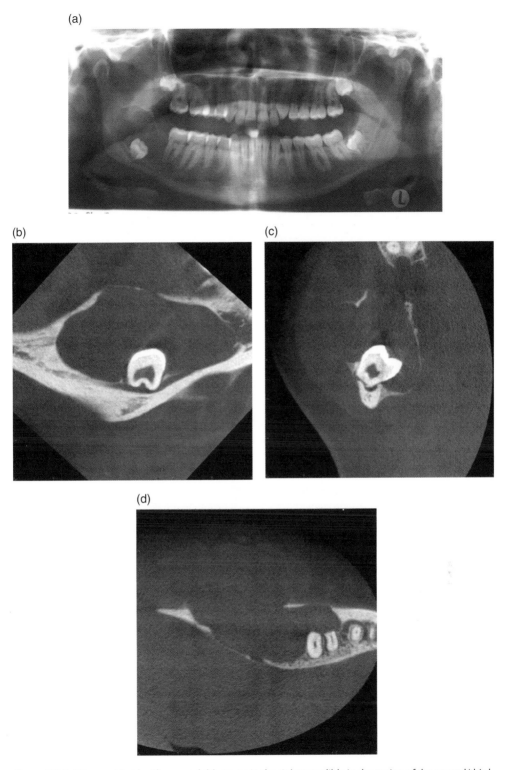

Figure 6.2.9 17-year old girl with an ameloblastoma in the right mandible in the region of the second/third molar and ascending ramus. The third molar is impacted and displaced towards the mandibular angle. The right mandibular canal is still partially visible in its course in the lower aspect of the lesion. (a) Panoramic view. (b) Sagittal CBCT image depicting the displaced third molar and aspects of the mandibular canal. (c) Coronal CBCT view again depicting the third molar, a compressed mandibular canal and a missing cortical demarcation of the lesion on the cranial and lingual aspects. (d) Axial CBCT cut through the lesion, exhibiting the extension of the lesion towards the submandibular fossa, as well as root resorption, especially on the mesial apex of tooth 47.

syndrome can also be associated with ocular abnormalities or cleft lips and palate (Bresler et al., 2016).

There are a number of different treatment approaches for syndromic and nonsyndromic odontogenic keratocysts. The most conservative is marsupialisation with decompression, whilst the most invasive is en bloc resection. Others include enucleation with or without the use of Carnoy's solution and the combination of a marsupialisation/decompression followed by enucleation (Antonoglou et al., 2014).

Ameloblastomas

Ameloblastomas are benign but locally aggressive tumours originating from the epithelium involved in tooth formation. The posterior mandible is the most affected site (Figure 6.2.9). If not discovered by chance during routine check-up, larger ameloblastoma can present as a firm swelling.

The unicystic ameloblastoma is found most often in Caucasian children. The clinical and radiographic features of this form are similar to those of a dentigerous cyst (Figure 6.2.9). To maintain quality of life in a younger population, a relatively conservative treatment plan (e.g. simple tumour enucleation with curettage but without resection) is favoured by various authors. Recurrence should not be considered a failure in a paediatric population (Jundt and Reichart, 2008; Seintou et al., 2014).

References

Allon, D. M., Allon, I., Anavi, Y., Kaplan, I., Chaushu, G. 2015. Decompression as a treatment of odontogenic cystic lesions in children. *Journal of Oral Maxillofacial Surgery*, **73**(4), 649–54.

Antonoglou, G. N., Sándor, G. K., Koidou, V. P., Papageorgiou, S.N. 2014. Non-syndromic and syndromic keratocystic odontogenic tumors: systematic review and meta-analysis of recurrences. *Journal of Craniomaxillofacial Surgery*, **42**(7), e364–71.

Bezerra, T. M., Monteiro, B. V., Henriques, Á. C., de Vasconcelos Carvalho, M., Nonaka, C. F., da Costa Miguel, M. C. 2016. Epidemiological survey of mucus extravasation phenomenon at an oral pathology referral center during a 43 year period. *Brazilian Journal of Otorhinolaryngology*, **82**(5), 536–42.

Bombeccari, G. P., Guzzi, G., Ruffoni, D., Gianatti, A., Mariani, U., Spadari, F. 2011. Mucosa-associated lymphatic tissue lymphoma of the lower lip in a child. *Journal of Pediatric Surgery*, **46**(12), 2414–16.

Bresler, S. C., Padwa, B. L., Granter, S. R. 2016. Nevoid basal cell carcinoma syndrome (Gorlin syndrome). *Head and Neck Pathology*, **10**(2), 119–24.

Brown, R. E., Harave, S. 2016. Diagnostic imaging of benign and malignant neck masses in children-a pictorial review. *Quantitative Imaging in Medicine and Surgery*, **6**(5), 591–604.

de Souza, L. B., Gordón-Núñez, M. A., Nonaka, C. F., de Medeiros, M. C., Torres, T. F., Emiliano, G. B. 2010. Odontogenic cysts: demographic profile in a Brazilian population over a 38-year period. *Medicina Oral, Patologia Oral Y Cirugia Bucal*, **15**(4), e583–90.

El-Naggar, A. K., Chan, J. K. C., Grandis, J. R., Takata, T., Slootweg, P. J. (eds). 2017. WHO classification of head and neck tumours. In: *WHO/IARC Classification of Tumors*, 4th edn, volume **9**. Lyon: IARC Press.

Giraddi, G. B., Saifi, A. M. 2016. Micro-marsupialization versus surgical excision for the treatment of mucoceles. *Annals of Maxillofacial Surgery*, **6**(2), 204–9.

Hidalgo Rivas, J. A., Horner, K., Thiruvenkatachari, B., Davies, J., Theodorakou, C. 2015. Development of a low-dose protocol for cone beam CT examinations of the anterior maxilla in children. *British Journal of Radiology*, **88**(1054), 20150559.

Jones, A. V., Craig, G. T., Franklin, C. D. 2006. Range and demographics of odontogenic cysts diagnosed in a UK population over a 30-year period. *Journal of Oral Pathology & Medicine*, **35**(8), 500–7.

Jundt, G., Reichart, P. A. 2008. Benign odontogenic ectomesenchymal tumors [in German]. *Pathologe*, **29**(3), 199–204.

Kaugars, G. E, Miller, M. E, Abbey, L. M. 1989. Odontomas. *Oral Surgery Oral Medicine Oral Pathology*, **67**(2), 172–6.

Kurabayashi, T., Ida, M., Yasumoto, M., Ohbayashi, N., Yoshino, N., Tetsumura, A., Sasaki, T. 2000. MRI of ranulas. *Neuroradiology*, **42**(12), 917–22.

La'porte, S. J., Juttla, J. K., Lingam, R. K. 2011. Imaging the floor of the mouth and the sublingual space. *Radiographics*, **31**(5), 1215–30.

Lin, H. P, Wang, Y. P, Chen, H. M, Cheng SJ, Sun A, Chiang CP. 2013. A clinicopathological study of 338 dentigerous cysts. *Journal of Oral Pathology and Medicine*, **42**(6), 462–7.

Lo Muzio, L., Mascitti, M., Santarelli, A., Rubini, C., Bambini, F., Procaccini, M., et al. 2017. Cystic lesions of the jaws: a retrospective clinicopathologic study of 2030 cases. *Oral Surgery Oral Medicine Oral Pathology Oral Radiology*, **124**(2), 128–38.

Martins-Filho, P. R, Santos, T. de S., da Silva, H. F., Piva, M. R, Andrade, E. S., da Silva, L. C. 2011. A clinicopathologic review of 138 cases of mucoceles in a pediatric population. *Quintessence International*, **42**(8), 679–85.

Moraes, P. de C., Teixeira, R. G, Thomaz, L. A, Arsati, F., Junqueira, J. L., Oliveira, L. B. 2012. Liquid nitrogen cryosurgery for treatment of mucoceles in children. *Pediatric Dentistry*, **34**(2), 159–61.

Mossaz, J., Kloukos, D., Pandis, N., Suter, V. G., Katsaros, C., Bornstein, M. M. 2014. Morphologic characteristics, location, and associated complications of maxillary and mandibular supernumerary teeth as evaluated using cone beam computed tomography. *European Journal of Orthodontics*, **36**(6), 708–18.

Ochsenius, G., Escobar, E., Godoy, L., Peñafiel, C. 2007. Odontogenic cysts: analysis of 2944 cases in Chile. *Medicina Oral, Patologia Oral Y Cirugia Bucal*, **12**(2), E85–91.

Oenning, A. C., Jacobs, R., Pauwels, R., Stratis, A., Hedesiu, M., Salmon, B.; DIMITRA Research Group. 2018. Cone-beam CT in paediatric dentistry: DIMITRA project position statement. *Pediatric Radiology*, **48**(3), 308–16.

Philipsen, H. P., Reichart, P. A., Slootweg, P. J., Slater, L. J. Neoplasms and tumour-like lesions arising from the odontogenic apparatus and maxillofacial skeleton. In: Barnes, L., Evenson, J. W., Reichart, P., Sidransky, D. (eds). 2005. *Pathology and Genetics of Head and Neck Tumours. World Health Organization Classification of Tumours*, 3rd edn, volume **9**. Lyon: IARC Press.

Qaisi, M., Eid, I. 2016. Pediatric head and neck malignancies. *Oral and Maxillofacial Surgery Clinics of North America*, **28**(1),11–19.

Romeo, U., Palaia, G., Tenore, G., Del Vecchio, A., Nammour, S. 2013. Excision of oral mucocele by different wavelength lasers. *Indian Journal of Dental Research*, **24**(2), 211–15.

Ryu, M., Han, S., Che, Z., Min, Y., Yoo, K. H., Koo, H. H., et al. 2009. Pediatric mucosa-associated lymphoid tissue (MALT) lymphoma of lip: a case report and literature review. *Oral Surgery Oral Medicine Oral Pathology Oral Radiology and Endodology*, **107**(3), 393–7.

Seintou, A., Martinelli-Kläy, C. P., Lombardi, T. 2014. Unicystic ameloblastoma in children: systematic review of clinicopathological features and treatment outcomes. *International Journal of Oral Maxillofacial Surgery*, **43**(4), 405–12.

Şen-Tunç, E., Açikel, H., Sönmez, I. S., Bayrak, Ş., Tüloğlu, N. 2017. Eruption cysts: a series of 66 cases with clinical features. *Medicina Oral, Patologia Oral Y Cirugia Bucal*, **22**(2), e228–32.

Shear, M., Speight, P. M. 2007. *Cysts of the Oral and Maxillofacial Regions*, 4th edn. Oxford: Blackwell Munksgaard.

Soluk Tekkesin, M., Tuna, E. B., Olgac, V., Aksakallı, N., Alatlı, C. 2016. Odontogenic lesions in a pediatric population: Review of the literature and presentation of 745 cases. *International Journal of Pediatric Otorhinolaryngology*, **86**, 196–9.

Thompson, L. D., Herrera, H. B., Lau, S. K. 2016. A clinicopathologic series of 685 thyroglossal duct remnant cysts. *Head and Neck Pathology*, **10**(4), 465–74.

Wright, J. M., Vered, M. 2017. Update from the 4th edition of the World Health Organization classification of head and neck tumours: odontogenic and maxillofacial bone tumors. *Head and Neck Pathology*, **11**(1), 68–77.

Wu, C. W., Kao, Y. H., Chen, C. M., Hsu, H. J., Chen, C. M., Huang, I. Y. 2011. Mucoceles of the oral cavity in pediatric patients. *Kaohsiung Journal of Medical Sciences*, **27**(7), 276–9.

Yagüe-García, J., España-Tost, A. J., Berini-Aytés, L., Gay-Escoda, C. 2009. Treatment of oral mucocele-scalpel versus CO_2 laser. *Medicina Oral, Patologia Oral Y Cirugia Bucal*, **14**(9), e469–74.

6.3

Oral Problems in Patients Undergoing Haematology or Oncology Treatment

Adrian M. Ramseier[1], Jakob Passweg[2] and Tuomas Waltimo[1]

[1] *Department of Oral Health & Medicine, University Center for Dental Medicine Basel, University of Basel, Basel, Switzerland*
[2] *Department of Hematology, University Hospital Basel, Basel, Switzerland*

Introduction

Uniquely, disruptions in the formation and function of circulating blood cells trigger changes in the immune system, blood clotting and oxygen transportation. Whilst there is a quite frequent occurrence of anaemia, it plays a rather minor role in dentistry, since normally it is only mildly severe and quickly remedied.

Haematological malignancies are rare, with an incidence of about 30/100 000 (Sant et al., 2010). The oral cavity is often affected in patients without functioning defence, and complications are common during dental intervention, especially when there is a lack of neutrophil granulocytes. In general, seriously ill haematological patients receive dental treatment at university centres.

Infections within the oral cavity may also be initial manifestation of a haematological disorder. This should in particular be considered when gingival bleeding occurs in otherwise healthy conditions and in the presence of petechiae.

Wanted and unwanted medicinal effects on blood clotting and infection defence occur very often, due to the wide spread of corresponding diseases. This is related to treatments like the application of corticosteroids or anticoagulation in connection with atrial fibrillation. The effects of these medications are acutely relevant for the choice of dental treatment. However, in children and adolescents, medicinal anticoagulation is seldom applied. This is why it is not addressed in this chapter. High-dose local irradiation is also rather seldom administered in the area of the mouth in children, and so it too is not discussed.

We begin by explaining the basic concepts, before looking at specific problems associated with the oral mucosa that are often encountered in connection with chemotherapy, total body irradiation and stem cell transplants.

Haemostasis

Stopping the blood flow from injured blood vessels is a complex process, in which a number of factors interact. Successful haemostasis consists in three steps: (i) vasoconstriction to reduce the blood flow; (ii) formation of a platelet plug by thrombocyte adherence, activation and aggregation; and (iii) plasmatic coagulation by a cascade of proteins, which forms a stable clot. When thrombocytes come in contact with collagen in the exposed connective tissue, they attach there by mediation of the von Willebrand factor, a protein that adheres both to collagen

Management of Dental Emergencies in Children and Adolescents, First Edition.
Edited by Klaus W. Neuhaus and Adrian Lussi.
© 2019 John Wiley & Sons Ltd. Published 2019 by John Wiley & Sons Ltd.
Companion website: www.wiley.com/go/neuhaus/dental_emergencies

and to thrombocytes. Thus, the thrombocytes are activated. By releasing cytokines, more thrombocytes are attracted, and the plasmatic coagulation cascade is initiated. Through several intermediate stages, prothrombin is transformed, both intrinsically (activation factors) and extrinsically (tissue factor in the injured subendothelial tissue), to thrombin, which in turn polymerises fibrinogen to fibrin. This results in a net incorporating aggregated thrombocytes as well as erythrocytes, and thus forming a stable blood clot. Other factors are responsible for preventing exaggerated or spontaneous thrombus formation.

Cellular Haemostasis Disorders (Thrombocytes)

Depressed platelet count (thrombocytopaenia) and dysfunction of the platelet count (thrombocytopahthies) can be either congenital or acquired. Table 6.3.1 provides an overview of possible causes of thrombocytopaenia.

The most commonly isolated thrombocytopaenia in children is the immune thrombocytopaenia (ITP) (Ishii, 2017). Thrombocytopaenia may also occur following a replacement of normal bone marrow with leukaemic cells (e.g. in acute leukaemia) or bone marrow failure, or it may be inherited.

Nonsteroidal anti-inflammatory drugs (NSAIDs) inhibit platelet aggregation. With aspirin, such aggregation is irreversible, except by the production of new thrombocytes.

Small petechial haemorrhages on skin and on the mucosa are the typical sign of marred thrombocytes; often, they occur on the lower extremities (gravity) or in the oral cavity. In case of severe thrombocytopaenia, they can become confluent (ecchymoses). Spontaneous bleeding starts only with a platelet count of $20–30 \times 10^9/l$ (Scully, 2014). Depending on the severity of the disorder, it can result from minor traumata, gingival bleeding or suffusions on the skin.

The normal platelet count is $150–450 \times 10^9/l$; a value of $>100 \times 10^9/l$ is thought to be ideal for surgical intervention. With values

Table 6.3.1 Causes of thrombocytopaenia (Hoffbrand and Moss, 2016).

Failure of platelet production
Selective megakaryocyte depression
Rare congenital defects
Drugs, chemicals, viral infections
Part of general bone marrow failure
Cytotoxic drugs
Radiotherapy
Aplastic anaemia
Leukaemia
Myelodysplastic syndromes
Myelofibrosis
Marrow infiltration (e.g. carcinoma, lymphoma, Gaucher's disease)
Multiple myeloma
Megaloblastic anaemia
HIV infection

Increased consumption of platelets
Immune
Autoimmune
Idiopathic
Associated with systemic lupus erythematosus, chronic lymphocytic leukaemia or lymphoma
Infections: *Helicobacter pylori*, human immunodeficiency virus (HIV), other viruses, malaria
Drug-induced, e.g. heparin
Post-transfusional purpura
Foeto-maternal alloimmune thrombocytopaenia
Disseminated intravascular coagulation
Thrombotic thrombocytopaenic purpura

Abnormal distribution of platelets
Splenomegaly, e.g. liver disease

Dilutional loss
Massive transfusion of stored blood to bleeding patients

$>50 \times 10^9/l$ and good functioning of the existing platelets, dentoalveolar surgery can normally be performed without bleeding complications (Henderson et al., 2001). Measures like compression, wound suture and local haemostatics are usually sufficient. With values of $<30 \times 10^9/l$, spontaneous bleeding can occur. In this situation, the indication of surgical treatment should be carefully considered, and surgery should be conducted in collaboration with haematology. Haemostasis can be improved by transfusion of thrombocyte concentrates. This is recommended during dentoalveolar intervention with a platelet count of $<50 \times 10^9/l$, as well as during maxillofacial intervention with a platelet count of $<100 \times 10^9/l$ (Scully, 2014).

The success of thrombocyte transfusions needs to be checked: it is essential to measure the platelet count prior to and after transfusion. Patients who do not adequately react to thrombocyte transfusions constitute a special problem. In such cases, therapeutic interventions can be performed whilst transfusion continues.

Plasmatic Coagulation Disorders

Congenital coagulation disorders include haemophilia A (factor VIII deficiency) and the much rarer haemophilia B (factor IX deficiency). Only the male gender is affected by haemophilia B. Spontaneous haemorrhaging and strong life-threatening postoperative bleeding may occur. Missing factors can be added; however, there is insufficient evidence from randomised controlled trials to assess the most effective and safe haemostatic treatment to prevent bleeding in people with haemophilia or other congenital bleeding disorders undergoing surgical procedures (Coppola et al., 2015; Spivakovsky et al., 2015).

In von Willebrand disease, the von Willebrand factor is missing or malfunctioning. Because of this, platelet function is impaired. Von Willebrand disease is classified into a number of subcategories, and is associated with slight to considerable bleeding disorders.

Disorders of the Immune System/Granulocytes

Defence comprises cellular elements, all of which belong to the leucocytes. The various cells evolved from one multipotent stem cell of haematopoiesis, which is capable of differentiating into different cell lines with various functions:

- Neutrophilic granulocytes are implicated in nonspecific immunity against bacteria and fungi. Basophilic granulocytes are involved in hypersensitivity reactions (asthma, urticaria, allergic rhinitis and anaphylaxis). Eosinophilic granulocytes play a role in the defence against parasites.
- Lymphocytes are subdivided into T-cells, which have the important function of differentiating between foreign and self, B-cells, which are amongst other things responsible for the production of antibodies (plasma cells, memory cells), and NK-cells, which play an essential role in protecting against virus cells and tumour cells.
- Monocytes migrate into tissue, where they become macrophages. They can recognise exogenous material, ingest it (phagocytosis), dissolve it and present it at their cell surface. This causes the activation of other defence cells (antigen presentation) (Kasper et al., 2015).

Causes

Haematological Disorders

Abnormalities in the immune response may have many different causes. There might be disturbances in the differentiation of individual or all cell lines. This can result in functional reduction of the cell line(s) affected, in a deficiency of these cells (lymphopaenia: T-cells and B-cells, neutropaenia) or in an overproduction, which can replace the production of other cell lines in the bone marrow. Table 6.3.2 provides a list of haematological disorders.

Disorders of the Immune System through Medication

Disorders of the immune system can occur as a wanted or unwanted effect of many chemotherapeutics and immunosuppressives. Particular emphasis must be given to glucocorticoids like dexamethasone and prednisone, but other immunosuppressives like cyclosporin A (Sandimmun), tacrolimus (Prograf) and the folic acid antagonist methotrexate (Methotrexat) can also have this effect.

Table 6.3.2 World Health Organization (WHO) Classification of Hematologic Malignancies (Abridged Version) (Aster and Bunn, 2017).

Subtype	Putative cell of origin
Myeloid neoplasms	
Acute myeloid leukemia (AML) AML with recurrent genetic aberrations AML without recurrent genetic aberrations AML following cytotoxic therapy	Early myeloid progenitor
Myeloproliferative neoplasms Chronic myeloid leukemia Polycythemia vera Essential thrombocythemia Chronic eosinophilic leukemia Primary myelofibrosis	Hematopoietic stem cell or early myeloid progenitor
Myelodysplastic syndromes	Early myeloid progenitor
Lymphoid neoplasms	
Immature B-cell and T-cell tumors B-cell acute lymphoblastic leukemia/lymphoma T-cell acute lymphoblastic leukemia/lymphoma	Early B-cell progenitor Early T-cell progenitor
Mature B-cell tumors Chronic lymphocytic leukemia/small lymphocytic lymphoma Mantle cell lymphoma Follicular lymphoma Burkitt lymphoma Diffuse large B-cell lymphoma	Post-germinal center B cell Naïve B cell Germinal center B cell Germinal center B cell Germinal center or post-germinal center B cell
Plasma cell tumors and related entities Multiple myeloma Lymphoplasmacytic lymphoma	Post-germinal center B cell Mature B-cell
Mature T-cell and natural killer cell tumors	Mature T-cell or natural killer cell
Hodgkin lymphoma	Germinal center or post-germinal center B cell

Physical Damage

Blood formation can be impaired by irradiation, either therapeutic or accidental. Stem cells and lymphocytes are especially vulnerable. Thus, a reduction in lymphocytes can be observed at a very early stage after irradiation, whilst the number of granolocytes, thrombocytes and erythrocytes decreases only as damage to the stem cells progresses.

Clinical Oral Appearance

Sometimes, haematological disorders can be discovered by the dentist. Manifestations of haematological disorders in the oral cavity can cause suspicion and suggest additional investigations:

- Bleeding of the oral mucosa that does not result from gingivitis may be an indication of coagulation abnormalities due to a variety of causes. Petechial haemorrhages, and haemorrhages at other places in the oral mucosa, are typical for thrombocytopaenia (Hoffbrand and Moss, 2016).
- In case of acute myeloid leukaemia, gingival swelling can be determined (Figure 6.3.1) (Kasper et al., 2015). Occasionally, this can also be seen after treatment with cyclosporine A and tacrolimus.

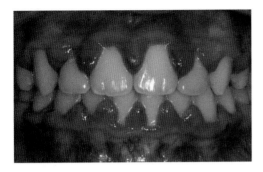

Figure 6.3.1 Gingival swelling and acute myeloid leukaemia.

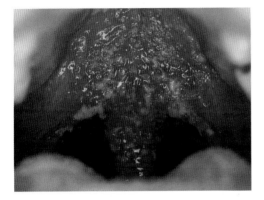

Figure 6.3.2 Thrush (Candida).

- Unusual infections in terms of frequency, manifestation or the occurrence of rare microbes are signs of possible immunosuppression. Candida infections are encountered quite often (Figure 6.3.2), and non-Candida albicans species (e.g. tropicalis, krusei and parapsilosis) are increasingly being seen. What should be noted is that these are often resistant to common therapeutics. Typical for leukaemias are virus reactivations of, for instance, herpes zoster and herpes simplex virus (HSV) (Ramseier et al., 2015). Intraoral ulcers and large aphtae are common manifestations of HSV. All of these infections can cause severe pain.
- Swelling of the lymph nodes and anaemia (recognisable by paleness of the mucosa) may point towards a haematological disorder. So might fever and night sweats recorded in the medical history.

Clinical Significance

When an immune deficiency exists, a possible haematogeneous spreading of microorganisms may be expected after intervention. Together with the haematologist or family doctor, it needs to be determined whether prophylactic antibiotics should be implemented or whether treatment should just be postponed.

A focus search should be conducted prior to haematological treatment by chemotherapy or haematopoietic stem cell transplantation (HSCT). Ideally, located infection foci are treated first; however, this is not always possible because of the already limited immune response and wound healing, or because of the urgency of treating the malignant tumours.

In patients who have received allogeneic stem cell transplantation, the current situation concerning immune response should always be clarified with the attending haematologist: when appropriate, prophylactic antibiotics should be given prior to tooth cleaning, deep scaling, caries treatment and extractions, or else the treatment must simply be postponed.

In chemotherapeutic treatment, which is sometimes accompanied by total body irradiation, hyposalivation occurs on a regular basis. The result may be increased susceptibility to caries, gingivitis, periodontitis, mucocutaneous diseases and fungal infections (Bagattoni et al., 2014; Buglione et al., 2016).

After allogeneic stem cell transplantation, acute and chronic rejection reactions may occur (graft-versus-host disease, GvHD). The oral mucosa shows typical lichenoid changes with or without erythematous lesions, ulcers or mucoceles. Often, hyposalivation takes place at the same time, combined with a correspondingly increased risk of caries, periodontitis and infections of the mucosa. Long-term effects include secondary malignant tumours of the oral mucosa. Because of this, the oral mucosa needs to be inspected regularly and thoroughly. The indication for biopsy sampling should be wide and generous for the exclusion and detection of malignancy, respectively (Elad et al., 2015).

Anaemia

Anaemia is defined by a reduction of the haemoglobin concentration in the blood. Common causes are vitamin B_{12}, folic acid and iron deficiencies caused by chronic bleeding, for instance due to excessive menstrual flow or chronic diseases like tumours. Other causes include innate haemoglobin synthesis disorders such as sickle-cell anaemia and thalassaemia.

Clinical Significance

Anaemias hardly have an effect on dental treatment. The following manifestations could indicate anaemia and necessitate further clarification with the family doctor: complaints about reduced performance, weakness, heart palpitations and dyspnoea under stress, as well as the occurrence of pale skin or mucosa. Angular cheilitis, burning tongue or dysphagia (Plummer–Vinson syndrome) may appear in case of iron deficiency. Vitamin B_{12} and folic acid deficiencies cause burning tongue with impaired sense of taste and trophic glossitis with disappearing papillae.

Mucositis

Mucositis is an inflammation of the mucous membranes of the gastrointestinal tract as a consequence of chemotherapy and radiation therapy. Patients who are receiving HSCT or irradiation in the area of the mouth are affected particularly often.

Oral mucositis is associated with erythema, and at times with ulcerations and violent pain. It is one of the most frequent side effects of cancer treatment, and is often the reason for reducing the treatment dose or for having to postpone treatment. It also may necessitate tube feeding or parenteral nutrition.

Pathogenesis has not yet been fully clarified, although considerable progress has been made in recent years. The procedure can be broken down into five stages: initiation, primary damage response, signal amplification, ulceration and healing (Sonis, 2004). It is a complex interaction of cells from the mucosa and submucosa that is regulated by cytokines such as tumour necrosis factor alpha (TNF-α), interleukins 6 (IL-6) and 1b (IL-1b) and cyclooxygenase 2 (COX-2). The oral microbiome also plays a role (Sonis, 2011; Al-Dasooqi et al., 2013; Villa and Sonis, 2015; Cinausero et al., 2017).

There are a variety of approaches to the treatment and prophylaxis of oral mucositis. Cryotherapy and low-level light therapy (LLLT) are recommended for children receiving chemotherapy or HSCT conditioning with regimens associated with a high rate of mucositis, whilst keratinocyte growth factor (KGF) is recommended for cooperative children receiving HSCT conditioning with regimens associated with a high rate of severe mucositis (Lalla et al., 2014; Villa and Sonis, 2016; Sung et al., 2017):

- Cryotherapy involves cooling the oral mucosa with ice whilst the patient receives chemotherapy by short infusion. Because of the vasoconstriction in the cooled mucosa, fewer cytotoxic substances are supposed to arrive there. Thus, the method is only suitable for chemotherapeutic agents which are administered in short infusion and have a short half-life. However, it is inexpensive and readily accessible (Sung et al., 2017).
- LLLT (also called photobiomodulation, PBM) is the therapeutic use of light (e.g. visible, near-infrared or infrared light), which is absorbed by endogenous chromophores and triggers nonthermal, noncytotoxic biochemical reactions by photochemical and photophysical effects, leading to physiological alterations (Bensadoun and Nair, 2012, 2015; Zecha

et al., 2016a,b). However, the method is laborious and is not available everywhere.

- KGF (e.g. Palifermin) is an epithelium growth factor. Since there are no studies on its use, and since there is the possibility of thickening the oral mucosa and causing long-term damage, it should only be applied in selected cases where there is a high risk of severe mucositis (Sung et al., 2017).

As with all children, good oral hygiene should be ensured. Professional tooth cleaning can reduce pain in case of mucositis (Kubota et al., 2015).

Graft-versus-Host Disease

Despite immunosuppressive treatment, GvHD occurs in almost 25% of cases following allogeneic HSCT, with the mouth being one of the most frequently affected organs (Flowers et al., 2002; Meier, 2011). It can significantly impair quality of life. Oral GvHD impresses by hyposalivation, lichenoid hyperkeratotic striae or plaque with or without erythematous changes (Figure 6.3.3). Additionally, ulcerations and superficial mucoceles may occur. The ulcerations can be very painful. In certain circumstances, severe

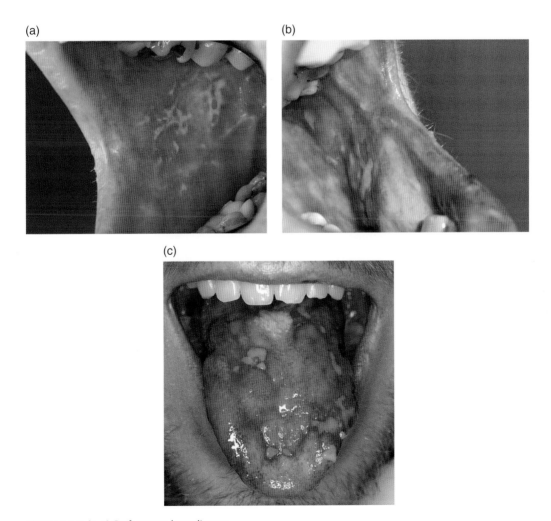

Figure 6.3.3 (a–c) Graft-versus-host disease.

sclerosis develops as a late effect, restricting mouth or jaw opening and reducing mobility of the tongue. Persistant chronic GvHD is associated with increased risk of squamous cell carcinomas. Viral factors like human papillomavirus (HPV) seem to be of significance in the aetiology and pathogenesis of this type of carcinoma.

Management

In case of existing abnormalities of the oral mucosa like aphthae and GvHD, products containing sodium lauryl sulphate or menthol frequently cannot be tolerated because they cause pain. Affected patients mostly avoid them, along with spicy food. They may have to use toothpaste that is free of sodium lauryl sulphate. Products with antimicrobial and protective effects on the oral mucosa are recommended for oral rinsing. Alleviating dry mouth with moisturising agents and covering open aphthae can help relieve the pain.

After allogeneic HSCT, regular examinations of the mucous membranes are essential, in order to discover secondary carcinoma early (Majhail et al., 2012). Secondary infections occur frequently in cases of poor oral hygiene, which may also increase the intensity of GvHD. Thus, maintaining good oral hygiene is very important. However, such lesions may hamper attempts in this direction, because of the pain. Depending on the condition, several dental hygiene treatments a year – including oral hygiene instructions – are recommended.

For oral GvHD, topical steroids (e.g. budesonide or dexamethasone) are recommended

as first-line therapy. Extracorporeal photopheresis is considered a second-line systemic therapy for steroid-refractory GvHD. Local anaesthetics may be helpful in pain control (Dignan et al., 2012).

All carious lesions should be restored. It is advisable to encourage patients to practise good oral hygiene and additional fluoridation (either by direct application or via fluoridation splints at home or in a dental practice).

Existing odontogenic infections should receive therapy, preferably prior to immunosuppression. In this way, systemic infections connected with blood stem cell transplants can be reduced by one-third, and the deaths of an additional 18/10 000 treated patients can be avoided (Elad et al., 2008). However, the extraction of teeth necessitates a long healing period (2 weeks), and there is often an urgent need for therapy, especially in leukaemia patients, so dental treatment must frequently be postponed until after blood stem cell transplantation. Due to the danger of haematogenic spread, dental treatments should be conducted by giving antibiotic prophylaxis.

Generally, in immunosuppressed patients, contact should be made with the attending physician as soon as is possible. At times, referral to university dental clinics is recommended, as they deal with immunosuppressed patients every day – including during inpatient treatment – and can meet all diagnostic needs. The objectives in giving dental treatment to immunosuppressed patients are prevention of infection, pain relief, maintenance of function, treatment of complications and improvement of quality of life.

References

Al-Dasooqi, N., Sonis, S. T., Bowen, J. M., Bateman, E., Blijlevens, N., Gibson, R. J., et al. 2013. Emerging evidence on the pathobiology of mucositis. *Supportive Care in Cancer*, **21**(11), 3233–41.

Aster, J. C., Bunn, H. F. 2017. *Pathophysiology of Blood Disorders*, 2nd edn. New York: McGraw-Hill.

Bagattoni, S., D'Alessandro, G., Prete, A., Piana, G., Pession, A. 2014. Oral health and dental late adverse effects in children in remission from malignant disease. A pilot case-control study in Italian children. *European Journal of Paediatric Dentistry*, **15**(1), 45–50.

Bensadoun, R. J., Nair, R. G. 2012. Low-level laser therapy in the prevention and treatment of cancer therapy-induced mucositis: 2012 state of the art based on literature review and meta-analysis. *Current Opinions in Oncology*, **24**(4), 363–70.

Bensadoun, R. J., Nair, R. G. 2015. Low-level laser therapy in the management of mucositis and dermatitis induced by cancer therapy. *Photomedicine and Laser Surgery*, **33**(10), 487–91.

Buglione, M., Cavagnini, R., Di Rosario, F., Sottocornola, L., Maddalo, M., Vassalli, L., et al. 2016. Oral toxicity management in head and neck cancer patients treated with chemotherapy and radiation: dental pathologies and osteoradionecrosis (part 1) literature review and consensus statement. *Critical Reviews in Oncology/Hematology*, **97**, 131–42.

Cinausero, M., Aprile, G., Ermacora, P., Basile, D., Vitale, M. G., Fanotto, V., et al. 2017. New frontiers in the pathobiology and treatment of cancer regimen-related mucosal injury. *Frontiers in Pharmacology*, **8**(8), 354.

Coppola, A., Windyga, J., Tufano, A., Yeung, C., Di Minno, M. N. 2015. Treatment for preventing bleeding in people with haemophilia or other congenital bleeding disorders undergoing surgery. *Cochrane Database of Systematic Reviews*, **9**(2), CD009961.

Dignan, F. L., Scarisbrick, J. J., Cornish, J., Clark, A., Amrolia, P., Jackson, G., et al. 2012. Organ-specific management and supportive care in chronic graft-versus-host disease. *British Journal of Haematology*, **158**(1), 62–78.

Elad, S., Thierer, T., Bitan, M., Shapira, M. Y., Meyerowitz, C. 2008. A decision analysis: the dental management of patients prior to hematology cytotoxic therapy or hematopoietic stem cell transplantation. *Oral Oncology*, **44**(1), 37–42.

Elad, S., Raber-Durlacher, J. E., Brennan, M. T., Saunders, D. P., Mank, A. P., Zadik, Y., et al. 2015. Basic oral care for hematology-oncology patients and hematopoietic stem cell transplantation recipients: a position paper from the joint task force of the Multinational Association of Supportive Care in Cancer/International Society of Oral Oncology (MASCC/ISOO) and the European Society for Blood and Marrow Transplantation (EBMT). *Supportive Care in Cancer*, **23**(1), 223–36.

Flowers, M. E., Parker, P. M., Johnston, L. J., Matos, A. V., Storer, B., Bensinger, W. I., et al. 2002. Comparison of chronic graft-versus-host disease after transplantation of peripheral blood stem cells versus bone marrow in allogeneic recipients: long-term follow-up of a randomized trial. *Blood*, **100**(2), 415–19.

Henderson, J. M., Bergman, S., Salama, A., Koterwas, G. 2001. Management of the oral and maxillofacial surgery patient with thrombocytopenia. *Journal of Oral and Maxillofacial Surgery*, **59**(4), 421–7.

Hoffbrand, A. V., Moss, P. A. H. 2016. *Hoffbrand's Essential Haematology*, 7th edn. Chichester, UK: Wiley-Blackwell.

Ishii, E. (ed.). 2017. *Hematological Disorders in Children, Pathogenesis and Treatment.* Singapore: Springer Nature.

Kasper, D. L., Fauci, A. S., Hauser, S. L., Longo, D. L., Jameson, J. L., Loscalzo, J. (eds). 2015. *Harrison's Principles of Internal Medicine*, 19th edn. New York: McGraw-Hill.

Kubota, K., Kobayashi, W., Sakaki, H., Nakagawa, H., Kon, T., Mimura, M., et al. 2015. Professional oral health care reduces oral mucositis pain in patients treated by superselective intra-arterial chemotherapy concurrent with radiotherapy for oral cancer. *Supportive Care in Cancer*, **23**(11), 3323–9.

Lalla, R. V., Bowen, J., Barasch, A., Elting, L., Epstein, J., Keefe, D. M., et al. 2014. MASCC/ISOO clinical practice guidelines for the management of mucositis secondary to cancer therapy. *Cancer*, **120**(10), 1453–61. Erratum in: *Cancer*, **121**(8), 1339.

Majhail, N. S., Rizzo, J. D., Lee, S. J., Aljurf, M., Atsuta, Y., Bonfim, C., et al. 2012. Recommended screening and preventive practices for long-term survivors after hematopoietic cell transplantation. *Biology of Blood and Marrow Transplantation*, **18**(3) 348–71.

Meier, J. K., Wolff, D., Pavletic, S., Greinix, H., Gosau, M., Bertz, H., et al. 2011. Oral chronic graft-versus-host disease: report from the International Consensus Conference on clinical practice in cGVHD. *Clinical Oral Investigations*, **15**(2), 127–39.

Ramseier, A. M., Filippi, A., Halter, J., Waltimo, T. 2015. Orale Manifestationen bei Immunsuppression. *Quintessenz*, **66**(1), 1–9.

Sant, M., Allemani, C., Tereanu, C., De Angelis, R., Capocaccia, R., Visser, O., et al. 2010. Incidence of hematologic malignancies in Europe by morphologic subtype: results of the HAEMACARE project. *Blood*, **116**(19), 3724–34.

Scully, C. 2014. *Scully's Medical Problems in Dentistry*, 7th edn. London: Churchill Livingstone Elsevier.

Sonis, S. T. 2004. The pathobiology of mucositis. *Nature Reviews Cancer*, **4**(4), 277–84.

Sonis, S. T. 2011. Oral mucositis. *Anti-Cancer Drugs*, **22**(7), 607–12.

Spivakovsky, S., Keenan, A. V., Congiusta, M., Spivakovsky, Y. 2015. Congenital bleeding disorders and dental surgery. *Evidence Based Dentistry*, **16**(3), 90–1.

Sung, L., Robinson, P., Treister, N., Baggott, T., Gibson, P., Tissing, W., et al. 2017. Guideline for the prevention of oral and oropharyngeal mucositis in children receiving treatment for cancer or undergoing haematopoietic stem cell transplantation. *BMJ Supportive & Palliative Care*, **7**(1), 7–16.

Villa, A., Sonis, S. T. 2015. Mucositis: pathobiology and management. *Current Opinion in Oncology*, **27**(3), 159–64.

Villa, A., Sonis, S. T. 2016. Pharmacotherapy for the management of cancer regimen-related oral mucositis. *Expert Opinion on Pharmacotherapy*, **17**(13), 1801–7.

Zecha, J. A., Raber-Durlacher, J. E., Nair, R. G., Epstein, J. B., Sonis, S. T., Elad, S., et al. 2016a. Low level laser therapy/ photobiomodulation in the management of side effects of chemoradiation therapy in head and neck cancer: part 1: mechanisms of action, dosimetric, and safety considerations. *Supportive Care in Cancer*, **24**(6), 2781–92.

Zecha, J. A., Raber-Durlacher, J. E., Nair, R. G., Epstein, J. B., Elad, S., Hamblin, M. R., et al. 2016b. Low-level laser therapy/ photobiomodulation in the management of side effects of chemoradiation therapy in head and neck cancer: part 2: proposed applications and treatment protocols. *Supportive Care in Cancer*, **24**(6), 2793–805.

Unit 7

Management of Non-infective Dental Conditions

7.1

Molar–Incisor Hypomineralisation

Jan Kühnisch[1] and Roswitha Heinrich-Weltzien[2]

[1] Department of Conservative Dentistry and Periodontology, Ludwig-Maximilians-University, Munich, Germany
[2] Department of Preventive and Paediatric Dentistry, Jena University Hospital, Jena, Germany

Introduction

Whilst caries in children and adolescents has been steadily decreasing in incidence in recent decades, a marked increase in developmental defects in the permanent teeth has been reported. Molar–incisor hypomineralisation (MIH) is the most common manifestation of this condition. According to national and international epidemiological trials, prevalence rates for MIH in children and adolescents range from 10 to 30% (Kühnisch et al., 2014a). Analyses of the dentition at the tooth level reveals that ~90% of all teeth affected by MIH have enamel opacities without enamel breakdown (Kühnisch et al., 2014a). Only about 10% of affected teeth (mainly posterior teeth) have enamel breakdown requiring extensive treatment.

With regard to clinical practice, two points should be emphasised: first, enamel defects have a heterogeneous appearance (Figures 7.1.1–7.1.5), and second, factors such as endodontic complications, the state of dental development and the child's ability to cooperate have a significantly influence on the treatment strategy. The aim of this chapter is to describe and assess critically treatment options for patients with MIH, and to derive recommendations for clinical practice.

Diagnosis of MIH

MIH is the diagnosis of developmental defects characterised by qualitative enamel mineralisation changes. MIH defects range from white to yellowish or brownish opacities of the enamel. If defects can be demarcated from the healthy enamel, the disturbance is classified as MIH. Since demarcated opacities might also be caused by dental trauma or as sequence of apical inflammations of the deciduous teeth, differential diagnosis is needed. Diffuse opacities, on the other hand, are frequently discussed as a cause of high fluoride exposure (dental fluorosis) and should not be misclassified as MIH.

Quantitative enamel defects (hypoplasia) are characterised by a reduction in the normal enamel thickness. In the case of MIH, pre-eruptive enamel breakdown or less-developed hypoplastic and hypomineralised enamel can be diagnosed in a distinct number of cases. Post-eruptive enamel breakdown, on the other hand, only occurs in association with functional loading. The occlusal surfaces of the (first) permanent molars are predisposed to post-eruptive enamel breakdown and may show signs of disintegration immediately after tooth eruption. Clinically, differentiation between mild (Figure 7.1.2), moderate

Management of Dental Emergencies in Children and Adolescents, First Edition.
Edited by Klaus W. Neuhaus and Adrian Lussi.
© 2019 John Wiley & Sons Ltd. Published 2019 by John Wiley & Sons Ltd.
Companion website: www.wiley.com/go/neuhaus/dental_emergencies

(a) (b)

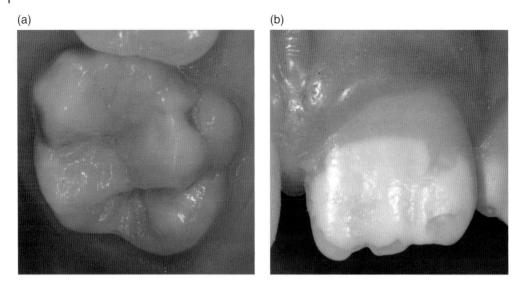

Figure 7.1.1 Hypomineralisation on (a) an occlusal and (b) a smooth surface without enamel breakdowns.

(a) (b)

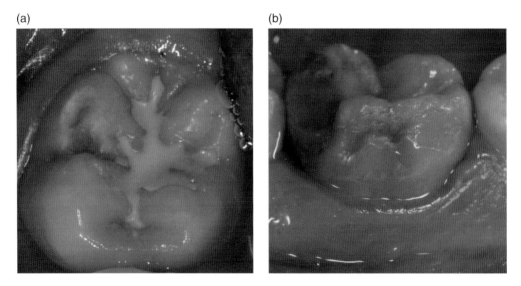

Figure 7.1.2 Mild, small-sized enamel breakdown on (a) a hypomineralised occlusal surface and (b) a smooth surface.

(Figure 7.1.3) and severe (Figure 7.1.4) enamel defects with dentin exposure is possible. The main clinical sign is hypersensitivity of the affected teeth to thermal, chemical and mechanical stimuli (Jälevik and Klingberg, 2002; Weerheijm, 2004). Hypersensitivity often makes adequate daily oral hygiene of hypomineralised teeth difficult, leading to an increased risk of caries in these teeth and these patients.

Different definitions are used for the diagnosis of MIH today. The most common one, favoured by the European Academy of Paediatric Dentistry (EAPD), involves the use of index teeth (Weerheijm et al., 2003; Lygidakis et al., 2010). At least one first permanent molar must be affected by hypomineralisation in order to establish the diagnosis of MIH. However, this definition has been criticised for various reasons. First, it is based

(a)

(b)

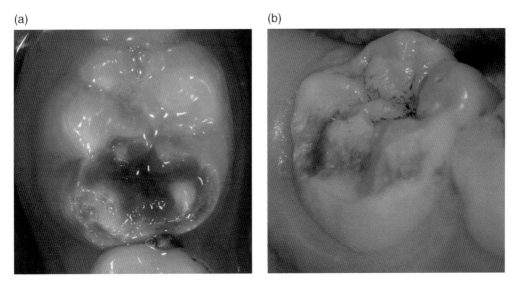

Figure 7.1.3 Moderate, medium-sized enamel breakdown on (a) a hypomineralised occlusal surface and (b) a smooth surface.

(a)

(b)

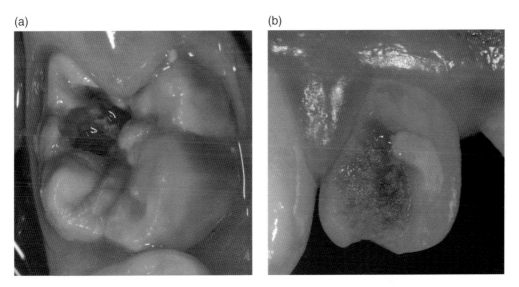

Figure 7.1.4 Severe enamel breakdown on (a) a hypomineralised occlusal surface and (b) a smooth surface. Due to the extensive disintegration of hard tissue, dentin is exposed.

solely on an empirical assumption that has yet to be validated (Weerheijm et al., 2001). Second, the occurrence of enamel defect is related to the exposure time, which can be variable. The implications for clinical practice are that, ultimately, all teeth of both dentitions can be affected, and index tooth-based diagnosis leads to underestimation of the true prevalence of MIH. Therefore, a shift from using index teeth to tooth- and tooth-surface-related registration of demarcated opacities, enamel breakdowns, atypical restorations and tooth extractions due to MIH is recommended (Kühnisch et al., 2014a). This methodological approach is comparable to the well-accepted dmf/DMF index.

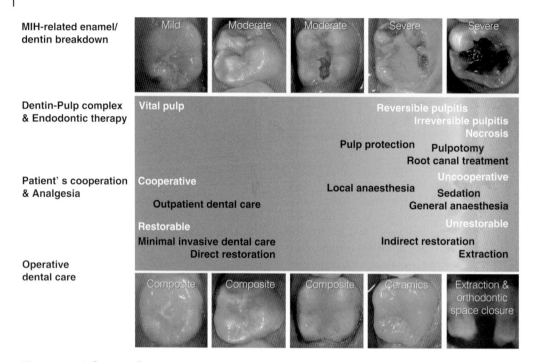

Figure 7.1.5 Influencing factors and possible treatment options in MIH-related tooth defects.

Aetiology of MIH

Both systemic and local factors seem to play a key role in the development of MIH or hypoplasia (Crombie et al., 2009; Alaluusua, 2010). There is consensus that systemic damage of the ameloblast cells must occur during tooth development. Various factors are discussed in the literature. These include exposure to the environmental contaminants bisphenol A (BPA) and dioxin, early childhood infections, antibiotic medications in early childhood, oxygen deficiency during childbirth, decreased serum vitamin D levels (Kühnisch et al., 2015), and disorders of calcium or phosphate metabolism. However, the exact etiologic chain of MIH is still unknown (Crombie et al., 2009; Alaluusua, 2010; Kühnisch et al., 2014b).

Prevention of MIH

In view of the lack of an evidence-based proof of the aetiological chain of MIH, there is currently no effective approach to its prevention. This underscores the need for further efforts to identify the causes of this enamel disorder.

Noninvasive Dental Care of MIH-Affected Teeth

In clinical practice, the most common feature of MIH is off-white to yellowish brown areas of hypomineralisation/opacity without enamel breakdown (Figure 7.1.1), associated with a varying degree of hypersensitivity. These teeth generally require no restorative treatment and should receive "classical" caries prevention measures, such as topical fluoride (Hellwig et al., 2013) and fissure sealant application (Kühnisch et al., 2017). The aim of topical fluoride application is to (re)mineralise hypomineralised tooth surfaces. Fluorides also help to counteract the problem of hypersensitivity. Sealants are applied to protect pits and fissures on molars affected by MIH. Recently, the use of (nano)hydroxylapatite products to stabilise enamel surfaces and reduce hypersensitivity in teeth with MIH defects has been suggested. However, scientific studies of this approach are lacking. In regard to casein phosphopeptide (CPP)- and amorphous calcium phosphate (ACP)- containing products (GC Toothmousse, GC Europe, Leuven, Belgium), Baroni and Marchionni (2011) reported that their use led to clinical improvement of the enamel structure and clinical symptoms of MIH. The use of a product containing calcium carbonate and arginine (Elmex Sensitive Professional, CP GABA, Hamburg, Germany) also led to a decrease in hypersensitivity (Bekes et al., 2017). However, the effects of topical products can only be expected on the outer enamel surface, and complete repair of hypomineralised enamel is still not possible. Another empirical observation in this context is that the initial hypersensitivity after tooth eruption decreases over the course of dentin maturation and tooth development in many cases.

Another aspect is that, when the vestibular surfaces of permanent anterior teeth are affected, patients frequently complain of impaired aesthetics (Fayle, 2003; Lygidakis, 2010; Lygidakis et al., 2010). A micro-invasive infiltration technology (ICON, DMG America, Hamburg, Germany) has been proposed as a treatment option for these cases. However, the success rates achieved in the few studies conducted to date are heterogeneous (Crombie et al., 2014; Kumar et al., 2017), meaning that infiltration treatments for MIH do not always result in satisfactory aesthetic results. Therefore, a restrictive approach to establishing the indication for these treatments is currently recommended.

Restorative Dental Care

If enamel breakdown has occurred, restorative treatment measures may be indicated (Lygidakis et al., 2003, 2010; Mejare et al., 2005). Whilst monitoring of teeth with minimal enamel defects is recommended, direct fillings are indicated for those with moderate to severe enamel breakdown. Indirect restorations are a treatment option, particularly in posterior teeth with extensive enamel defects. Adhesively bonded restorations are preferentially used in all cases. Restorability and the absence of pulpitis symptoms are crucial to preserving hypomineralised teeth via the direct-filling technique. Direct restorations are also indicated in patients with extensive dentin exposure, associated with hypersensitivity and pain during chewing or the performance of daily tooth brushing. In these cases, the treatment goals are to preserve chewing function, prevent endodontic complications and promote the healing of any reversible pulpitis. However, in making the decision to restore, the dentist must meet the requirements for long-lasting, high-quality dental restorations, which is necessary to avoid costly and time-consuming repeat treatments and maintain the child's ability to cooperate. From the perspective of materials science, the use of adhesively bonded composite materials is preferred. Because these cavities do not offer much retentiveness but are occlusion-bearing, the use of amalgam and glass ionomer cements (GICs) should be restricted.

There are clinical limitations on the direct restorability of multisurface enamel defects with composite materials, especially in the posterior region. Although the placement of multisurface, occlusion-bearing composite fillings is technically possible, it must be borne in mind that the probability of partial or complete loss increases with increasing restoration size. Therefore, indirect restorations represent a functional and long-lasting treatment alternative in cases with complete (or near-complete) involvement of the occlusal surface (Manhart et al., 2004). The strategic importance of the (first) permanent molars to dentition development and masticatory function justifies this approach. Today, indirect restorations are recommended for the treatment of hypomineralised molars (Koch and García-Godoy, 2000; Feierabend et al., 2012). The main advantages of placing indirect restorations are that tooth preparation can be performed (congruent to the margins of hypomineralised defects in an enamel-preserving manner) and no additional retention is needed.

The clinical and laboratory effort required for indirect restoration is high, however, and often exceeds the paediatric or adolescent patient's ability to cooperate. The availability of chairside dental CAD/CAM technologies that enable the rapid production of indirect restorations in a single appointment (Wittneben et al., 2009) is increasingly challenging the dogma that indirect restoration is contraindicated in children and adolescents. As with the treatment of adults, it requires good cooperation on the part of the patient or the use of general anaesthesia (Pfisterer et al., 2016). Although long-term data on the proposed treatment in children and adolescents are currently unavailable, the clinical experience gained in similar case studies suggests that it has a good long-term prognosis (Millet et al., 2015; Zimmermann et al., 2016).

From our point of view, prefabricated stainless-steel crowns, which are commonly used in paediatric dentistry, should no longer be a treatment option in MIH-affected molars. Although easy to perform, non-technique-sensitive, long-lasting and protective against further enamel fractures and defects (Zagdwon et al., 2003; Kotsanos et al., 2005), this approach has major disadvantages when it comes to performing later indirect restoration. Whilst teeth need to be prepared tangentially for stainless-steel crowns, the preparation margins usually run subgingival to the interproximal surfaces. This substantially restricts the adhesive placement of definite indirect restorations. Therefore, we believe that placement of prefabricated crowns should only be performed on permanent teeth without any circumferential preparation, which increases the risk of overhanging crown margins. Periodontal complications due to non-individualised crown margins have also been described (Guelmann et al., 1988). Overhanging crown margins might possibly impede the eruption of adjacent teeth. Moreover, many patients (and their parents/guardians) find the aesthetic unsatisfactory. Because of these disadvantages, prefabricated crowns for restoration of the permanent dentition should be used in a restrictive manner.

Cavity Preparation

The issue of whether and to what extent the removal of structurally damaged enamel is necessary is a matter of discussion. The answer will depend on the size of the defect and the cooperation of the paediatric patient. In many cases, hypomineralised enamel is stable enough to withstand the mechanical forces of mastication in spite of its defects. This means that it is not necessary to remove all of the hypomineralised enamel, and a defect-related approach should be routinely used, particularly in paediatric patients. Therefore, small to medium-sized defects can often be treated using a non- or minimally invasive cavity preparation followed by adhesive restoration management. When treating larger defects with dentin involvement, it is important to design a sufficiently contoured cavity in order to reduce the risk of partial or total losses. From the clinical perspective, both the removal of hypomineralised hard tissue and the location of the cavity margins in sound enamel play an important role. If an indirect restoration is to be used, strict adherence to the aforementioned preparation principles is crucial.

Treatment of the Dentin–Pulp Complex

Extensive enamel loss on dentin exposure due to MIH may be comparable to (deep) dentinal caries where microbial infection and dentinal destruction occur, leading to similar responses of the dentin–pulp complex (Rodd et al., 2007). Moreover, the risk of pulpitis increases as infectious processes progresses towards the pulp. Clinical key features are thermal hypersensitivity of the teeth and pain during food intake. Whilst reversible inflammation signs dominate in the initial stages, the risk of an irreversible pulpitis or pulp necrosis increases as the disease spreads, or where it is located near the pulp. Spontaneous and nocturnal complaints are clinical key markers of an irreversible inflammatory process. This must be distinguished from teeth with percussion and biting sensitivity, which are associated with apical periodontitis.

Regarding the diagnostic spectrum of the disease, two treatment strategies should be discussed (Figure 7.1.6). In case of reversible inflammation, protection of the dentin–pulp

(a)

(b)

(c)

(d)

(e)

(f)

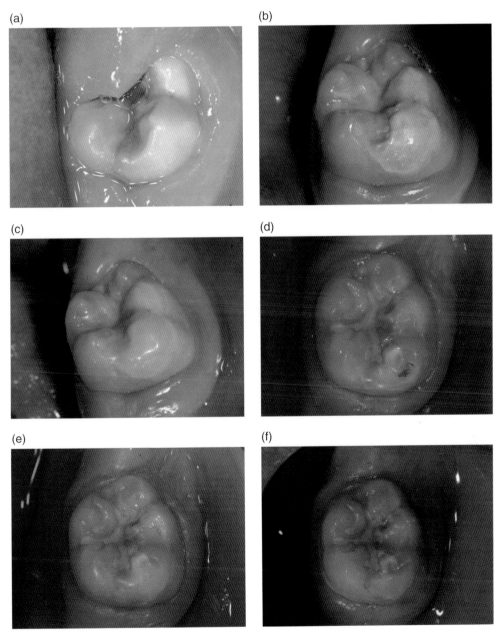

Figure 7.1.6 Clinical management of a moderate enamel breakdown on an occlusal surface over an observation period of 13 years. Just after (a) tooth eruption, (b) an enamel disintegration was diagnosed, which was covered with (c) an adhesively bonded flowable composite restoration. Nearly 1 year later, the restoration was (d) worn and had to be (e) repaired. The clinical situation at the ages of (f) 11, (g) 12, (h) 13, (i) 14 and (j) 19 years was basically stable. Nevertheless, the composite restoration was renewed at the age of 14 (i).

(g) (h)

(i) (j)

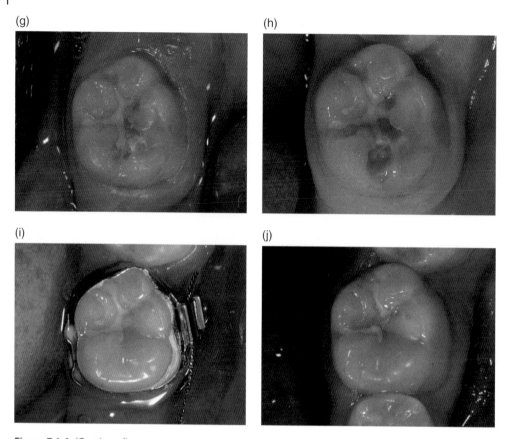

Figure 7.1.6 (Continued)

complex is the primary focus of clinical attention. This is achieved by removing the bacterial biofilm and sealing the cavity with a restoration (Kidd, 2004). The range of treatment options may also include direct pulp capping or pulpotomy, particularly in teeth with incomplete root growth. If the history and clinical examination show signs of irreversible pulpitis, pulpal necrosis or apical periodontitis, trepanation, cleaning, irrigation, disinfection, shaping and temporary or permanent filling of the root canal system is indicated. Especially in such cases, tooth extraction followed by orthodontic space closure may be justified from a pragmatic point of view, as the prognosis of the tooth is difficult to assess in children and adolescents.

Extraction and Orthodontic Space Closure

Extraction followed by orthodontic space closure is a further treatment option for MIH-affected molars (Jälevik and Möller, 2007). In the authors' opinion, extraction should be limited to individual cases, since it is always associated with extensive follow-up measures, which may require general anaesthesia in paediatric patients and pose additional challenges to the patient's family, dentist and orthodontist. Indications for extraction include molars with extensive destruction and endodontic complications like apical periodontitis. Orthodontic aspects (e.g. dental crowding) and the age of the patient also play a role in the indication for extraction. Ideally, a first permanent molar should not be extracted until immediately before the eruption of the second permanent molar, in order to prevent possible growth inhibition associated with early extraction (Eichenberger et al., 2015). This approach allows physical mesial migration of the second permanent molar. For these reasons, the correct timing of tooth extraction can significantly promote the orthodontic space-closure procedure. However, this strategy generally requires temporarily preservation of the affected tooth until the time of extraction. In routine clinical practice, this means that patients must receive adequate restorative treatment and probably even temporary endodontic care between the ages of 6 and 11 years.

Interim Management until Adolescence or Adulthood

When children of early school age first present with MIH, tooth-related problems such as hypersensitivity and marked enamel defects are at the forefront of treatment. Both factors affect the ability to cooperate during restorative treatment (Jälevik and Klingberg, 2002). In cases with a correctly established treatment indication and prognosis, experience has shown that simple measures are more successful. More invasive and challenging treatments can then be postponed until adolescence, when the patient is better able to cooperate. Coverage of enamel defects with universal adhesive and (flowable) composite without tooth preparation is an effective simple measure to achieve defect sealing and hypersensitivity reduction. These restorations may be more prone to wear, which is a disadvantage of the simplified procedure. As a rule of thumb, it can be said that the risk of repeated restoration increases proportionally with the defect size and occlusal stress. Based on clinical experience, early definitive treatment seems more advisable in case of children and adolescents with extensive or multisurface enamel defects, and compromise treatments consisting in temporary solutions are not recommended. This is supported by the observation that repeated dental treatments exhaust the patient's ability to cooperate, so that, ultimately, rehabilitation can only be achieved under general anaesthesia. Thus, providing adequate pain relief and establishing a treatment plan that takes into account the patient's cooperation are important facets of patient management during early dental treatment (Figure 7.1.6).

Implications for Dental Practice

The concepts presented in this chapter illustrate the challenges and limitations of the available treatment options for the management of children and adolescents with MIH (Figure 7.1.6). Since effective local anaesthesia is often difficult to achieve, sedation or general anaesthesia is required in order to perform extensive invasive treatment procedures in paediatric patients with limited ability to cooperate. Direct adhesive restoration is the tooth-conserving treatment of choice for teeth with mild to moderate enamel breakdown. In cases of hypomineralisation with severe enamel and dentin defects, the dentist may choose between an adhesive and an indirect restoration. The latter can help lengthen restoration cycles and improve the cooperation and quality of life of affected children and adolescents. The extraction of MIH-affected molars with subsequent orthodontic space closure is reserved for teeth with extensive destruction of the clinical crown and is relatively rarely indicated.

References

Alaluusua, S. 2010. Aetiology of molar-incisor hypomineralisation: a systematic review. *European Archives of Paediatric Dentistry*, **11**, 53–8.

Baroni, C., Marchionni, S. 2011. MIH supplementation strategies: prospective clinical and laboratory trial. *Journal of Dental Research*, **90**, 371–6.

Bekes, K., Heinzelmann, K., Lettner, S., Schaller, H. G. 2017. Efficacy of desensitizing products containing 8% arginine and calcium carbonate for hypersensitivity relief in MIH-affected molars: an 8-week clinical study. *Clinical Oral Investigations*, **21**(7), 2311–17.

Crombie, F., Manton, D., Kilpatrick, N. 2009. Aetiology of molar-incisor hypomineralization: a critical review. *International Journal of Paediatric Dentistry*, **19**, 73–83.

Crombie, F., Manton, D., Palamara, J., Reynolds, E. 2014. Resin infiltration of developmentally hypomineralised enamel. *International Journal of Paediatric Dentistry*, **24**, 51–5.

Eichenberger, M., Erb, J., Zwahlen, M., Schätzle, M. 2016. The timing of extraction of non-restorable first permanent molars: a systematic review. *European Journal of Paediatric Dentistry*, **16**, 272–8.

Fayle, S. A. 2003. Molar incisor hypomineralisation: restorative management. *European Journal of Paediatric Dentistry*, **4**, 121–6.

Feierabend, S., Halbleib, K., Klaiber, B., Hellwig, E. 2012. Laboratory-made composite resin restorations in children and adolescents with hypoplasia or hypomineralization of teeth. *Quintessence International*, **43**, 305–11.

Guelmann, M., Matsson, L., Bimstein, E. 1988. Periodontal health at first permanent molars adjacent to primary molar stainless steel crowns. *Journal of Clinical Periodontology*, **15**, 531–3.

Hellwig, E., Schiffner, U., Schulte, A. 2013. S2k-Leitlinie: Fluoridierungsmaßnahmen zur Kariesprophylaxe. Available from http://www.awmf.org/leitlinien/detail/ll/083-001.html (last accessed 30 January 2019).

Jälevik, B., Klingberg, G. A. 2002. Dental treatment, dental fear and behaviour management problems in children with severe enamel hypomineralization of their permanent first molars. *International Journal of Paediatric Dentistry*, **12**, 24–32.

Jälevik, B., Möller, M. 2007. Evaluation of spontaneous space closure and development of permanent dentition after extraction of hypomineralized permanent first molars. *International Journal of Paediatric Dentistry*, **17**, 328–35.

Kidd, E. A. M. 2004. How "clean" must a cavity be before restoration? *Caries Research*, **38**, 305–13.

Koch, M. J., García-Godoy, F. 2000. The clinical performance of laboratory-fabricated crowns placed on first permanent molars with developmental defects. *Journal of the American Dental Association*, **131**, 1285–90.

Kotsanos, N., Kaklamanos, E. G., Arapostathis, K. 2005. Treatment management of first permanent molars in children with molar-incisor hypomineralisation. *European Journal of Paediatric Dentistry*, **6**, 179–84.

Kühnisch, J., Heitmüller, D., Thiering, E., Brockow, I., Hoffmann, U., Neumann, C., et al. 2014a. Proportions and extent of manifestation of molar-incisor-hypomineralisations according to different phenotypes. *Journal of Public Health Dentistry*, **74**, 42–9.

Kühnisch, J., Mach, D., Thiering, E., Brockow, I., Hoffmann, U., Neumann, C., et al. 2014b. Respiratory diseases are associated with molar-incisor hypomineralizations. *Swiss Dental Journal*, **124**, 286–93.

Kühnisch, J., Thiering, E., Kratzsch, J., Heinrich-Weltzien, R., Hickel, R., Heinrich, J., et al. 2015. Elevated serum 25(OH)-vitamin D levels are negatively correlated with MIH. *Journal of Dental Research*, **94**, 381–7.

Kühnisch, J., Reichl, F. X., Hickel, R., Heinrich-Weltzien, R. 2017. S3-Leitlinie: Fissuren- und Grübchenversiegelung. Available from: http://www.awmf.org/leitlinien/detail/ll/083-002.html (last accessed 30 January 2019).

Kumar, H., Palamara, J. E., Burrow, M. F., Manton, D. J. 2017. An investigation into the effect of a resin infiltrant on the micromechanical properties of hypomineralised enamel. *International Journal of Paediatric Dentistry*, **27**(5), 399–411.

Lygidakis, N. A. 2010. Treatment modalities in children with teeth affected by molar-incisor enamel hypomineralisation (MIH): a systematic review. *European Archives of Paediatric Dentistry*, **11**, 65–74.

Lygidakis, N. A., Chaliasou, A., Siounas, G. 2003. Evaluation of composite restorations in hypomineralised permanent molars: a four year clinical study. *European Journal of Paediatric Dentistry*, **4**, 143–8.

Lygidakis, N. A., Wong, F., Jälevik, B., Vierrou, A. M., Alaluusua, S., Espelid, I. 2010. Best clinical practice guidance for clinicians dealing with children presenting with molar-incisor-hypomineralisation (MIH): an EAPD policy document. *European Archives of Paediatric Dentistry*, **11**, 75–81.

Manhart, J., Chen, H., Hamm, G., Hickel, R. 2004. Buonocore Memorial Lecture. Review of the clinical survival of direct and indirect restorations in posterior teeth of the permanent dentition. *Operative Dentistry*, **29**, 481–508.

Mejare, I., Bergman, E., Grindefjord, M. 2005. Hypomineralized molars and incisors of unknown origin: treatment outcome at age 18 years. *International Journal of Paediatric Dentistry*, **15**, 20–8.

Millet, C., Duprez, J. P., Khoury, C., Morgon, L., Richard, B. 2015. Interdisciplinary care for a patient with amelogenesis imperfecta: a clinical report. *Journal of Prosthodontics*, **24**, 424–31.

Pfisterer, J., Kessler, A., Kühnisch, J. 2016. Einzeitige CAD/CAM-Seitenzahnrestauration bei einem 8-Jährigen mit Molaren-Inzisiven-Hypomineralisation (MIH). *Quintessenz*, **68**, 7–16.

Rodd, H. D., Boissonade, F. M., Day, P. F. 2007. Pulpal status of hypomineralized permanent molars. *Pediatric Dentistry*, **29**, 514–20.

Weerheijm, K. L. 2004. Molar incisor hypomineralization (MIH): clinical presentation, aetiology and management. *Dental Update*, **31**, 9–12.

Weerheijm, K. L., Jälevik, B., Alaluusua, S. 2001. Molar-incisor hypomineralisation. *Caries Research*, **35**, 390–1.

Weerheijm, K. L., Duggal, M., Mejare, I., Papagiannoulis, L., Koch, G., Martens, L. C., Hallonsten, A. L. 2003. Judgement criteria for molar incisor hypomineralization (MIH) in epidemiologic studies: a summary of the European meeting on MIH held in Athens, 2003. *European Journal of Paediatric Dentistry*, **4**, 110–13.

Wittneben, J. G., Wright, R. F., Weber, H. P., Gallucci, G. O. 2009. A systematic review of the clinical performance of CAD/CAM single-tooth restorations. *International Journal of Prosthodontics*, **22**, 466–71.

Zagdwon, A. M., Fayle, S. A., Pollard, M. A. 2003. A prospective clinical trial comparing preformed metal crowns and cast restorations for defective first permanent molars. *European Journal of Paediatric Dentistry*, **4**, 138–42.

Zimmermann, M., Koller, C., Hickel, R., Kühnisch, J. 2016. Chairside treatment of amelogenesis imperfecta, including establishment of a new vertical dimension with resin nanoceramic and intraoral scanning. *Journal of Prosthetic Dentistry*, **116**, 309–13.

7.2

Dentine Hypersensitivity

Thiago Saads Carvalho and Samira Helena João-Souza

Department of Restorative, Preventive and Pediatric Dentistry, School for Dental Medicine, University of Bern, Bern, Switzerland

What is Dentine Hypersensitivity?

Pain is a very common problem in the daily dental practice. It leads to anxiety and stress in patients, eventually causing a negative impact on their quality of life. Since pain is a subjective condition, it can be difficult to assess its precise state and intensity, especially when dealing with children, who are still learning to express themselves.

Amongst the different kinds of oral pain, we most commonly find in the clinic those related to dental caries, pulpitis, fractured teeth and restorations, cracked tooth syndrome (CTS), molar–incisor hypominerali-sation (MIH), post-restorative sensitivity, marginal leakage, vital bleaching and gingival inflammation. If a particular pain cannot be assigned to any of these conditions, it might be related to dentine hypersensitivity (DH). By definition, DH is a diagnosis of exclusion, and it is characterised as a sharp pain, with short duration, arising from different stimuli on exposed dentine, occurring when no other form of dental defect or disease is identified (Holland et al., 1997; Canadian Advisory Board, 2003).

How Does DH Occur?

The most common factors leading to DH are gingival recession and loss of dental hard tissue. Gingival recession is a change of the gingival position from the cement–enamel junction to a more apical location. It may occur due to the use of orthodontic devices, traumatic toothbrushing or periodontitis and its treatment, amongst other causes (Smith, 1997). Loss of dental hard tissue (known as erosive tooth wear, ETW) occurs when erosion and abrasive forces continually impact the tooth surface, which can completely wear away the enamel, expose the underlying dentine and leave the dentine tubules patent to the oral environment (Lussi and Carvalho, 2014; Carvalho et al., 2015). Figure 7.2.1 shows a deciduous molar with ETW lesions, exposed dentine and patent tubules. If the erosive and abrasive forces occur in an area of gingival recession, it can lead to a wedge-shaped defect on the cervical area of the tooth and expose the underlying dentine.

The feeling of pain in DH arises because the dentinal tubules are open to the oral environment and the dental pulp. The fluid

Management of Dental Emergencies in Children and Adolescents, First Edition.
Edited by Klaus W. Neuhaus and Adrian Lussi.
© 2019 John Wiley & Sons Ltd. Published 2019 by John Wiley & Sons Ltd.
Companion website: www.wiley.com/go/neuhaus/dental_emergencies

(a) (b) (c)

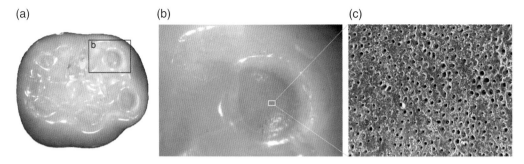

Figure 7.2.1 Deciduous molar with (a) ETW lesions on the occlusal surface, exhibiting (b) exposed dentine. (c) Scanning electron microscopy (SEM) image showing the patent dentine tubules.

within the tubules is free to move throughout the whole extent of the dentine. This movement changes the flow direction and pressure of the dentinal fluid, resulting in a shift in the pulpal pressure, which stimulates the pulpal nerves and causes a sharp pain sensation (Brännström et al., 1967). This means that any number of stimuli occurring in the exposed tubules will trigger a sharp movement of the dentinal fluid and cause pain. These stimuli can be thermal, evaporative, tactile, osmotic or chemical, but epidemiological data show that cold (thermal) is the main trigger for DH (Brännström et al., 1967; Amarasena et al., 2011).

Prevalence of DH in Children and Adolescents

ETW is an important factor in DH, especially in young adults, whose chances of experiencing pain from DH increase at least threefold when ETW is present (West et al., 2013). In children and adolescents, the prevalence of ETW can reach 79–100%, whilst the prevalence of DH varies in the range 4.7–45.2% (Table 7.2.1). Amongst studies reporting DH in children and adolescents (Table 7.2.1), practically none shows specific prevalence data for children, but most present some for adolescents. In general, premolars and incisors are the most commonly affected teeth, and patients typically complain that the pain is triggered by a cold stimulus or that toothbrushing causes DH discomfort.

Given the scarce epidemiological evidence on this condition in children, it is difficult to pinpoint specific prevalence values in this age group or to describe how the condition shifts as a function of age. However, studies show that DH is already a concern for some adolescent patients.

Clinical Aspects of DH in Children and Adolescents

When a patient complains of pain, dental professionals should meticulously analyse his or her dental history and carry out a thorough clinical examination to identify its source and location, and all possible factors that could be driving the process of dentine exposure.

In the clinic, the assessment of pain is commonly made with an air blast or tactile stimulus, but the patient's perception of pain and their reported history are also important sources of information (Canadian Advisory Board, 2003). In general, the assessment of DH-related pain is not easy, given the subjective nature of the pain. Whilst older children and adolescents can communicate and express themselves without extreme influence of any cognitive, emotional or situational factors (von Baeyer and Spagrud, 2007), younger children have difficulty in precisely expressing their sensations. They are highly influenced by previous unpleasant dental experiences, and they may present an anxious response to clinical tests. Proper

Table 7.2.1 Studies reporting the prevalence of DH in children and adolescents.

Study	Study type	Number of volunteers	Age group (years)	Prevalence of DH (%)
Fischer et al. (1992)	Clinical and questionnaire	635	13–87	17.0[a] 25.0[b]
Rees (2000)	Clinical	3593	15–83	3.8
Clayton et al. (2002)	Questionnaire	228	17–58	**45.2[c]**
Rees and Addy (2002)	Clinical	4841	16–82	4.1
Rees et al. (2003)	Clinical	226	12–82	**<25.0[c]**
Rees and Addy (2004)	Clinical	5477	15–80	2.8
Chi and Milgrom (2008)	Questionnaire	45	14–28	52.6
Bamise et al. (2010)	Questionnaire	1019	14–41	**4.7[c]**
Amarasena et al. (2011)[d]	Clinical	12 692	<20 to >60	**4.7[c]**
Oderinu et al. (2011)	Questionnaire	382	17–37	**40.9[c]**
Bahsi et al. (2012)	Clinical	1368	13–71	1.6
Çolak et al. (2012)	Questionnaire	1463	17–33	8.4
Shitsuka et al. (2015)	Case–control	48	4–9	**41.0[c]**
Haneet and Vandana (2016)	Clinical	404	16–55	**39.2[c]**

[a] Prevalence value obtained from the clinical assessment.
[b] Prevalence value obtained from the questionnaires.
[c] Prevalence values specific for children and adolescents (<20 years old).
[d] Reference found after searching for (dentin OR dentine) AND (sensitivity OR hypersensitivity) AND (prevalence). A literature search was performed on PubMed using the terms (dentin OR dentine) AND (sensitivity OR hypersensitivity) AND (child OR children OR adolescent OR adolescents OR teenager OR teenagers) AND (prevalence). The search resulted in a total of 83 studies, amongst which only 13 involved children or adolescents (<20 years old), one of which (Shitsuka et al., 2015) was specifically on children. Another study (Amarasena et al., 2011) was later added after using a broader search term.[d]

assessment of pain location and intensity in these young patients is thus challenging.

Once the location and source of pain are established, the dental professional should determine which factors are associated with the DH in their patient. Gingival recession is one of the most common factors in DH, and it is frequently observed in adolescents. Its prevalence increases with age, and it is most commonly observed in buccal surfaces of canines, premolars and first molars (Ainamo et al., 1986). Most of the prevalence studies in Table 7.2.1 associate DH with gingival recession. Its causes are mainly soft-tissue trauma (e.g. from toothbrushing) and orthodontic therapy.

In addition to gingival recession, dental professionals should also bear in mind the factors related to ETW (Shitsuka et al., 2015). Frequent consumption of acidic foods or drinks is highly associated to ETW (Carvalho et al., 2014; Lussi and Carvalho, 2014). The constant presence of acids in the oral cavity is not only related to the loss of dental hard tissue and dentine exposure, but also maintains the dentinal tubules constantly open, thus sustaining the conditions for pain related to DH. For this reason, dental professionals should assess the daily diet of their patients (and their families, in case of children). This can be done using a food diary, where the patient must take note of any food or beverage consumed over the course of 4 days, including one weekend day. Using this diary, dental professionals can identify the substances related to ETW and establish individual-tailored advice for their patients on reducing the frequency of acid intake.

Acids from gastro-esophageal reflux disease (GERD) are important factors for this condition, too. Children as young as 3–4 years who reportedly suffer from GERD present higher rates of ETW with dentine exposure on deciduous teeth (Murakami et al., 2011). Patients reporting GERD should be referred to their medical doctor or gastroenterologist for check-up. Occasionally, a patient may present ETW lesions and have no apparent GERD symptoms. Such patients may be suffering from silent reflux, and they should also be referred to their doctor. Silent reflux occurs when a patient is not aware that they suffer from reflux, but still present some subtle clinical signs of ETW related to GERD, such as asymmetric ETW lesions. These lesions are slightly more discernible in one side of the mouth than the other. If GERD is not treated, the condition can persist into the teenage years and adulthood, sustaining the ETW and possibly act as the driving force for DH on permanent teeth. Furthermore, eating disorders such as anorexia and bulimia can arise during the teenage years and early adulthood. These disorders will likewise influence the development of ETW lesions, which, in turn, can be related to DH.

In addition to determining the factors associated with gingival recession and ETW, it is also important to assess the patient's oral hygiene and behavioural characteristics, especially those related to drinking habits (swishing or holding erosive drinks in the mouth). Follow-up assessments and monitoring of these patients can help achieve the best diagnosis and clinical management of DH.

Clinical Management of DH

First and foremost, dental professionals must provide a clinical management individually tailored to their patients. This should begin with the least invasive procedures, such as the use of homecare products like toothpastes and mouthrinses. Products containing specific desensitising agents (e.g. potassium, stannous fluoride, calcium sodium phosphosilicate, arginine) are capable of reducing DH in adults (Bae et al., 2015). They act by hindering the nervous response or by blocking the opening of the tubules, where they precipitate and thus reduce fluid movement. These products should be considered as the first treatment choice for DH, although there are still a limited number of studies regarding their use in children.

For an extra degree of safety, in-office desensitising agents can be applied. Amongst the products available for in-office use, fluoride varnishes are a good option for children (Miller and Vann, 2008). These varnishes form a layer over the dentine surface, which serves as a physical barrier against external stimuli and acts as a source of fluoride. They should be considered as an initial treatment option for use in DH, but they provide only an immediate and short-term pain relief. If the pain persists, other minimally invasive options (e.g. sealants) should be considered.

Sealants such as glass ionomer, resin-based sealants and adhesives can provide a physical barrier over the exposed dentine. These materials have shown successful results in the treatment of DH, with pain relief lasting several months (Veitz-Keenan et al., 2013; West et al., 2014; Madruga et al., 2017). Sealants can be used in DH cases where treatment with fluoride varnishes has not been successful. However, when the loss of dental hard tissue is so substantial that a restoration is required, further treatment is advocated. As a rule, all restorative treatments should follow the principles of minimally invasive treatment, preferably using adhesive materials such as composites. Moreover, restorative treatment should always be carried out in conjunction with continuous preventive management, to reduce the effect of the predisposing factors related to gingival recession and ETW (Carvalho et al., 2015).

Conclusion

Despite the lack of studies on DH in children, recent findings show that the condition is becoming increasingly frequent in younger patients. If children or adolescents complain about oral pain, dental professionals are urged to carry out a full clinical assessment, and to verify whether the pain is related to exposed dentine. Children who present exposed dentine in their deciduous teeth are more likely to present dentine exposure in their permanent ones. So, staying alert to the clinical signs related to DH allows the dental professional to establish and implement preventive managements as early as possible.

References

Ainamo, J., Paloheimo, L., Nordblad, A., Murtomaa, H. 1986. Gingival recession in schoolchildren at 7, 12 and 17 years of age in Espoo, Finland. *Community Dentistry and Oral Epidemiology*, **14**(5), 283–6.

Amarasena, N., Spencer, J., Ou, Y., Brennan, D. 2011. Dentine hypersensitivity in a private practice patient population in Australia. *Journal of Oral Rehabilitation*, **38**(1), 52–60.

Bae, J. H., Kim, Y. K., Myung, S. K. 2015. Desensitizing toothpaste versus placebo for dentin hypersensitivity: A systematic review and meta-analysis. *Journal of Clinical Periodontology*, **42**(2), 131–41.

Bahsi, E., Dalli, M., Uzgur, R., Hamidi, M., Olak, H. 2012. Clinical features of dentine hypersensitivity. *European Review for Medical and Pharmacological Sciences*, **16**(8), 1107–16.

Bamise, C. T., Kolawole, K., Oloyede, E., Esan, T. 2010. Tooth sensitivity experience among residential university students. *International Journal of Dental Hygiene*, **8**(2), 95–100.

Brännström, M., Lindén, L. A., Aström, A., 1967. The hydrodynamics of the dental tubule and of pulp fluid. A discussion of its significance in relation to dentinal sensitivity. *Caries Research*, **1**(4), 310–17.

Canadian Advisory Board on Dentin Hypersensitivity. 2003. Consensus-based recommendations for the diagnosis and management of dentin hypersensitivity. *Journal of the Canadian Dental Association*, **69**(4), 221–6.

Carvalho, T. S., Lussi, A., Jaeggi, T., Gambon, D. 2014. Erosive tooth wear in children. *Monographs in Oral Science*, **25**, 262–78.

Carvalho, T. S., Colon, P., Ganss, C., Huysmans, M. C., Lussi, A., Schlueter, N., et al. 2015. Consensus report of the European Federation of Conservative Dentistry: erosive tooth wear – diagnosis and management. *Clinical Oral Investigations*, **19**(7), 1556–61.

Chi, D., Milgrom, P. 2008. The oral health of homeless adolescents and young adults and determinants of oral health: preliminary findings. *Special Care in Dentistry*, **28**(6), 237–42.

Clayton, D. R., McCarthy, D., Gillam, D. G. 2002. A study of the prevalence and distribution of dentine sensitivity in a population of 17–58-year-old serving personnel on an RAF base in the Midlands. *Journal of Oral Rehabilitation*, **29**(1), 14–23.

Çolak, H., Aylikçi, B.U., Hamidi, M. M., Uzgur, R. 2012. Prevalence of dentine hypersensitivity among university students in Turkey. *Nigerian Journal of Clinical Practice*, **15**(4), 415–19.

Fischer, C., Fischer, R. G., Wennberg, A. 1992. Prevalence and distribution of cervical dentine hypersensitivity in a population in Rio de Janeiro, Brazil. *Journal of Dentistry*, **20**(5), 272–6.

Haneet, R. K., Vandana, L. K. 2016. Prevalence of dentinal hypersensitivity and study of associated factors: a cross-sectional study based on the general dental population of Davangere, Karnataka, India. *International Dental Journal*, **66**(1), 49–57.

Holland, G. R., Narhi, M. N., Addy, M., Gangarosa, L., Orchardson, R. 1997. Guidelines for the design and conduct of clinical trials on dentine hypersensitivity. *Journal of Clinical Periodontology*, **24**(11), 808–13.

Lussi, A., Carvalho, T. S., 2014. Erosive tooth wear: a multifactorial condition of growing concern and increasing knowledge. *Monographs in Oral Science*, **25**, 1–15.

Madruga, M. M., Silva, A. F., Rosa, W. L. O., Piva, E., Lund, R. G. 2017. Evaluation of dentin hypersensitivity treatment with glass ionomer cements: a randomized clinical trial. *Brazilian Oral Research*, **31**, e3.

Miller, E. K., Vann, W. E. Jr. 2008. The use of fluoride varnish in children: a critical review with treatment recommendations. *Journal of Clinical Pediatric Dentistry*, **32**(4), 259–64.

Murakami, C., Oliveira, L. B., Sheiham, A., Corrêa, M. S. N. P., Haddad, A. E., Bönecker, M. 2011. Risk indicators for erosive tooth wear in Brazilian preschool children. *Caries Research*, **45**(2), 121–9.

Oderinu, O. H., Savage, K. O., Uti, O. G., Adegbulugbe, I. C. 2011. Prevalence of self-reported hypersensitive teeth among a group of Nigerian undergraduate students. *Nigerian Postgraduate Medical Journal*, **18**(3), 205–9.

Rees, J. S. 2000. The prevalence of dentine hypersensitivity in general dental practice in the UK. *Journal of Clinical Periodontology*, **27**, 860–5.

Rees, J. S., Addy, M. 2002. A cross-sectional study of dentine hypersensitivity. *Journal of Clinical Periodontology*, **29**(11), 997–1003.

Rees, J. S., Addy, M. 2004. A cross-sectional study of buccal cervical sensitivity in UK general dental practice and a summary review of prevalence studies. *International Journal of Dental Hygiene*, **2**(2), 64–9.

Rees, J. S., Jin, L. J., Lam, S., Kudanowska, I., Vowles, R. 2003. The prevalence of dentine hypersensitivity in a hospital clinic population in Hong Kong. *Journal of Dentistry*, **31**(7), 453–61.

Shitsuka, C., Mendes, F. M., Corrêa, M. S. N. P., Leite, M. F. 2015. Exploring some aspects associated with dentine hypersensitivity in children. *Scientific World Journal*, **2015**, 764905.

Smith, R. G. 1997. Gingival recession. Reappraisal of an enigmatic condition and a new index for monitoring. *Journal of Clinical Periodontology*, **24**(3), 201–5.

Veitz-Keenan, A., Barna, J. A., Strober, B., Matthews, A. G., Collie, D., Vena, D., et al. 2013. Treatments for hypersensitive noncarious cervical lesions. *Journal of the American Dental Association*, **144**(5), 495–506.

von Baeyer, C. L., Spagrud, L. J. 2007. Systematic review of observational (behavioral) measures of pain for children and adolescents aged 3 to 18 years. *Pain*, **127**(1–2), 140–50.

West, N. X., Sanz, M., Lussi, A., Bartlett, D., Bouchard, P., Bourgeois, D. 2013. Prevalence of dentine hypersensitivity and study of associated factors: a European population-based cross-sectional study. *Journal of Dentistry*, **41**(10), 841–51.

West, N., Seong, J., Davies, M. 2014. Dentine hypersensitivity. *Monographs in Oral Science*, **25**, 108–22.

7.3

Cracked Tooth Syndrome

Renata Chałas[1] and Stefan Hänni[2,3]

[1] *Department of Conservative Dentistry and Endodontics, Medical University of Lublin, Lublin, Poland*
[2] *Department of Preventive, Restorative and Pediatric Dentistry, School for Dental Medicine, University of Bern, Bern, Switzerland*
[3] *Private endodontic office, Bern, Switzerland*

What is Cracked Tooth Syndrome?

The American Association of Endodontists (AAE) categorises tooth fractures into five types: type I, craze line; type II, cuspal fracture; type III, cracked tooth; type IV, split tooth; and type V, vertical root fracture (AAE, 2008). The term "cracked tooth syndrome" (CTS), describing a symptomatic cracked tooth (type III), was introduced to the field of dentistry by Caryl Cameron when he applied it to a clinical condition characterised by an incomplete fracture of a vital posterior tooth, originating from the coronal dentin, which may progress into the pulp or periodontal ligament (Cameron, 1964; Türp and Gobetti, 1996). Since then, CTS has become a well-documented entity in clinical practice. It is also known as cuspal fracture odontalgia (Ellis 2001; Hasan et al. 2015).

Epidemiology

The occurrence of CTS is unknown, but an incidence rate of 34–74% has been documented (Hasan et al., 2015). Although it occurs more frequently in individuals within the age range of 30–50 years (Hood, 1991), with a female predilection (Homewood, 1998; Udoye and Jafarzadeh, 2009), it can be seen in younger patients, too. In the past few years the number of reported cases of CTS has increased suggesting that the risks and complications associated with a popularity of tongue piercings may lead to cracked-tooth syndrome in the lower first molar teeth (Ziebolz et al., 2012; Plastargias and Sakellari, 2014). Another aspect is the inability to diagnose during the early course of the lesion which causes frustration to both, the dentist, and the patient because of the difficulty to localise the pain (Jurczykowska et al., 2015).

In descending order, the most commonly involved teeth are the mandibular molars, maxillary premolars, maxillary molars and mandibular premolars (Homewood, 1998). In adolescents, special attention should be given to the mandibular first molars, because they are usually the first permanent teeth to erupt into the dental arch, and hence are more prone to dental caries and subsequent restorative intervention (Lubisich et al., 2010; Ratcliff et al., 2001). Thus, they are more susceptible to cracks. But there is insufficient information on the dynamics of crack propagation and no established correlation

Management of Dental Emergencies in Children and Adolescents, First Edition.
Edited by Klaus W. Neuhaus and Adrian Lussi.
© 2019 John Wiley & Sons Ltd. Published 2019 by John Wiley & Sons Ltd.
Companion website: www.wiley.com/go/neuhaus/dental_emergencies

between the presence of incomplete tooth fracture and the occurrence of CTS-specific symptoms. The "wedging effect" on the lower first molars from the prominent mesiopalatal cusp of the maxillary first molars may also be contributory (Hamouda and Shehata, 2011).

Aetiology

The aetiology of CTS has a multifactorial character. In normal conditions, teeth are apt to withstand physiological functional loads. But in pathological situations, the following factors predispose to CTS (Figure 7.3.1). These should be understood before undertaking any interventions in adolescents (Banerji et al., 2010a,b).

Individual risk of crack formation is modified by morphological factors:

- deep cusp-fossa intercuspation;
- occlusal interferences; and
- tooth malposition (open bite, cross bite);

and, more importantly, by iatrogenic factors:

- cavity preparation;
- filling materials and techniques;
- posts, pins and screws; and
- overloading of pillar teeth.

Recent evidence shows that grinding or localised enamel hypoplasia may contribute to microcrack initiation and propagation in deciduous teeth, which might then serve as a pathway for bacteria entering the teeth (Ranjitkar et al., 2015).

Clinical Picture

A fracture line in CTS usually runs in the mesio-distal direction on the occlusal surface of the tooth (Figure 7.3.2) – unlike a vertical root fracture, which runs in the bucco-oral direction (Luebke, 1984). The depth of the crack and its orientation through the tooth structure are not evident. The fracture may involve the pulp, root dentin or cementum communicating with the periodontal space.

Clinically, pain is the main complaint of CTS patients. A thorough pain history (where, how, since when, how often, for how long, how strong, triggers and attendant symptoms) ought to be taken during dental examination (Brynjulfsen et al., 2002). Whilst giving the pain history, the patient usually reports pain during biting, especially in the case of foods that contain a hard component, such as cereals, nuts, whole bread and any meal containing grains. Moreover, pain may occur with changes of temperature. Increased reaction is observed in the case of cold thermal stimuli. Hypersensitivity pain may occur in the case of sweet foods intake (Sadasiva et al., 2015). It is also important in taking a history to determine whether a patient has had an earlier incidence of CTS. The teeth

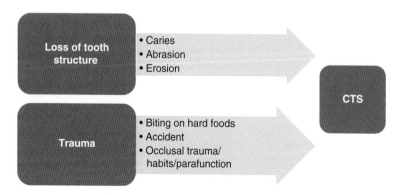

Figure 7.3.1 CTS-predisposing factors.

affected by the CTS can be sensitive to percussion, particularly where the stimulus is acting in an apical direction. Patients then feel prolonged pain, which may be radiating (Kahler, 2008).

Diagnosis

The diagnosis of CTS can be challenging to a dental practitioner, especially with young patients, as the condition presents an incomplete history, nonspecific symptoms and unidentifiable signs during clinical examination and standard radiographic imaging (Banerji et al., 2010a,b). That's why CTS is a diagnostic challenge for even the most experienced dentist. A careful and early diagnosis is very important in preventing the progression of CTS (Figure 7.3.3).

One should remember that a crack is a finding, not a symptom – symptoms arise from pulpal or periodontal involvement. Cardinal symptoms for CTS are:

- Erratic pain on mastication.
- Pain on release of biting pressure.

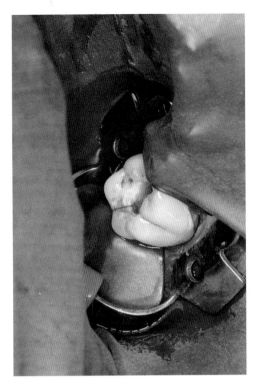

Figure 7.3.2 Cracked line visible in the distal region of the occlusal surface of a first mandibular molar after removal of an old restoration.

Figure 7.3.3 Diagnosis of CTS.

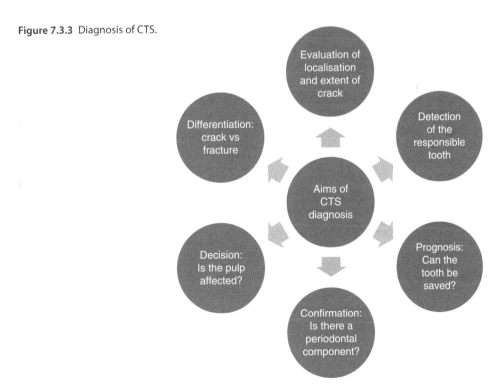

- Thermal or osmotic hypersensibility.
- Sudden occurrence of pain on an unrestored or only slightly restored tooth.

The basis of an effective diagnosis is a careful history-taking, including an extensive pain history. The subsequent clinical inspection is carried out on the cleaned and dried teeth, using some kind of magnification aid (Clark et al., 2003).

Detection of the Affected Tooth

In the detection of the affected tooth, a biting test is helpful. The patient is asked to gradually increase the pressure on a cotton roll and then quickly release it. In case of pain during the sudden release, the suspected CTS is confirmed.

Evaluation of the Localisation and Extent of the Crack

To narrow the search for a cracked cusp, a biting test using a small wooden wedge can be performed. The wedge should be placed consecutively on each of the tooth cusps when biting. The patient's pain is evaluated upon closing and opening, with pain upon release usually indicative of a cracked tooth. Other available tools for assisting in the diagnosis of CTS are tools like Fracfinder (Figure 7.3.4) and Tooth Slooth II. These can be used in the same way as a wedge – to help find a cracked cusp – and their usage definitely saves time. The use of transillumination (Figure 7.3.5) and ultimately the removal of an existing restoration may help assess the course and extent of the crack (Jurczykowska et al., 2015).

Differentation: Crack versus Fracture

Wedging forces are used to determine if the parts of the tooth are mobile, where no mobility indicates a crack, whilst mobile parts indicate a cusps fracture or split tooth.

Is the Pulp Affected?

If the crack divides the tooth into two halves (i.e. passes through two marginal ridges with the assumption of pulp involvement) then the prognosis is unfavourable. At the onset of irreversible pulpitis symptoms, endodontic treatment should be initiated. Chronic pulpitis with mild clinical symptoms may be seen as a result of microleakage of bacterial byproducts and toxins. Cracks with pulpal involvement may result in pulpal and periodontal symptoms.

Is there a Periodontal Component?

Clinical examination with isolated deep probing may reveal the occurrence of localised periodontal defects where cracks extend subgingivally. The localised periodontal defect is the result of a fracture line extending below the gingiva (Zimet and Endo, 2000).

Can the Tooth be Saved?

As for the decision whether a tooth can be preserved or not, there is little hard data. Experts agree that as soon as a crack involves the root canal, prognosis is reduced, and that teeth showing cracks that cross the furcal floor should be considered hopeless. In the worst-case scenario, a cracked tooth cannot be repaired (Toure et al., 2011).

Clinical Management

In general, one should focus on the prevention of crack formation through timely recognition of at-risk teeth and adequate cavity preparation. Treatment aims are as follows:

- Preservation and stabilisation of the remaining tooth structure.
- Resolution of pain.
- Preservation of tooth vitality.

There are many treatment options according to the course of the infraction and the severity of the symptoms. For example, if the crack is detected at an early stage, adhesive procedures may be used. When the crack is larger, treatment aims to protect the remaining structure through more extensive restorations

(a)

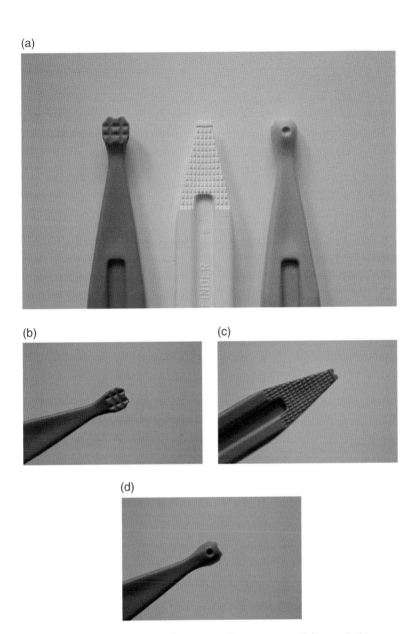

(b)

(c)

(d)

Figure 7.3.4 (a–d) Fracfinder – different sizes of instruments and diagnostic tips.

Figure 7.3.5 Transillumination of the tooth can help detect cracks.

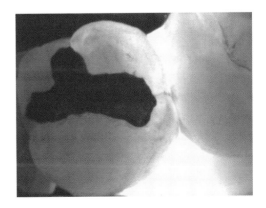

(Liu and Sidhu, 1995; Bader et al., 1996). When the destruction is severe, a complete crown may be indicated. However, all treatment options have their pros and cons, and there is only very limited clinical evidence in the dental literature to substantiate the use of any of them. What's more, clinical studies have not resolved which has the highest success rate (Banerji et al., 2010a,b).

be a difficult and complicated condition to manage in adolescents, even though it is not a very common problem in this age group. When appearing in the dental office with nontypical tooth pain, children should be diagnosed in the direction of CTS to avoid any complications and provide early therapeutic procedures.

Conclusion

CTS as a non-infective dental condition with a variety of signs and symptoms can

Acknowledgements

Thanks to Klaus W. Neuhaus and Paweł Maksymiuk for support with the images.

References

American Association of Endodontists (AAE). 2008. Endodontics: Colleagues for Excellence Newsletter, Summer 2008. American Association of Endodontics. Cracking the Cracked Tooth Code: Detection and Treatment of Various Longitudinal Tooth Fractures. Available from: https://www.aae. org/specialty/wp-content/uploads/ sites/2/2017/07/ecfesum08.pdf (last accessed 30 January 2019).

Bader, J. D., Shugars, D. A., Robertson, T. M. 1996. Using crowns to prevent tooth fracture. *Community Dentistry Oral Epidemiology*, **24**(1), 47–51.

Banerji, S., Mehta, S. B., Millar, B. J. 2010a. Cracked tooth syndrome. Part 1: Aetiology and diagnosis. *British Dental Journal*, **208**(10), 459–63.

Banerji, S., Mehta, S. B., Millar, B. J. 2010b. Cracked tooth syndrome. Part 2: Restorative options for the management of cracked tooth syndrome. *British Dental Journal*, **208**(11), 503–14.

Brynjulfsen, A., Fristad, I., Grevstad, T., Hals-Kvinnsland, I. 2002. Incompletely fractured teeth associated with diffuse longstanding orofacial pain: diagnosis and treatment outcome. *International Endodontic Journal*, **35**(5), 461–6.

Cameron, C. E. 1964. Cracked-tooth syndrome. *Journal of the American Dental Association*, **68**(3), 405–11.

Clark, D. J., Sheets, C. G., Paquette, J. M. 2003. Definitive diagnosis of early enamel and dentine cracks based on microscopic evaluation. *Journal of Esthetic and Restorative Dentistry*, **15**(7), 391–401.

Ellis, S. G. 2001. Incomplete tooth fracture – proposal for a new definition. *British Dental Journal*, **190**(8), 424–8.

Hamouda, I. M., Shehata, S. H. 2011. Fracture resistance of posterior teeth restored with modern restorative materials. *Journal of Biomedical Research*, **25**(6), 418–24.

Hasan, S., Singh, K., Salati, N. 2015. Cracked tooth syndrome: overview of literature. *International Journal of Applied Basic Medical Research*, **5**(3), 164–8.

Homewood, C. I. 1998. Cracked tooth syndrome – incidence, clinical findings and treatment. *Australian Dental Journal*, **43**(4), 217–21.

Hood, J. A. 1991. Biomechanics of the intact, prepared and restored tooth: some clinical implications. *International Dental Journal*, **41**(1), 25–32.

Jurczykowska, M., Munoz-Sandoval, C., Szabelska, A., Chałas, R. 2015. Cracked tooth syndrome as a major issue of today's patients – review of literature. *Journal of Stomatology*, **68**(5), 579–90.

Kahler, W. 2008. The cracked teeth conundrum: terminology, classification, diagnosis and management. *American Journal of Dentistry*, **21**(5), 275–82.

Liu, H. H., Sidhu, S. K. 1995. Cracked teeth – treatment rational and case management: case reports. *Quintessence International*, **26**(7), 485–92.

Lubisich, E. B., Hilton, T. J., Ferracane, J. 2010. Cracked teeth: a review of literature. *Journal of Esthetic and Restorative Dentistry*, **22**(3), 158–67.

Luebke, R. G. 1984. Vertical crown-root fractures in posterior teeth. *Dental Clinics of North America*, **28**(4), 883–94.

Plastargias, I., Sakellari, D. 2014. The consequences of tongue piercing on oral and periodontal tissues. *International Scholarly Research Notices Dentistry*, **2014**, Article ID 876510.

Ranjitkar, S., Cheung, W., Yong, R., Deverell, J., Packianathan, M., Hall, C. 2015. Odontogenic facial swelling of unknown origin. *Australian Dental Journal*, **60**, 426–33.

Ratcliff, S., Becker, I. M., Quinn, L. 2001. Type and incidence of crack in posterior teeth. *Journal of Prosthetic Dentistry*, **86**(2), 168–72.

Sadasiva, K., Ramalingam, S., Rajaram, K., Meiyappan, A. 2015. Cracked tooth syndrome: a report of three cases. *Journal of Pharmacy and BioAllied Sciences*, **7**(Suppl. 2), S700–3.

Toure, B., Faye, B., Kane, A. W., Lo, C. M., Niang, B., Boucher, Y. 2011. Analysis of reason for extraction of endodontically treated teeth: a prospective study. *Journal of Endodontics*, **37**(11), 1512–15.

Türp, J. C., Gobetti, J. P. 1996. The cracked tooth syndrome: an elusive diagnosis. *Journal of the American Dental Association*, **127**(10), 1502–7.

Udoye, C. I., Jafarzadeh, H. 2009. Cracked tooth syndrome: characteristics and distribution among adults in a Nigerian teaching hospital. *Journal of Endodontics*, **35**(3), 334–6.

Ziebolz, D., Hildebrand, A., Proff, P., Rinke, S., Hornecker, E., Mausberg, R. F. 2012. Long-term effects of tongue piercing – a case control study. *Clinical Oral Investigations*, **16**(1), 231–7.

Zimet, P. O., Endo, C. 2000. Preservation of the roots-management and prevention protocols for cracked tooth syndrome. *Annals of the Royal Australasian College of Dental Surgeons*, **15**, 319–24.

Index

Page locators in **bold** indicate main articles. Page locators in *italics* indicate figures. This index uses letter-by-letter alphabetization.

Management of Dental Emergencies in Children and Adolescents, First Edition.
Edited by Klaus W. Neuhaus and Adrian Lussi.
© 2019 John Wiley & Sons Ltd. Published 2019 by John Wiley & Sons Ltd.
Companion website: www.wiley.com/go/neuhaus/dental_emergencies